PROLACTIN

Edited by **György M. Nagy** and **Bela E. Toth**

Prolactin
http://dx.doi.org/10.5772/2950
Edited by György M. Nagy and Bela E. Toth

Contributors

Kambadur Muralidhar, Jaeok Lee, Hideya Takahashi, Hiroki Kudose, Chiyo Takagi, Shunsuke Moriyama, Tatsuya Sakamoto, I.V. Lazebnaya, O.E. Lazebny, S.R. Khatami, G.E. Sulimova, Lorenza Díaz, Mauricio Díaz-Muñoz, Leticia González, Saúl Lira-Albarrán, Fernando Larrea, Isabel Méndez, Weijiang Zhao, Flavio Mena, Nilda Navarro, Alejandra Castilla, Edyta Molik, Tomasz Misztal, Dorota A. Zieba, Toru R. Saito, Márk Oláh, Misao Terada, György M. Nagy, Gokalp Oner, Viktória Reinhoffer, Márk Oláh, Miklós Vecsernyés, Béla E. Tóth, György M. Nagy, Erika Ginsburg, Christopher D. Heger, Paul Goldsmith, Barbara K. Vonderhaar, Miguel Ángel Castaño López, José Luís Robles Rodríguez, Marta Robles García

Published by InTech

Janeza Trdine 9, 51000 Rijeka, Croatia

Publishing Process Manager Viktorija Zgela
Technical Editor InTech Prepress, Novi Sad
Cover InTech Design team

Additional hard copies can be obtained from orders@intechopen.com

Prolactin, Edited by György M. Nagy and Bela E. Toth
p. cm.
ISBN 978-953-51-0943-3

For EU product safety concerns:
IN TECH d.o.o., Prolaz Marije Krucifikse Kozulić 3, 51000 Rijeka, Croatia,
info@intechopen.com or visit our website at intechopen.com.

Meet the editors

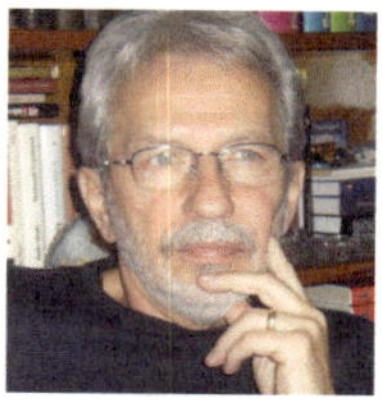

György M. Nagy, MD, PhD, DSc graduated from the Medical University in Pécs in 1974. He started his work at the Semmelweis University in 1974 at the 2nd Department of Anatomy led by Prof. Béla Halász. He obtained his PhD in Neuroendocrinology in 1992 and his Doctor of Science Degree in 1995. He worked in Birmingham (University of Alabama at Birmingham, USA) as a Research Fellow from 1984 to 1987 in the laboratory of Jimmy D. Neill. He also spent two years (from 1989 till 1991) as a visiting professor in Charleston, SC at the Medical University of South Carolina, USA, in the laboratory of Steve L. Frawley and one year (between 1997-1998) at the Florida State University, Tallahassee, FL, USA in Marc E. Freeman's laboratory. At present, he is a Professor of The Ross University, Department of Anatomy, Commonwealth of Dominica. His main interests are the hypothalamic regulation of pituitary prolactin secretion and the molecular aspects of the function of mammotrope cells. The title of his best cited article is "Prolactin: Structure, function and regulation of secretion", written by Freeman ME, Kanyicska B, Lerant A, and Nagy GM (Physiological Reviews 80: 1523-1631, 2000)

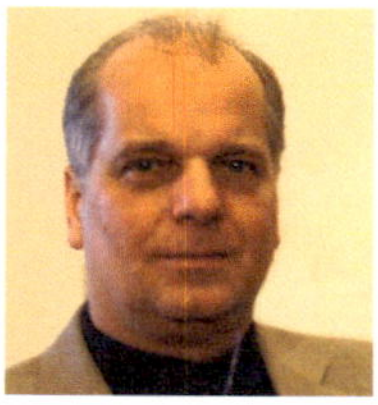

Bela Ernest Toth Dipl. Eng, MD, PhD started his education with School of Engineering, (Dipl. Eng), graduated as a Medical Doctor (MD), and completed PhD in Neuroscience. He worked as a lecturer for graduate and postgraduate education at Medical School and also at Faculties of Bioengineering and Healthcare Sciences. His scientific background is based on university appointments and academic collaborations (Semmelweis University Budapest, Neuroendocrine Research Group Hungarian Academy of Sciences, Rudolph Magnus Institute of Pharmacology, University of Utrecht; Dept. of Molecular and Cell Biology Penn State University, USA; University of Veterinary Sciences, Hungary). Dr. Toth's research interest on circadian rhythms of PRL secretion started during the university years. He later continued to focus on biology of nutrition, development and regulation of immune cell response, and function of DA in neuroendocrine regulation. Lately, his interests are involving pre-clinical research. Dr. Toth continues his work as an expert in clinical trials for pharmaceutical drug development.

Contents

Preface XI

Chapter 1 **Prolactin and Angiogenesis: Biological Implications of Microheterogeneity 1**
Kambadur Muralidhar and Jaeok Lee

Chapter 2 ***In vitro* Effects of the Prolactin, Growth Hormone and Somatolactin on Cell Turnover in Fish Esophagus: Possible Mode of Opposite Osmoregulatory Actions of Prolactin and Growth Hormone 21**
Hideya Takahashi, Hiroki Kudose, Chiyo Takagi, Shunsuke Moriyama and Tatsuya Sakamoto

Chapter 3 **Use of the Bovine Prolactin Gene (*bPRL*) for Estimating Genetic Variation and Milk Production in Aboriginal Russian Breeds of *Bos taurus* L. 35**
I.V. Lazebnaya, O.E. Lazebny, S.R. Khatami and G.E. Sulimova

Chapter 4 **Prolactin in the Immune System 53**
Lorenza Díaz, Mauricio Díaz-Muñoz, Leticia González, Saúl Lira-Albarrán, Fernando Larrea and Isabel Méndez

Chapter 5 **Neuregulin-1 (Nrg1): An Emerging Regulator of Prolactin (PRL) Secretion 83**
Weijiang Zhao

Chapter 6 **Autocrine and Paracrine Regulation of Prolactin Secretion by Prolactin Variants and by Hypothalamic Hormones 97**
Flavio Mena, Nilda Navarro and Alejandra Castilla

Chapter 7 **The Effect of Physiological and Environmental Factors on the Prolactin Profile in Seasonally Breeding Animals 121**
Edyta Molik, Tomasz Misztal and Dorota A. Zieba

Chapter 8 **The Role of Prolactin in the Regulation of Male Copulatory Behavior 139**
Toru R. Saito, Márk Oláh, Misao Terada and György M. Nagy

Chapter 9 **Prolactin and Infertility 147**
Gokalp Oner

Chapter 10 **The Regulation of Pituitary Prolactin Secretion: Hypothalamic, Intrapituitary and Intracellular Factors and Signaling Mechanisms 167**
Viktória Reinhoffer, Márk Oláh, Miklós Vecsernyés, Béla E. Tóth and György M. Nagy

Chapter 11 **Prolactin Receptor Isoforms in Human Breast Cancer 195**
Erika Ginsburg, Christopher D. Heger, Paul Goldsmith and Barbara K. Vonderhaar

Chapter 12 **Physiological and Pathological Hyperprolactinemia: Can We Minimize Errors in the Clinical Practice? 213**
Miguel Ángel Castaño López, José Luís Robles Rodríguez and Marta Robles García

Preface

Prolactin is a polypeptide hormone that is synthesized in and secreted from the lactotrophs of the anterior pituitary gland. The name of the hormone was originally given 80 years ago based on the fact that bovine pituitary extract causes growth of the crop sac and stimulate the elaboration of crop milk in pigeons[1]. Nowadays, we already know that prolactin plays multiple pivotal roles in control of general homeostasis[2-5]. Without giving a detailed list, rather some of them will be highlighted here. The classical role can be seen in mammals where prolactin stimulates the mammary glands to produce milk during lactation and the development of corpus luteum of the ovary to secrete its hormone i.e. progesterone.

Its osmoregulatory role is also well defined. It has a critical role in fish, so it is also called a "freshwater-adapting" hormone[6]. Plasma prolactin levels may follow the changes of environmental milieu, i.e. be lower in seawater fish, but increased in freshwater.

During the last two decades we have learned that prolactin has a prominent and well defined role in the regulation of immune function[7,8]: as an immune modulator it enhances the proliferative response, but also has a role in certain autoimmune diseases as a pathoclinical indicator in multi-organ and organ specific autoimmune diseases (e.g. in lupus erythematosus (SLE), rheumatoid arthritis (RA), Sjogren's syndrome, Hashimoto's thyroiditis, multiple sclerosis (MS), psoriasis, etc)[9, 10, 11]. Prolactin may also participate in the development of immune tolerance between the fetus and the maternal organism during pregnancy[12]. Several experimental and also clinical evidences confirming the relationship between prolactin and the immune system have required to open new "sub-folder" for the role of prolactin in "immune-biology", "immune-endocrinology" and "neuroimmune-modulation", as well as for non-clinical and clinical contributions to the search for potential new drugs in the development process.

The physiological role of prolactin is still important in the classical fields of reproduction. Prolactin seems to be involved in the central control of sexual behavior and activity. There is a brief and sudden elevation of prolactin during orgasm indicating that it may have a role in the "gratification" during sexual acts as well[13]. On the other hand, a nondrug related female sexual dysfunction (FSD), affecting up to 1 in 10 US women, manifested with a decreased sexual desire could also be associated with increased prolactin levels [14]. A chronic hyperprolactinemia is clinically associated with hypogonadotropic hypogonadism and sexual dysfunction as well, while treatment of hyperprolactinemia restores normal sexual function both in men and women[15].

Moreover, prolactin levels and our behavior are potentially also connected. Prolactin is higher during periods of nursing in some species, but also in human during "maternal" as well as "paternal" behavior: fathers of infants have elevated prolactin levels [16].

Prolactin stimulates proliferation of oligodendrocyte precursor cells (they are cells that differentiate into oligodendrocytes, and they are responsible for the formation of myelin sheet of axons in the central nervous system (CNS)[17,18]. Interestingly, high prolactin levels stimulate the proliferation of olfactory epithelium[19].

Prolactin can also be found in amniotic fluid and contributes to surfactant synthesis of fetal lungs at the end of pregnancy[20].

Since pituitary prolactin is under a close and mainly inhibitory control of hypothalamic dopaminergic system, it is predictable that drugs attenuating pathological neurotransmitter levels (like in schizophrenia, mood disturbances, etc) may have potential side effect resulting in clinical signs associated with or caused by hyperprolactinemia. Some of the effective antipsychotic treatments may have medication related adverse drug reactions appear in more than two-thirds of the patients [21, 22, 23], indicating the continuous need to search for prolactin-sparing solutions.

Furthermore, we are now aware that synthesis and secretion of prolactin is not restricted to the anterior lobe of the pituitary gland, but other organs and individual cells can also produce it. Indeed, the multiple roles and sources of prolactin had led Bern and Nicoll *(1968)*, to suggest renaming it to "omnipotin" or "versatilin" [24]. This book provides the headlines to follow a course of cumulated knowledge on prolactin research during the last two-three decades and it may also help us understand some of the concerns that we face today.

György M. Nagy and **Dr Bela Ernest Toth**

References

[1] Riddle O, Bates RW, Dykshorn SW *(1933)* The preparation, identification and assay of prolactin—a hormone of anterior pituitary. *Am J Physiol* 105:191–216.

[2] MacLeod RM. Influence of norepinephrine and catecholamine-depleting agents on the synthesis and release of prolactin and growth hormone. Endocrinology. 1969; 85: 916-23.

[3] Neill JD, Nagy GM. Prolactin secretion and its control. In: Knobil E, Neill J.D., eds. Physiology of Reproduction. New York: Raven Press; 1994. p. 1833-60.

[4] Freeman ME, Kanyicska B, Lerant A, Nagy G. Prolactin: structure, function, and regulation of secretion. Physiol Rev.2000; 80: 1523-631.

[5] MacLeod RM. Regulation of prolactin secretion. In: Martini L, Ganong WF, eds. Frontiers in Neuroendocrinology. New York: Raven Press; 1976. p. 169-94.

[6] McCormick SD, Bradshaw D. Hormonal control of salt and water balance in vertebrates. Gen Comp Endocrinol.2006; 147: 3-8.

[7] Berczi I. The role of the growth and lactogenic hormone family in immune function. Neuroimmunomodulation.1994; 1: 201-16.

[8] Dorshkind K, Horseman ND. Anterior pituitary hormones, stress, and immune system homeostasis. Bioessays.2001; 23: 288-94.

[9] Shelly S, Boaz M, Orbach H. Prolactin and autoimmunity. Autoimmun Rev. 2012 May;11(6-7):A465-70. doi: 10.1016/j.autrev.2011.11.009. Epub 2011 Dec 2. Review. PubMed PMID: 22155203.

[10] Jara LJ, Medina G, Saavedra MA, Vera-Lastra O, Navarro C. Prolactin and autoimmunity. Clin Rev Allergy Immunol. 2011 Feb;40(1):50-9. doi: 10.1007/s12016-009-8185-3. Review. PubMed PMID: 19911311.

[11] Orbach H, Shoenfeld Y. Hyperprolactinemia and autoimmune diseases. Autoimmun Rev. 2007 Sep;6(8):537-42. Epub 2006 Dec 1. Review. PubMed PMID: 17854745.

[12] Zen M, Ghirardello A, Iaccarino L, Tonon M, Campana C, Arienti S et al. Hormones, immune response, and pregnancy in healthy women and SLE patients. Swiss Med Wkly.2010; 140: 187-201.

[13] Kruger TH, Hartmann U, Schedlowski M. Prolactinergic and dopaminergic mechanisms underlying sexual arousal and orgasm in humans. World J Urol.2005; 23: 130-138.

[14] Simon JA. Low sexual desire--is it all in her head? Pathophysiology, diagnosis, and treatment of hypoactive sexual desire disorder. Postgrad Med. 2010 Nov;122(6):128-36.

[15] Corona G, Ricca V, Bandini E, Mannucci E, Lotti F, Boddi V, Rastrelli G, Sforza A, Faravelli C, Forti G, Maggi M. Selective serotonin reuptake inhibitor-induced sexual dysfunction. J Sex Med. 2009 May;6(5):1259-69. doi: 10.1111/j.1743-6109.2009.01248.x. PubMed PMID: 19473282.

[16] Gettler LT, McDade TW, Feranil AB, Kuzawa CW. Prolactin, fatherhood, and reproductive behavior in human males. Am J Phys Anthropol. 2012 Jul;148(3):362-70. doi: 10.1002/ajpa.22058. Epub 2012 May 11. PubMed PMID: 22576125.

[17] Gregg C, Shikar V, Larsen P, Mak G, Chojnacki A, Yong VW et al. White matter plasticity and enhanced remyelination in the maternal CNS. J Neurosci.2007; 27: 1812-23.

[18] Gregg C. Pregnancy, prolactin and white matter regeneration. J Neurol Sci.2009; 285: 22-27.

[19] Orita S, Yoshinobu J, Orita Y, Tsujigiwa H, Kakiuchi M, Nagatsuka H, Nomiya S, Nagai N, Nishizaki K. Prolactin may stimulate proliferation in the olfactory epithelium of the female mouse. Am J Rhinol Allergy. 2009 Mar-Apr;23(2):135-8. doi: 10.2500/ajra.2009.23.3282.

[20] Mendelson CR, Boggaram V. Hormonal control of the surfactant system in fetal lung. Annu Rev Physiol.1991; 53: 415-40.

[21] Carroll RW, Christodoulou P, Baynes KC, Kahn DA. Hyperprolactinemia in a patient with a pituitary adenoma receiving antipsychotic drug therapy. J Psychiatr Pract. 2012 Mar;18(2):126-9.

[22] Gallego JA, Nielsen J, De Hert M, Kane JM, Correll CU. Safety and tolerability of antipsychotic polypharmacy. Expert Opin Drug Saf. 2012 Jul;11(4):527-42. doi: 10.1517/14740338.2012.683523. Epub 2012 May 8.

[23] Inder WJ, Castle D. Antipsychotic-induced hyperprolactinaemia. Aust N Z J Psychiatry. 2011 Oct;45(10):830-7. doi: 10.3109/00048674.2011.589044. Epub 2011 Jun 30. Review. PubMed PMID: 21714721.

[24] Bern HA, Nicoll CS. The comparative endocrinology of prolactin. Recent Prog Horm Res. 1968;24:681-720. Review.

Chapter 1

Prolactin and Angiogenesis: Biological Implications of Microheterogeneity

Kambadur Muralidhar and Jaeok Lee

Additional information is available at the end of the chapter

http://dx.doi.org/10.5772/54318

1. Introduction

Prolactin (PRL) was discovered in 1928. It is found in all vertebrates including humans. The name 'prolactin' is derived from its established role, in female mammals, in mammopoiesis. That raised the first mystery regarding its role in the human male and in non-mammalian vertebrates. More than 300 effects have been produced by injecting PRL into animals of all phylogenic groups. That raised the second mystery i.e. absence of any reliable and relevant bio assay for PRL till today. Following the approaches of Reductionist Biology, prolactin has been purified and characterized from a number of vertebrate groups. That raised the third mystery i.e. extensive microheterogeneity in structure and its doubtful relevance to physiology. The mechanism of action of prolactin has been studied extensively and that gave rise to the fourth mystery as to why it does not follow the second messenger model in signaling pathways, as in the case of other membrane receptor acting hormones like epinephrine or Luteinizing hormone (LH) or FSH etc. Prolactin behaves more like a cytokine and growth factor than like a hormone! In spite of exhibiting multiple physiological effects on a variety of tissues like brain (behavior), gonadal and mammary tissues, accessory sex organs like ventral prostate, immune system of phagocytes and lymphocytes etc, no disease whose origin can be ascribed to mutations in PRL or PRL receptor genes has yet been discovered. That is the fifth mystery. There is no known clinical model of prolactin deficiency. Hyperprolactinemia due to tumors of pituitary lactotrophs is the only known pathological condition. Long term hyperprolactinemia can lead to amenorrhea in women, loss of libido in men and infertility in both.

2. Relevant biochemistry and biology of prolactin

The first observation related to prolactin was made in 1928 (Stricker and Grueter, 1928). These French scientists injected a bovine pituitary extract into pseudopregnant rabbits and observed that such rabbits started lactating. Thereafter Riddle et al (1933) reported that the crude extract could stimulate the production of "milk" by the crop sac of pigeons. Later it was established that the same pituitary principle was responsible for both the crop "milk" production and mammary gland secretion. The same component of pituitary was purified using a pigeon crop sac development as bioassay from bovine pituitary and termed as "Prolactin" (Riddle et al 1933). Thirty years after its discovery, the first amino acid sequence of ovine Prolactin was completed in 1970 (Li et al. 1970). Prolactin from different species of fishes to mammals has since been sequenced (Sinha, 1995).

Prolactin and growth hormone from buffalo pituitaries have been purified and characterized in our laboratory (Muralidhar, et al., 1994; Khurana and Muralidhar, 1997; Maithal et al, 2001). The molecular size of buPRL monomer was 22,664 Da as determined by MALDI-TOF analysis (Panchal and Muralidhar, 2008). Enhancement of Nb2 rat lymphoma cell proliferation by the hormone has been studied (Khurana and Muralidhar, 1997). Prolactin from number species of different classes of vertebrate has been purified and characterized. Primary structure of PRL from about 45 species is known either by protein sequence directly or deduction from gene sequence or cDNA sequence (Sinha, 1995). In most of the mammalian species prolactin contains three intra-disulfide bridges between Cysteine residues 4-11, 58-174 and 191-199. Teleost PRLs, however, lack the amino terminal disulfide loop (Sinha, 1995).

The major role of prolactin in eutherians and marsupials is regulation of milk secretion and growth of mammary gland. The binding specificity of prolactin receptors does vary between species, however (Amit et al, 1997). Prolactin also plays other roles in mammals, like in immunomodulation, osmoregulation and control of parental behavior and it may be that variation in the relative importance of one or more of these provide the drive for adaptive change (Wallis, 2000).

Prolactin is biosynthesized as a larger precursor protein but processed into a ~23 kDa protein in most of the species. Many different molecular size isoforms as well as forms of PRL with post translational modifications like glycosylation, phosphorylation and sulfation have been described in literature. Dimerisation and polymerization of prolactin or aggregation with binding proteins, such as immunoglobulins, by covalent and non covalent bonds may result in high-molecular-weight forms. In general, the high-molecular weight forms have reduced biological activity (Sinha, 1995). The role of prolactin-IgG macromolecular complex in the detection and differential diagnosis of different prolactinemias is targeted primarily in clinical studies (Cavaco et al 1995).

Tyrosine sulfation is not a very common post-translational modification. Recently a review on this modification has listed 62 proteins which have been identified as tyrosine sulfated. For the majority of these, a role for sulfation in the function(s) of the proteins has not been described. In some cases sulfation is important in optimal receptor-ligand interactions (e.g.chemokine receptor binding), optimal proteolytic processing (e.g. gastrin processing), and proteolytic activation of extra cellular proteins (e.g. factor V and VIII activation) (Moore 2003).

There is only one pituitary hormone known to have sulfation of tyrosine and this is prolactin. It was found that a prolactin containing fraction had very high radioactivity when pituitary cells were incubated with radio labeled sulfate. Later it was proved that prolactin was the protein which was containing this radioactivity. Chemical analysis proved the sulfation is on the tyrosine residue/s of prolactin. Role of this tyrosine sulfated prolactin is still an unanswered question (Kohli et al 1987, Kohli et al 1988). Thus the key feature of PRL is structural microheterogeneity in various forms. The microheterogeneous isoforms of prolactin and growth hormone have been reported by our laboratory earlier. These isoforms reported included tyrosine sulphated prolactin (Kohli, et al., 1987; 1988; Chadha, et al., 1991), lower sized (19 kDa and 13 kDa) iso forms (Khurana and Muralidhar, 1997) and glycosylated isoforms (Khurana and Muralidhar, 1997) in buPRL. Similar size and charge isoforms of buffalo growth hormone have also been reported by our laboratory earlier (Maithal et al, 2001) However, the unique biological functions of the heterogeneous forms, if any, are not known yet. To serve as a frame work for investigations, we postulated two hypotheses with regard to biological significance of microheterogeneity in PRL. One was that microheterogeneous forms have different potencies in a given bioassay during ontogeny. Two, that microheterogeneous forms exhibit different biological activities in different phylogenic groups of animals during phylogeny. It was observed that the non-glycosylated isoform of buPRL was 4-5 times more potent than the glycosylated isoform of buPRL in the Nb2 rat lymphoma cell growth assay *in vitro* (Khurana and Muralidhar, 1997). Similarly it was observed that the PRL with higher isoelectric point (i.e. more basic isoform) had a higher potency than the PRL isoform with lower isoelectric point (i.e. more acidic isoform) in the same assay.

2.1. Prolactin from peripheral tissues

The cells of the anterior pituitary gland which synthesize and secrete prolactin were initially described by light microscopy using conventional staining techniques (Herlant 1964). These cells designated lactotrophs or mammotrophs comprise 20-50% of the cellular population of the anterior pituitary gland depending on the sex and physiological status of the animal. The first observation that prolactin is produced in the brain was by Fuxe (Fuxe et al 1977) who found prolactin immuno reactivity in hypothalamic axon terminals. Prolactin immuno reactivity was subsequently found in the telencephalon in the cerebral cortex, hippocampus amygdala, septum (Devito 1988), caudate putamen (Emanuele et al 1992), brain stem (Devito 1988), cerebellum (Seroogy et al 1988), spinal cord (Siaud et al 1989), choroids plexi, and the circum ventricular organs (Thompson 1982).

Several approaches have been taken to prove that prolactin is found in the hypothalamus and that it is synthesized locally, independent of prolactin synthesis in the pituitary gland. Indeed, hypophysectomy has no effect on the amount of immuno reactive prolactin in the male hypothalamus and only diminishes but does not abolish the quantity of immuno reactive prolactin in the female rat hypothalamus (Devito 1988). With the use of conventional peptide mapping and sequencing of a polymerase chain reaction (PCR) product of hypothalamic cDNA from intact and hypophysectomized rats (Wilson et al 1992), it has been established that the primary structure of prolactin of hypothalamic origin is identical to that of the prolactin of the anterior pituitary (Wilson et al 1992). The deciduas produce a prolactin-like molecule that is indistinguishable from pituitary prolactin in human (Andersen 1990, Riddick et al 1978), Finally, the non pregnant uterus has been shown to be a source of prolactin as well. Indeed a decidual-like prolactin, indistinguishable from pituitary prolactin (Gellersen et al 1989) has been identified in the myometrium of nonpregnant rats (Ben-Jonathan et.al, 2008). In addition to uptake of prolactin from the blood, the mammary epithelial cells of lactating animals are capable of synthesizing prolactin. The presence of prolactin mRNA (Kurtz et al 1993) as well as synthesis of immunoreactive prolactin by mammary epithelial cells of lactating rats has been described (Lkhider et al 1996). A great deal of evidence suggests that lymphocytes can be a source of prolactin as well (Gala et al 1994, Montgomery et al 1990).

2.2. Receptors to Prolactin (PRLR)

The PRLR was identified as a specific, high-affinity, membrane–anchored protein (Kelly et al 1974). The cDNA encoding the rat PRLR has been prepared. As is true for their respective ligands, receptors for PRL and GH (GHR) are also closely related (Boutin et al 1988, Kelly et al 1991). Both are single–pass transmembrane chains and despite a relatively low degree (~30%) of sequence identity, they share several structural and functional features (Kelly et al 1991, Goffin et al 1998). The gene encoding human PRLR is located on chromosome 5 (p13-14) and contains at least 10 exons for an overall length exceeding 100 kb (Arden et al 1990). multiple isoforms of membrane-bound PRLR resulting from alternative splicing of the primary transcript have been identified in several species (Boutin et al 1988)..

3. Prolactin and angiogenesis

Angiogenesis has been described well. A number of factors regulate this process in the body (Iyer and Acharya, 2002). We report here that naturally occurring lower size isoforms of buPRL, Cathepsin derived peptide fragments of prolactin and synthetic peptide from the internal sequence of both prolactin and growth hormone were found to exhibit anti-angiogenic activity in endothelial cell migration and CAM assays. Further using in silico methods, the three dimensional structure of buffalo prolactin was arrived at including the location of the anti angiogenic peptide sequence. A 16 K PRL as a newly generated N-terminal 16 K fragment resulting from the proteolysis of rat PRL by acidified mammary extracts was discovered and reported in 1980 (Mittra 1980a and 1980b). Since then, this PRL fragment has received considerable attention from the scientific community. The protease responsible for the cleavage of rat PRL into 16K was identified as Cathepsin D, The 16K PRL was shown to have lost PRL receptor binding ability but otherwise to have acquired the ability to specifically bind another membrane receptor (Clapp and Weiner 1992) through which it exerts antiangiogenic activity (Clapp et al 1993). Although this receptor is still not identified, some of its downstream signaling targets have been elucidated (D'Angelo et al 1999, Corbacho et al 2000).However; many questions related to the biology of 16K PRL remain unanswered. First, although the majority of investigations have used rat 16K PRL, results are much less clear for other species, especially humans, in which PRL was recently reported to be resistant to Cathepsin D (Khurana et al 1999a and 1999b). This contrasts with the findings indicating that hPRL yields partial, but reproducible, proteolysis leading to N-terminal 16K like PRL fragments when incubated with this protease. Second, because it may be generated both centrally (Clapp et al 1994) and at the periphery, such as in pulmonary fibroblasts (Corbacho et al 2000) and endothelial cells (Corbacho et al 2000), the site/s of 16K PRL generation remains to be clearly identified. Hence, whether all sites of extra pituitary PRL synthesis can generate 16K PRL from endogenous 23K PRL or alternatively, whether circulating PRL is internalized before the proteolyzed form is exported (or both) remains open to investigation. Also, the sub-cellular compartment/s in which appropriate proteolysis conditions are found remain/s to be identified, although one can not discard the possibility that the cleavage of takes place in extra cellular milieu. In humans, although various recombinant forms of 16K hPRL were shown to be antiangiogenic, no insight into the biological relevance of hPRL *in vivo* was provided. It is relevant to ask also whether, the effects of PRL on tumors *in vivo* should be viewed from a new angle, considering a balance between the mitogenic and angiogenic (pro-tumor) activities of full-length PRL versus the antiangiogenic (anti tumor) activity of 16K-PRL (Goffin et al 1999).

3.1. Purification of buffalo PRL monomer from a discarded acid pellet

Buffalo pituitary prolactin in monomeric form can be prepared (Panchal and Muralidhar, 2008). The lower size isoforms of buffalo PRL can be separated from the monomer as well as the higher sized isoforms by differential alcohol fractionation (Panchal and Muralidhar, 2008) This lower size isoform containing fraction was designated as (AP) P-190-70. The APP-I, a semi-pure buPRL from buffalo pituitaries (Chaudhary, et al., 2004), has higher sized forms (>34.9 kDa, 34.9 kDa and 25.9 kDa (26 K)) and lower sized forms (18.4 kDa (18 K), 14.5 kDa (14 K) and <14.5 kDa) as well as buPRL monomer (23.4 kDa). The lower sized forms, approximately 18 K and 14 K under non-reducing conditions transform into 19 K and 13 K bands under reducing conditions (Khurana and Muralidhar, 1997). The 26 K PRL under non-reducing condition is probably the isoform nicked in the large loop of intact form but with intact disulfide bonds (Mittra I, 1980a; 1980b). Khurana and Muralidhar (1997) reported that 25 K buPRL (under non-reducing condition of SDS-PAGE) disappeared under reducing condition of the gel. The size isoform mixture, APP-I could be separated by differential alcohol precipitation. APP-I 70 (higher sized form mixture) and APP-I 90-70 (lower sized form mixture) were checked by SDS-PAGE analysis. The lower sized form mixture, APP-I 90-70, was confirmed to be free from higher sized forms by immunoblotting analysis. The reason for the successful separation is that the two different sized mixtures had different pI. Buffalo PRL monomer has pI 5.1~5.45 (Chadha, et al., 1991). The higher sized forms and monomer are probably soluble in the alkaline ethanol. The buPRL lower sized peptides had opposite property.

3.2. Anti-angiogenic activity of (AP) P-I 90-70 fraction, lower size isoforms mixture

It has been known that N-terminal 16K PRL fragment had an inhibitory effect on angiogenesis i.e. the formation of new blood vessels (Folkman and Shing 1992), in rat (Ferrara, et al 1991) and in human (Clapp, et al 1993) both *in vitro* and *ex vivo*. Thus, it was of interest to know whether the lower size forms mixture including 18K and 14K size forms i.e. naturally occurring PRL peptides, have the anti-angiogenic activity or not. Hence (AP) P-I 90-70 fraction was tested with endothelial cell migration assay (*in vitro*) and chick egg yolk membrane assay (*ex vivo*) (Figure 1). Approximately 7 % inhibition of cell migration compared to control was observed after 4 hrs and 8 hrs, when 30 pg/ml of (AP)P-I 90-70 was added to human immortalized umbilical vein endothelial cells, EAhy926. The exact amount of the active peptide(s) in this mixture is difficult to estimate. It is, therefore, clearly proved that the physiologically cleaved buPRL fragments (i.e. naturally occurring lower size isoforms) had an anti-angiogenic function. The C-terminal 16 K hPRL does not appear to have the anti angiogenic activity (Khurana et al 1999). Extrapolating this fact to buffalo PRL, the present PRL lower size isoforms have to be mostly N-terminal fragments. If C-terminal fragments were in the mixture of isoforms, their presence is much less than that of N-terminal ones. Or those fragments may include specific anti-angiogenic active site. This (AP)P-I 90-70 fraction needs to be further characterized. Struman et al. (1999) reported that intact human PRL, GH and PL exhibited angiogenic activity. However, our results indicate unequivocally that the buPRL monomer had no significant stimulatory or inhibitory effect on blood vessel formation in CAM and endothelial cell migration assays.

3.3. Peptides derived from buffalo PRL by enzymatic digestion have anti angiogenic activity

Most of the studies about the antiangiogenic N-terminal fragment cleaved by Cathepsin D (CD) have been done in the case of rat and human PRLs (Ferrara et al. 1991). It was therefore hypothesized that buffalo pituitary PRL can be cleaved by Cathepsin D, and that the fragment could inhibit angiogenesis via endothelial interference. Here, we demonstrate that buPRL size isoform produced by CD have an inhibitory action on angiogenesis. However, it was not clear which sequence in the N-terminal fragment plays a role in antiangiogenesis. Highly pure buPRL monomer was obtained from pituitary glands with the protocol standardized in our laboratory designed with differential ethanol extractions to separate both different sized forms followed by a single Sephacryl S-200 chromatography (Panchal and Muralidhar, *2008*). The selected fractions after S-200 gel filtration showed more than 95% size homogeneity of buPRL as determined by 15% SDS-PAGE and densitometry.

The purified buPRL monomer, intact form, was confirmed to be free from protease contamination especially from the acidic protease treatment. Intact buPRL was incubated

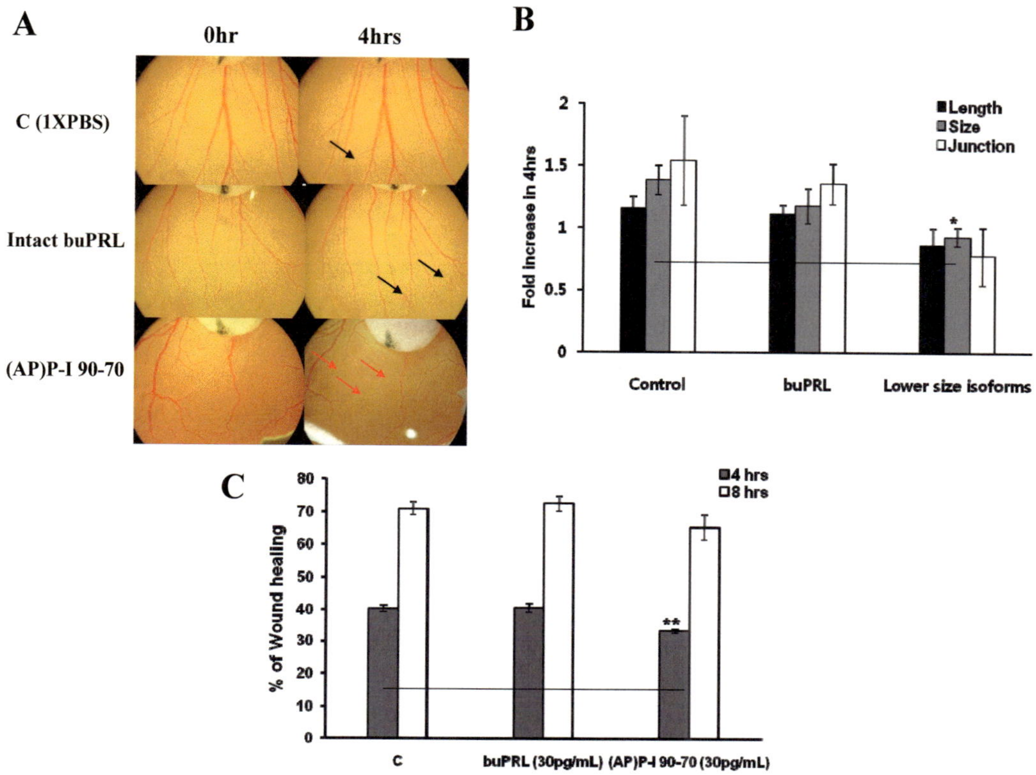

Figure 1. Antiangiogenic activity by *ex vivo* and *in vitro* assays. A, Results of CAM assay. Eggs at 6th day of incubation were used for the assay. B, Analysis of the results of A. C, Results of endothelial cell migration assay. Values are means ± SEM. P < 0.05 vs control. **Significantly different from control cells (P < 0.001).

with distilled water and 20 mM citrate/phosphate buffer including salt (i.e. pH 3.0) at 37°C, respectively, and then analyzed by electrophoresis at frequent intervals. When the intact buPRL was incubated in distilled water for 6 h, no lower-sized fragments were detected in SDS-PAGE either under non-reducing or reducing conditions. However, when the intact buPRL was incubated under the acidic conditions, a lower-sized form, approximately 21 kDa, was observed in SDS-PAGE under reducing conditions.. The lower form did not significantly increase in type and quantity during the incubation time, up to 12 h. Protease-free intact buPRL was incubated with bovine spleen CD (the ratio of substrate vs enzyme = 100:1) in acidic condition (pH 3.0) 37°C,and then the peptide mixture was separated in a 15% SDS-PAGE under reducing conditions.. Results indicated that the intact buPRL was cleaved by CD at pH 3.0 and the molecular weight of cleaved peptides were approximately 18.39 kDa (18K), 14 kDa (14K), 11.16 kDa (11K) and 7.47 kDa (7K). These sizes were identified by immunological analysis using buPRL antiserum (Figure 2B). The mixture did not show a significant contamination of CD (42.12 kDa and 29 kDa) (Fig. 2A) This enzymatic cleavage was confirmed when in the presence of pepstatin A (Marks et al. 1973), a known acidic protease inhibitor, CD did not generate lower-sized peptides from the monomer under non-reducing conditions to just below monomer under reducing conditions (Fig.2D and 2E, L1). The amount of cleaved isoform under non-reducing condition decreased at 6 h incubation (Fig. 2D, L6).

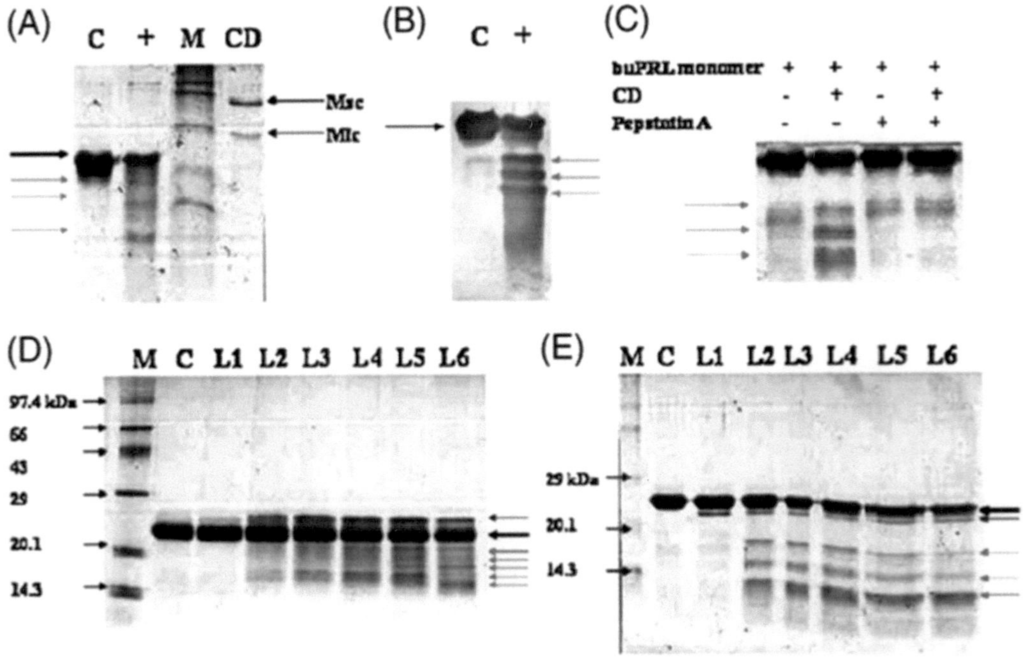

Figure 2. (**A**) Results of SDS-PAGE analysis after colloidal Coomassie blue staining. Lane C, buPRL monomer (5 µg); Lane +, buPRL monomer (5 µg) incubated with CD; Lane M, molecular weight marker; Lane CD, Cathepsin D (7.49 µ g); Msc, mature single chain (42.12 kDa); Mlc, mature large chain (29 kDa). (**B**) Immunoblot of **A** with anti-buPRL serum indicating the cleaved fragments of buPRL by CD. (**C**) Effect of pepstatin A on buPRL cleavage by CD. (**D**) Time course of action by CD on buPRL monomer. L1–L6 represent analysis of reaction mixture by SDS-PAGE under non-reducing conditions after 0 and 30 min, and 1, 2, 3 and 6 h, respectively. Lane C is the control where no enzyme was added; Lane M represents marker. (**E**) Same as **D** except that the gel was run under the reducing conditions. (Taken from Jaeok Lee et al 2011 with permission).

Cell migration analysis by wound healing assay was performed in EAhy926. The cell line expresses factor VIII-related antigen and has the same morphological distribution as primary endothelial cells with a doubling time of 12 h (Edgell et al. 1983).

A dose-dependent (3.3 pg/mL to 330 µg/mL) inhibition by buPRL peptide mixture including intact form on migration of EAhy926 cells was observed. Hence, 33 pg/mL of the peptide mixture was used for early stage (on the day 4) CAM assay, one of the *ex vivo* methods to study angiogenesis (Ribatti et al.1996).The blood vessel generation reduced with the dose of the peptide mixture in a time-dependent fashion. These studies were done with the peptide mixture which was not separated from the undigested PRL, if any. This meant that in our hands the PRL monomer had neither antiangiogenic nor angiogenic activity. Further intact

PRL was not binding to the putative receptors to which the peptides were supposed to bind and exhibit their antiangiogenic activity. Prolactin is known to bind to PRL- specific receptors. Hence it can also be concluded, tentatively at least, that Cathepsin digested PRL – derived peptides do not work through PRL receptors for their anti angiogenic activity.

3.4. The peptide mixture separated from PRL retains antiangiogenic activity

The results described above were confirmed when the peptide mixture was separated from the undigested intact PRL on an FPLC column and then tested for antiangiogenic activity (Jaeok Lee et al 2011). It is interesting to note the cleavage pattern of prolactins from different species when exposed to Cathepsin D is different. For example, the sizes of fragments obtained by CD from buffalo prolactin are different from the sizes of cleaved fragments of PRL from : rat pituitary (16K and 8K) (Mittra, 1980a, b), mouse pituitary (16K and 8K) (Sinha and Gilligan, 1984), and human pituitary (17K, 16.5K, 15K, 11K, 8K and 5K) (Piwnica et al. 2006) PRL (Fig.3) These different patterns of cleavage could be due to micro-variation in the primary structure among species. Comparing the cleaved sequences between human and rat PRLs, Tyr147-Pro148-Val149-Trp150-Ser151 of human and Tyr145-Leu146-Val147-Trp148-Ser149 of rat are homologous (Piwnica et *al.* 2006) (Fig.3B). The presence of Pro148 and Leu132 controls the cleavage pattern in hPRL (Piwnica et al 2006). Pro148 prevented high cleavage efficiency at 147–148 and 150–151 sites, while Leu132 produced the additional cleavage at 132–133 sites (Piwnica et al. 2006). Buffalo PRL has the same sequence at 147–151 site as in hPRL, but not at residue 132 (Fig. 3B). The Pro148 in buPRL also seems to link to a specific cleavage pattern. Hence, 18K and 14K of buPRL were considered homologous to 17K and 15K of hPRL, respectively. We could not detect a fragment similar to the 16.5K fragment of hPRL.

Angiogenesis, the process of developing new blood vessels from preexisting vessels, is crucial to reproduction, growth and wound healing (Folkman and Shing 1992). In the last two decades, numerous studies reported novel angiogenic regulators (Iyer and Acharya, 2002). Among the angiogenic regulators, hPRL fragment is one of the very paradoxical molecules. Its intact form has pro-angiogenic action (Struman et al. 1999), inducing cell proliferation and motility, and relates to breast carcinogenesis (Clevenger et al. 2003). The PRL fragments as well as intact PRL were are also known to be secreted from vascular endothelial cells (Ochoa et al. 2001). The antiangiogenic and anti mitogenic effects of peptide fragments were observed in BBBE and HUVE cells, even in the presence of PRL antibody. This suggested the possibility that they act as autocrine regulators of angiogenesis, (Clapp et al. 1998; Corbacho et al. 2000).

3.5. Buffalo pituitary PRL derived peptides are active at pico gram level

In the present study, the antiangiogenic activity of buPRL-derived peptides was demonstrated *in vitro* and ex *vivo*. Endothelial cell migration is fundamental to angiogenesis (Lamalice et al. 2007), because endothelial cells, derived from meso dermal cells, form capillary blood and lymphatic vessels (Venes and Thomas 2001).

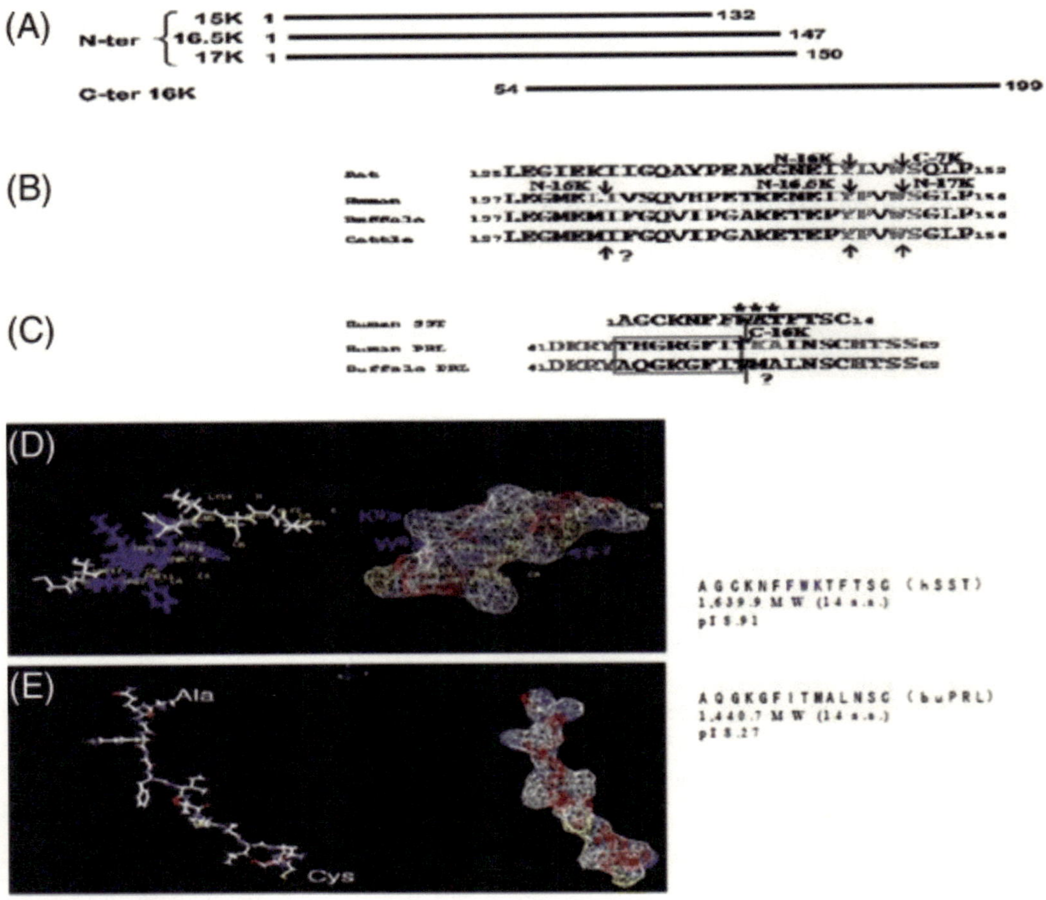

Figure 3. CD and thrombin cleavage site in the primary sequences of rat, human, buffalo and cattle PRLs. (**A**) In human PRL three N-termini by CD and C-terminus by thrombin (figure from Piwnica, et al. 2004). (**B**) CD cleavage sites in rat, human, buffalo and cattle PRLs. (**C**) The SST aligned sequences of buPRL and buGH are partially or completely involved in the sequence of N-terminus fragment known as antiangiogenic factor. Triple * in hSST is the specific binding site to SSTRs. The square window indicates the considered sequence has an antiangiogenic action. Arrows indicate the cleavage sites. (**D**) hSST in SWISS-Pdb viewer 4.0. Blue arrows and alphabets represent SST receptor binding sites. (**E**) The synthetic peptide derived from buPRL. Molecular size and pI of each peptide were gained from ExPASy Proteomics tools. (Taken from Jaeok Lee et al, 2011 with permission)

Earlier reports found antiangiogenic activity of r16K (Ferrara et al. 1991) and recombinant h16K (Clapp et.al. 1993; D'Angelo et.al. 1999) in micromolar concentrations. The present study demonstrates that buPRL-derived peptides have an antiangiogenic activity in nanomolar concentration. Even the cleaved fragments mixed with intact buPRL, considered a pro-angiogenic factor (Struman et al. 1999), are effective at the lower concentration level. The results of our study prove that buPRL peptides cleaved by CD have the antiangiogenic action, and these peptides must have come from N-terminal side. Mechanistic studies were undertaken and it was observed that the peptide mixture obtained by Cathepsin D digestion of prolactin was capable of antagonizing the action of Bradykinin (BK) in terms of NO production.

NO, produced by NO synthase (NOS), is a second messenger in the regulation of physiological and pathophysiological process in the cardiovascular, nervous and immune systems (Moncada and Higgs 1993; Nathan and Xie 1994). NO is involved in cell migration and cell protection (Lee et al. 2005; Kolluru et al. 2008). NO-mediated pathway is a well known signaling mechanism of angiogenesis, vasopermeability and vasorelaxation in relation to VEGF (Ferreira and Henzel, 1989; Ishikawa *et al.* 1989), BK (Regoli and Barabe 1980; Ferreira et al. 1992) and Acetyl choline (Ach) actions (Palmer et al. 1989). Gonzalez et al. (2004) reported that human and rat 16K PRL fragments inhibited NOS activation induced not only by VEGF and BK but also by Ach, in endothelial cells. Buffalo PRL fragments seem not to be correlated to the pathway stimulated by Ach in EAhy926 (Jaeok Lee et al, 2011). Moreover, the buPRL peptides were more effective in inhibiting the BK-mediated NO mechanism than that by VEGF. It is not known, however, how this peptide blocks the NO pathway. We envisage two possible mechanisms. One is that the peptides act as receptor antagonists of angiogenic factors, and the other is that the peptides induce another pathway to inhibit NO production driven by these angiogenic factors. Besides, the role of individual amino acid residues in the antiangiogenic action is not yet clear.

It has been observed that these proteolytically derived peptides from buffalo PRL are more potent than Somatostatin (Jaeok Lee et al, 2011). Somatostatin, a small peptide (14 amino acids) secreted from hypothalamus, is a negative regulator of growth hormone (GH) release (Norman 1997). Widely distributed throughout the body, SST binds to five different subtypes of its cognate receptors (SSTR1-5), one of them being a G-protein-coupled receptor present on the cell membrane (Patel *et al.* 1990; Lahlou *et al.* 2004). While the five SSTRs bind the natural peptide, SSTR2, SSTR3, and SSTR5 can bind its synthetic analogues (Lahlou et al. 2004). SST and its analogues inhibit angiogenesis and also the production and secretion of angiogenic factors including VEGF (Barrie *et al.* 1993). It was reported that SST blocked Kaposi sarcoma (KS) cells (KS-Imm), isolated from a kidney-transplanted, immuno suppressed patient and also highly angiogenic, xenografts into nude (nu/nu) mice through angiostasis (Albini et al. 1999). SST also induced cell death of human somatotrph tumor cells (SSTR2) (Ferrante *et al.* 2006). In the study with vascular endothelial cell (dominated by SSTR3) by Reisine and Bell 1995), SST inhibited cell proliferation through blocking of both endothelial NOS (eNOS) and MAPK activations. SST is a powerful anti-tumour angiostatic agent. The results of our work confirm that SST and 14K buPRL are significant antiangiogenic factors, and 14K is more effective than SST in the antiangiogenesis assays. The antiangiogenesis brought about by buPRL fragment seems to be related to the inhibition of vasopermeability of endothelial cells.

It is interesting to note that a synthetic peptide corresponding to the Somatostatin sequence within the amino acid sequence of buffalo pituitary Growth hormone is capable of antagonizing Bradykinin induced angiogenesis in terms of nitric oxide production (Syamantak Majumder et al, 2009). To what receptors do these lower size isoforms of buPRL bind in their antiangiogenic activity? In our hands, intact buffalo PRL had neither pro- nor anti- angiogenic activity. The peptides may act through PRL receptors or through other receptors like those to Bradykinin or VEGF. They may also have their own distinct receptors. As they are capable of inhibiting VEGF or Bradykinin induced angiogenesis, it can be safely concluded that the peptides might work through VEGF or Bradykinin receptors rather than PRL- specific receptors.

3.6. Antiangiogenic activity of the Synthetic peptides

Generally, the conformation of the cleaved fragment is either new and unstable or native-like which is less stable than that of the original (Creighton, 1993). No experimental details are available on the conformation of the cleaved fragment. Nevertheless, a significant difference in the N-terminal 14K PRL structure from the intact PRL was that the loop between the first and the second α-helices were loosened and more opened to the environment. In the intact form, the loop was close to the fourth α-helix.

The disulfide bond between the loop and the fourth α-helix, between Cys58 and Cys174, in the centre of the loop might be giving more compact configuration.

We have cloned and expressed cDNA for buffalo prolactin in E.coli and the bacterially expressed buffalo prolactin was biologically active in stimulating Nb2 rat lymphoma cells in vitro to divide (Manoj Panchal and Muralidhar, 2010). From the nucleotide sequence of the cDNA, the aminoacid sequence was deduced and from the available 3- dimensional structure of human prolactin, the 3-dimensional structure of buffalo prolactin was obtained by homology modelling. Somatostatin is a known inhibitor of angiogenesis. Using bioinformatics tool of BLAST search, we could locate a similar peptide in both prolactin and growth hormone. The peptides were synthesized through commercial sources. It was observed that the synthetic peptides, both the 13-mer and the 14-mer were active in pictogram range in all the *in vitro* and *ex vivo* bioassays.

Small ligands tend to bind, relatively speaking, the interior of globular proteins, while linear ligands tend to bind in clefts on the surface of proteins (Creighton *1993*). The small and linear structure of the synthesized peptide (Figure 3E) enables it to bind to both the interior of putative receptors and to the clefts on the surface of receptors. The synthetic peptide, Ala45-Gly47-Lys48-Gly49-Phe50-Ile51-Thr52-Met53-Ala54-Leu55-Asn56-Ser57-Cys58, also showed more active than SST in the antiangiogenic action. This SST-matching sequence peptide had a structure (linear) different from SST, which had α-helix structure (Figure 3D). This active motif for antiangiogenesis is not involved in binding to the PRLR sites, especially the second half of loop 1 (His59, Pro66 and Lys69) of site 1 (Goffin et al. 1992). This result also demonstrates that Ala45 to Met53 can be the active sites for angiostatic function. The C-terminal 16K peptide (54–199 residues) of hPRL does not appear to have the function of antiangiogenesis (Khurana et al. 1999b). In the C-terminal 16K fragment of hPRL, the fourth helix is still close to the partial second loop, which becomes exposed to environment in the N-terminal 16K fragment of hPRL. Because of this, the C-terminal 16K fragment of hPRL may not have antiangiogenic action. Three residues, Phe7-Trp8-Lys9, in SST sequence appear to have the crucial role in binding with high affinity to all SST receptors, SSTR1 to SSTR5 (Poitout et al. *2001*). However, in the synthetic sequence derived from buPRL, Ala1-Gln2-Gly3-Lys4-Gly5-Phe6-Ile7-Thr8-Met9-Ala10-Leu11-Asn12-Ser13-Cys14, 'Ile7-Thr8-Met9' is found instead of 'Phe7-Trp8-Lys9'. In the SST-matching sequence of hPRL, 'Ile51-Thr52-Lys53' replaces the SST tri-peptide sequence ('Phe7-Trp8-Lys9') positions (Figure 3C). This leads to the question of whether buPRL fragments bind to SSTR3 or not, and if the fragments bind to SSTR3, which residues in the sequence of the fragments bind to the receptor and mediate the antiangiogenic action? In the PRL fragments- and SST-mediated inhibition of the angiogenesis, there are similar mechanistic patterns. Both factors blocked VEGF-induced cell proliferation, which is known to be through the MAPK pathway in vascular endothelial cells (D'Angelo *et* al. 1999).

The hPRL and hGH tilted peptides (14-amino-acid sequence) consisting of 9 hydrophobic amino acids induce endothelial cell apoptosis and inhibit endothelial cell proliferation and capillary formation (Nguyen et al. 2006). The tilted peptide has been known to destabilize membrane and lipid core and is characterized by an asymmetric distribution of hydrophobic residues along the axis when helical. However, the synthetic tilted peptides derived from hPRL and hGH show 4 times and 32 times less activity, respectively, than the 16K hPRL *in vitro* (Nguyen et al. 2006). The synthetic peptide related to buPRL represents differences in structure and functional sensitivity from those of the tilted peptides. This peptide has similar sensitivity with 14K buPRL in the inhibition of angiogenesis *in vitro* and *ex vivo*. Although the peptide includes 9 hydrophobic amino acids, it does not form a helix (Figure 3E). These differences imply that the synthetic peptide related to buPRL has a receptor-binding mediated antiangiogenic function, rather than protein-membrane-interaction-mediated function.

4. Summary and speculation

The present study suggests that naturally occurring size iso forms of buPRL have antiangiogenic activity. Further, buPRL gives upon Cathepsin digestion a 16K-like fragment, but of 14K size and more cleaved fragments which have an antiangiogenic action. The antiangiogenic action of the fragments is, at least, related to the initial part of the sequence of the second loop between first and second α-helices. Furthermore, the synthetic peptide (derived by hSST matching area of buPRL) can be a potential anticancer therapeutic agent as well as for treatment of vascular, rheumatoid and other diseases whose etiology necessarily involves angiogenesis (Folkman 1995). Confirming the relevance of this idea requires demonstrating whether the buPRL fragments have N-terminal structure, and whether there are other sequences between Thr1 and Tyr44 having anti angiogenic action. Further work is required to explore whether SSTR3 is the specific receptor for 14K and other cleaved peptides, and if not, what is the specific receptor to the peptides, and what sequence part plays a crucial role in this antiangiogenic action? The biology of PRL is fascinating but very intriguing. More than 300 biological activities have been ascribed to PRL from various species. We have proposed two hypotheses to guide research on this hormone with regard to the significance of microheterogeneous isoforms. Our work has provided experimental evidence in support of these two hypotheses. Much more work needs to be done to understand and demystify prolactin actions.

Author details

Kambadur Muralidhar and Jaeok Lee
Hormone Research Laboratory, Department of Zoology, University of Delhi, Delhi, India

5. References

Albini A, Florio T, Giunciuglio D, Masiello L, Carlone S, Corsaro A, Thellung S, Cai T, Noonan DM and Schettini G (1999). Somatostatin controls Kaposi's sarcoma tumor growth through inhibition of angiogenesis; *FASEB J*.13: 647– 655.

Amit T, Dibner C, Barkey RJ (1997). Characterization of prolactin- and Growth hormone-binding proteins in milk and their diversity among Species. *Mol Cell Endocrinol* 130:167–180.

Andersen JR.(1990).Studies of decidual and amniotic prolactin in normal and pathological pregnancy *Dan Med Bull* 37: 154-165,1990.

Arden KC, Boutin JM, Djiane J, Kelly PA, Cavenee WK. (1990). The receptors for prolactin and growth hormone are localized in the same region of human chromosome 5. *Cytogenet Cell Genet*. 53 (2-3):161–165

Barrie R, Woltering EA, Hajarizadeh H, Mueller C, Ure T and Fletcher WS (1993). Inhibition of angiogenesis by somatostatin and somatostatin-like compounds is structurally dependent; *J. Surg. Res.* 55: 446-450.

Ben-Jonathan, N., La Pensee,C.R., and La Pensee, E.W (2008) What can we learn from rodents about prolactin in humans? *Endocrine Rev* 29: 1-41.

Boutin J-M, Jolicoeur C, Okamura H, Banville D, Dusanter-Fourt I, Djiane J & Kelly PA (1988). Cloning and expression of the rat prolactin receptor, a member of the growth hormone/prolactin receptor gene family. *Cell* 53: 69–77.

Boutin J-M, Edery M, Shirota M, Jolicoeur C, Lesueur L, Ali S, Gould D, Djiane J & Kelly PA (1989). Identification of a cDNA encoding a long form of prolactin receptor in human hepatoma and breast cancer cells. *Molecular Endocrinology* 3: 1455–1461.

Cavaco B , V Leite, M A Santos, E Arranhado, and L G Sobrinho (1995).Some forms of big big prolactin behave as a complex of monomeric prolactin with an immunoglobulin G in patients with macroprolactinemia or prolactinoma. *JCEM* 80: 2342-6;

Chadha N., Kohli R., Kumari G.L. and Muralidhar K. (1991) Physico-chemical and immunological characteristics of pituitary prolactin from water buffaloes (*Bubalus bubalis*). *Mol. Cell Biochem*. 105: 61-71.

Chaudhary R., Lee J.O. and Muralidhar K. (2004) Simultaneous isolation of prolactin and growth hormone from "discarded acid pellet" obtained from buffalo pituitaries. *Prep. Biochem. Biotech.* 34: 331-343.

Clapp C (1987): Analysis of the proteolytic cleavage of prolactin by the mammary gland and liver of the rat: Characterization of the cleaved and 16K forms; *Endocrinology* 121: 2055-2064.

Clapp C & Weiner RI (1992). A specific, high-affinity, saturable binding site for the 16-kiloDalton fragment of prolactin on capillary endothelial cells. *Endocrinology* 130: 1380–1386.

Clapp C, Martial JA, Guzman RC, Rentier-Delrue F and Weiner RI (1993). The 16-kilodalton N-terminal fragment of human prolactin is a potent inhibitor of angiogenesis. *Endocrinology* 133: 1292-1299.

Clapp, C.,Turner, L., Gutie'rrez-ospina, G., Alca'ntara, E., et al (1994). The prolactin gene is expressed in the hypothalamic neurohypophyseal system and the protein is processed into a14-kDa fragment with activity like 16-kDa prolactin. *Proc. Natl. Acad. Sci* (US) 91: 10384-10388.

Clapp C, López-Gómez FJ, Nava G, Corbacho A, Torner L, Macotela Y, Dueñas Z, Ochoa A, Noris G, Acosta E, Garay E and Martínez de la Escalera (1998). Expression of prolactin mRNA and of prolactin-like proteins in endothelial cells: evidence for autocrine effects. *J. Endocrinol.* 158: 137–144.

Clevenger CV, Furth PA, Hankinson SE and Schuler LA (2003).The role of prolactin in mammary carcinoma. *Endocr. Rev.* 24: 1-27.

Corbacho AM, Macotela Y, Nava G, Torner L, Dueñas Z, Noris G, Morales MA, Martínez de la Escalera and Clapp C (2000). Human umbilical vein endothelial cells express multiple prolactin isoforms, *J. Endocrinol.* 166: 53–62.

Creighton TE (1993). The folded conformations of globular proteins; in Creighton TE, "Proteins: Structures and Molecular properties (2nd edn), New York, WH Freeman and Company, pp 201-260.

D'Angelo G, Martini J-F, Iiri T, Fantl WJ, Martial J and Weiner RI (1999). 16K human prolactin inhibits vascular endothelial growth factor-induced activation of Ras in capillary endothelial cells. *Mol. Endocrinol.* 13: 692-704.

DeVito WJ (1988) Distribution of Immunoreactive Prolactin in the Male and Female Rat Brain: Effects of Hypophysectomy and Intraventricular Administration of Colchicine. *Neuroendocrinology* 47:284–289.

Edgell C-JS, McDonald CC and Graham JE (1983). Permanent cell line expressing human factor VIII-related antigen established by hybridization; *Natl. Acad. Sci. USA* 80: 3734-3737.

Emanuel N.V., Jurgens J.K., Halloran M.M., Tentler J.J., Lawerence A.M. and Kelley M.R. (1992). The rat prolactin gene is expressed in brain tissue: detection of normal and alternatively spliced prolactin messenger RNA. *Mol. Endocrinol.* 6: 35-42.

Ferrante E, Pellegrini C, Bondioni S, Peverelli E, Locatelli M, Gelmini P, Luciani P, Peri A, Mantovani G, Bosari S, Beck-Peccoz P, Spada A and Lania A (2006). Octreotide promotes apoptosis in human somatotroph tumor cells by activating somatostatin receptor type 2. *Endocr. Relat. Cancer* 13: 955-962.

Ferrara N, Clapp C and Weiner R (1991). The 16K fragment of prolactin specifically inhibits basal or fibroblast growth factor stimulated growth of capillary endothelial cells. *Endocrinology* 129: 896-900.

Ferreira N and Henzel WJ (1989). Pituitary follicular cells secrete a novel heparin-binding growth factor specific for vascular endothelial cells. *Bichem. Biophys. Ras. Commun.* 161: 851-858.

Ferreira MA, Andrade SP, Pesquero JL, Feitosa MH, Oliveira GM, Rogana E, Nogueira JC and Beraldo WT (1992). Kallikrein-kinin system in the angiogenesis; *Agents Actions Suppl.* 38: 165-174.

Folkman J and Shing Y (1992). Angiogenesis; *J. Biol. Chem.* 267: 10931–10934.

Folkman J (1995). Angiogenesis in cancer, vascular, rheumatoid and other disease; *Nature Medicine* 1: 27–31.

Fuxe, K., Lofstrom, A., Agnati, L., Eneroth, P., Gustavsson, J.A., Hokfelt, T. & Skett, P (1977).Central monoaminergic pathways. Their role in control of lutotropin, follitropin and prolactin secretion. In Endocrinology, vol. 1, ed. Turner, V.H.T., pp. 136-143. Amsterdam and Oxford: Excerpta Medica.

Gala RR, and E.M Shevach (1994).Evidence for the release of prolactin like substance by mouse lymphocytes and macrophages. *Proc. Soc.Exp. Biol. Med,* 205: 12-19.

Gellersen B., DiMattia G.E., Friesen H.G. and Bohnet H.G. (1989) Prolactin (PRL) mRNA from human deciduas differs from pituitary PRL mRNA but resembles the IM-9-P3 lymphoblast PRL transcript. *Mol. Cell. Endocrinol.* 64: 127-130.

Goffin V, Norman M and Martial JA (1992). Alanine-scanning mutagenesis of human prolactin: importance of the 58-74 regions for bioactivity; *Mol. Endocrinol.* 6: 1381–1392.

Goffin V., Bouchard B., Ormandy C.J., Weimann E., Ferrag F., Touraine P., Bole-Feysot C., Maaskant R.A., Clement-Lacroix P., Edery M., Binart N. and Kelly P.A. (1998) Prolactin: a hormone at the crossroads of neuroimmunoendocrinology. *Ann. NY. Acad. Sci.,* 840: 498–509.

Goffin V., Touraine P., Pichard C., Bernichtein S. and Kelly P.A. (1999) Should prolactin be reconsidered as a therapeutic target in human breast cancer? *Mol. Cell. Endocrino.* 151: 79–87.

Gonzalez C, Corbacho AM, Eiserich JP, Garcia C, Lopez-Barrera F, Morales-Tlalpan V, Barajas-Espinosa A, Diaz-Munoz M, Rubio R, Lin S-H, de la Escalera GM and Clapp C (2004). 16K-prolactin inhibits activation of endothelial nitric oxide synthase, intracellular calcium mobilization and endothelium-dependent vasorelaxation; *Endocrinology* 145: 5714–5722.

Herlant , M. (1964).The cells of the adenohypophysis and their functional significance. *Int. Rev. Cytol.,* 17: 299-382

Ishikawa F, Miyazone K, Hellman U, Drexler H, Wernstedt C, Hagiwara K, Usuki K, Takaku F, Risau W and Heldin CH (1989). Identification of angiogenic activity and the cloning and expression of platelet-derived endothelial cell growth factor; *Nature* 338 557-562

Iyer S and Acharya KR (2002) Angiogenesis: What we know and do not know; *Proc. Indian Natn. Sci. Acad.* B68 415-478.

Jaeok Lee, Syamantak Majumder, Suvro Chatterjee and Kambadur Muralidhar (2011) Inhibitory activity of the peptides derived from buffalo prolactin on angiogenesis *J.Biosci* 36(2): 341-354.

Kelly PA, Bradley C, Shiu RP, Meites J, Friesen HG.(1974). Prolactin binding to rat mammary tumor tissue. *Proc. Soc.Exp Biol Med.* 146:816-819.

Kelly PA , Djiane J,postel-vinay MC, Edery M.(1991). The prolactin/Growth hormone receptor family.*Endocr. Rev* 12: 235-251.

Khurana, S., and K.Muralidhar (1997) Heterogeneity in buffalo pituitary prolactin. *Mol. Cell. Biochem.* 173: 1-15.

Khurana S, Kuns R and Ben-Jonathan N (1999a) Heparin-binding property of human prolactin: A novel aspect of prolactin biology; *Endocrinology* 140: 1026-1029.

Khurana S, Liby K, Buckley AR and Ben-Jonathan N (1999b). Proteolysis of human prolactin: Resistance to cathepsin D and formation of a nonangiostatic, C-terminal 16K fragment by thrombin; *Endocrinology* 140: 4127-4132.

Kohli R., Chadha N. and Muralidhar K. (1987) Are sheep and buffalo prolactins sulfated? *Biochem. Biophys. Res. Commun.*, 149: 515-522.

Kohli R., Chadha N. and Muralidhar K. (1988) Presence of tyrosine-o-sulfate in sheep pituitary prolactin. *FEBS Lett.* 242: 139-143.

Kolluru GK, Tamilarasan KP, Rajkumar AS, Priya AG, Rajaram M, Saleem NK, Majumder S, Jaffar Ali, BM, Illavazagan G and Chatterjee S (2008). Nitric oxide/cGMP protects endothelial cells from hypoxia-mediated leakiness; *Europ. J. Cell Biol.* 87: 147-161.

Kurtz A, Bristol LA, Toth BE, Lazar-Wesley E, Takacs L and Kacsoh B.(1993). Mammary epithelial cells of Lactating rat express prolactin messenger ribonucleic acid. *Biol Reprod.* 48: 1095-1103.

Lahlou H, Guillermet J, Hortala M, Vernejoul F, Pyronnet S, Bousquet C and Susini C (2004). Molecular signaling of somatostatin receptors; *Ann. N. Y. Acad. Sci.* 1014: 121-131

Lamalice L, Boeuf FL and Huot J (2007). Endothelial cell migration during angiogenesis; *Circ. Res.* 100 782-794.

Lee JS, Decker NK, Chatterjee S, Yao J, Friedman S and Shah V (2005). Mechanisms of nitric oxide interplay with Rho GTPase family members in modulation of actin membrane dynamics in pericytes and fibroblasts; *Am. J. Pathol.* 166: 1861-1870.

Li, C.H., Dixon, J.S., Lo,T.B., Schmidt, K.D., and Pankov, Y.A. (1970) : Studies on pituitary lactogenic hormone.XXX. The primary structure of the sheep hormone. *Arch. Biochem. Biophys.*, 141: 705-737.

Lkhider, M., Delpal, S. and Ollivier-Bousquet, M. (1996). Rat prolactin inserum, milk and mammary tissue: characterisation and intracellularlocalisation. *Endocrinology* 137: 4969-4979.

Maithal, K., Krishnamurthy, H.G., and K. Muralidhar (2001) Physico-chemical characterization of growth hormone from water buffaloes (*Bubalus bubalis*). *Indian J. Biochem. Biophys.*. 38: 375-383.

Manoj Panchal and K. Muralidhar (2010). Purification and biological characterization of bacterially expressed recombinant buffalo Prolactin. *Prep. Biochem. Biotechnol.* 40 (4): 276-285.

Marks N, Grynbaum A and Lajtha A (1973). Pentapeptide (pepstatin) inhibition of brain acid protease. *Science* 181: 949-951.

Mittra I (1980a) A novel "cleaced PRL" in the rat pituitary: Part I biosynthesis, characterization and regulatory control; *Biochem. Biophusic. Res. Commun.* 95: 1750-1759.

Mittra I (1980b) A novel "cleaced PRL" in the rat pituitary: Part II in vivo mammary mitogenic activity of its N-terminal 16K moiety; *Biochem. Biophusic. Res. Commun.* 95: 1760-1780.

Moncada S and Higgs A (1993). The L-arginine-nitric oxide pathway; *N. Engl. J. Med.* 329: 2002-2012.

Montgomery, D.W. LeFevre, J.A.. Ulrich, E.D., Adamson, C'.R. and Zukoski. CF. (1990) Identification of prolactin like proteins synthesized by normal murine lymphocytes. *Endocrinology* 127: 2601- 2603.

Moore K.L. (2003). The biology and enzymology of protein tyrosine *O*-sulfation. *J. Biol. Chem.*, 278: 24243-24246.

Muralidhar, K., Kumar,T.R., Chadha, N., Khurana, S., Khanna,T., and Sharma, H.P. (1994) Strategies for purification of four reproductive hormones from the same batch of buffalo(*Bubalus bubalis*) pituitaries. *Indian J. Expt. Biology*. 32: 73-80.

Nathan C and Xie Q (1994). Nitric oxide synthase: roles, tolls, and controls; *Cell* 78: 915-918.

Nguyen NQN, Tabruyn SP, Lins L, Lion M, Cornet AM, Lair F, Rentier-Delrue F, Brasseur R, Martial JA and Struman I (2006). Prolactin/growth hormone-derived antiangiogenic peptides highlight a potential role of tilted peptides in angiogenesis. *Proc. Natl. Acad. Sci. (US)* 103 14319-14324.

Norman W (1997). Hormones (2nd edn), Academic Press, London.

Ochoa A, Montes de OP, Rivera JC, Dueñas Z, Nava G, Martínez de la EG and Clapp C (2001). Expression of prolactin gene and secretion of prolactin by rat retinal capillary endothelial cells; *Invest Ophthalmol. Visual Sci.* 42: 1639–1645.

Panchal M. and Muralidhar K. (2008) Purification of monomeric prolactin charge isoform from buffalo pituitaries. *Prep. Biochem. Biotechnol* 38: 99-109.

Papkoff H, Gospodarowicz D, Candiotti A and Li CH (1965). Preparation of ovine interstitial cell-stimulating hormone in high yield; *Arch. Biochem. Biophys.* 111: 431-438.

Palmer RMJ, Ferrige AG and Moncada S (1989). Nitric oxide release accounts for the biological activity of endothelium-derived relaxing factor; *Nature* 327: 524-526.

Panchal M and Muralidhar K (2008). Purification of monomeric prolactin charge isoform from buffalo pituitaries; *Prep. Biochem. Biotech.* 38: 94-104.

Patel YC, Murthy KK, Escher EE, Banville D, Spiess J and Srikant CB (1990). Mechanism of action of somatostatin: an overview of receptor function and studies of the molecular characterization and purification of somatostatin receptor proteins; *Metabolism* 39: 63-69.

Piwnica D, Fernandez I, Binart N, Touraine P, Kelly PA and Goffin V (2006). A new mechanism for prolactin processing into 16K PRL by secreted cathepsin D; *Mol. Endocrinol.* 20: 3263-3278.

Poitout L, Roubert P, Contour-Galcera MO, Moinet C, Lannoy J, Pommier J, Plas P, Bigg D and Thurieau C (2001). Identification of potent non-peptide somatostatin antagonists with sst3 selectivity; *J. Med. Chem.* 44: 2990-3000.

Regoli D and Barabe J (1980). Pharmacology of bradykinin and related kinins; *Pharmacol. Rev.* 32: 1-46.

Reisine T and Bell GI (1995) Molecular biology of somatostatin receptors; *Endocr. Rev.* 16: 427-442.

Ribatti D, Vacca A, Roncali L and Dammacco F (1996). The chick embryo chorioallantoic membrane as a model for in vivo research on angiogenesis. *Int. J. Dev. Biol.* 40: 1189-1197.

Riddick, D.H., Luciano, A.A., Kusmik, W.F. and Maslar, LA. (1978). De novo synthesis of prolactin by human decidua.*Life Sci.* 23, 1913-1922.

Riddle O., Bates,RW., and Dykshorn, S.W.(1933): The preparation, identification and assay of prolactin- a hormone of the anterior pituitary. *Am.J. Physiol*, 105:191-216.

Seroogy K. Tsruo Y.Hokfelt T. Walsh J Fahrenkrug J. Emson PC and Goldstein M (1988). Further analysis of presence of peptides in dopamine neurons Cholecystokinin peptide histidine–isoleucine/vaso active intestinal polypeptide and substance P in rat supera mammillary region and mesencephelon. *Exp Brain Res* 72: 523-534.

Siaud, P., Manzoni, O., Balmefrezol, M., Barbanel, G., Assenmacher, I. & Alonso, G. (1989). The organization of prolactin-like-immunoreactive neurons in the rat central nervous system. *Cell and Tissue Research* 255: 107-115.

Sinha YN and Gilligan TA 1984 A cleaved form of PRL in the mouse pituitary gland: Identification and comparison of in vitro synthesis a release in strains with high and low incidence of mammary tumors; *Endocrinology* 114: 2046-2053.

Sinha, Y.N., (1995) Structural Variants of Prolactin: Occurrence and physiological significance. *Endocr. Rev.*, 16: 354-369.

Stricker,P., and Grueter, P (1928): Action du lobe anterieur de l'hypophyse sur la montee laiteuse. *C.R. Soc. Biol*, 99: 1978-1980.

Struman I., Bentzien F., Lee H., Mainfroid V., D'Angelo G., Goffin V., Weiner R.I. and Martial J.A. (1999) Opposing actions of intact and N-terminal fragments of the human prolactin/growth hormone family members on angiogenesis: novel mechanism for the regulation of angiogenesis. *Proc. Natl. Acad. Sci. (US)*, 96: 1246-1251.

Syamantak Majumder, Suvro Chatterjee, Jaeok Lee and Kambadur Muralidhar (2009). Antiangiogenic Activity of Buffalo Growth hormone *Science & Culture* 75: (9-10) 369-371.

I, Bentzien F, Lee H, Mainfroid V, D'Angelo G, Goffin V, Weiner RI and Martial JA (1999) Opposing actions of intact and N-terminal fragments of the human prolactin/growth hormone family members on angiogenesis: novel mechanism for the regulation of angiogenesis; *Proc. Natl. Acad. Sci. (US)* 96: 1246-1251

Thompson SA (1982).Localizatio of immuno reactive prolactin in ependyma and curcum ventricular organs of rat brain *Cell Tissue Res* 225: 79-93.

Venes D and Thomas CL (2001).Taber's Encyclopedic Medical Dictionary (19th edn), London, FA Davis Company.

Wilson DM, Emanuele NV III, Jurgens JK and Kelly MR.(1992). Prolactin message in brain and pituitary of adult male rats is identical: PCR cloning and sequencing of hypothalamic prolactin cDNA fromintact and hypophysectomized adult male rats. *Endocrinology* 131: 2488-2490.

Wallis M (2000).Episodic evolution of protein hormones: molecular evolution of pituitary prolactin. *J Mol Evol*. 50: 465-473.

Chapter 2

In vitro Effects of the Prolactin, Growth Hormone and Somatolactin on Cell Turnover in Fish Esophagus: Possible Mode of Opposite Osmoregulatory Actions of Prolactin and Growth Hormone

Hideya Takahashi, Hiroki Kudose, Chiyo Takagi,
Shunsuke Moriyama and Tatsuya Sakamoto

Additional information is available at the end of the chapter

http://dx.doi.org/10.5772/53867

1. Introduction

Growth hormone, prolactin and somatolactin belong to the same hormone family and have a similar structure in teleost fishes [1]. Each of these three hormones appear to have opposite or specific functions in electrolyte balance in teleosts [2]. Teleost fish in freshwater environment face two primary challenges: preventing the loss of ions to the external hypoosmotic environment and preventing the influx of water. Prolactin plays a central role in these activities during the adaptation of fish to fresh water, as evidenced by its ability to increase plasma ion concentrations (primarily Na^+ and Cl^-) and decrease the permeability of osmoregulatory organs, such as gill, kidney and intestine [3]. In seawater environment, in contrast, diffusive water loss is counteracted by drinking seawater and actively taking up Na^+, Cl^- and water across the gastrointestinal tract, and the gill actively secretes Na^+ and Cl^- through chloride cells. Growth hormone activates these gill chloride cells with ion transporters (e.g., Na^+, K^+-ATPase and the Na^+,K^+,$2Cl^-$ cotransporter) involved in secretion of Na^+ and Cl^- across the branchial epithelium [3], and appears to stimulate the intestinal absorption [4]. On the other hand, somatolactin is proposed to be involved in regulation of acid-base, calcium and phosphate levels in several species [2, 3, 5-7], but the role of somatolactin in the intestine is unknown. Although the presence of receptors for these hormones in ion-transporting organs has been reported in a variety of teleost species [8-14] and several studies have investigated the direct effects of the teleost hormones on osmoregulatory organs [5, 15-18], the modes of action of the hormones are still unclear. In particular, the opposite *in-vitro* effects of growth hormone and prolactin have not been reported, and there is little information on the cellular and biochemical mechanisms of the osmoregulatory actions of these hormones.

In our *in-vivo* studies on esophagi from euryhaline fish, prolactin stimulated cell proliferation in the epithelium [14, 19]. This effect seems to be related to increased cell proliferation for the stratified epithelium to reduce permeability in fresh water [20]. We have also found the increased apoptosis for the simple epithelium to give high permeability in seawater [14, 19]. A large number of reported effects of prolactin are associated with cell proliferation and/or apoptosis [21]. Thyroid-hormone induced apoptosis of the metamorphosing amphibian tail is directly prevented by prolactin and enhanced by glucocorticoid [22]. Using recently developed techniques for the culture of esophagus from the euryhaline medaka, *Oryzias latipes*, we have demonstrated that cortisol directly induced both cell proliferation and apoptosis [23]. In this study, we compared the effects of prolactin, growth hormone and somatolactin in this system, and found the first evidence that prolactin and growth hormone have opposite effects on the osmoregulatory organ *in vitro*.

2. Materials and methods

2.1. Animals

Adult medaka (*Oryzias latipes*, 0.1-0.2 g in weight) of both sexes were kept in indoor freshwater tanks at 27 ± 2°C and fed on Tetrafin flakes (Tetra Werke, Melle, Germany) daily for more than two weeks. Osmoregulation, differentiation of gill chloride cells, hormonal status during adaptation to different salinities, and the *in-vivo* effects of osmoregulatory hormones in this species have been described in our previous reports [23, 24]. Fish were exposed to 0.1% Fungizone (Amphotericin B, Invitrogen, Tokyo, Japan) for two days without food to avoid contamination before isolation of the esophagus. All fish were handled, maintained, and used in accordance with the Guidelines for Animal Experimentation established by Okayama University in accordance with international standards on animal welfare and in compliance with national regulations.

2.2. Tissue culture

As previously described [23], esophagi were gently sliced open along the long axis and cut into halves. Each explant was placed in a individual well of 96-well culture plates containing preincubation medium (MEM with Hanks' salts, 25 mM HEPES, 5 mg/ml BSA, 250 U/ml penicillin G, and 250 μg/ml streptomycin sulfate, adjusted to pH 7.8 at 25°C). After several hours, the medium was replaced with MEM containing Earle's salts, 4 mg/ml BSA, 292 μg/ml L-glutamine, 50 U/ml penicillin G and 50 μg/ml streptomycin sulfate adjusted to pH 7.8 when saturated with 99% O_2 / 1% CO_2. The medium osmolarity was adjusted to 300 mOsm/kg with NaCl. Explants were randomly assigned to control and treatment groups (*N* = 4-6), and incubated at 27°C in an airtight humidified chamber and gassed daily. Chum salmon prolactin, growth hormone and somatolactin was (1, 10, 100 ng/ml) or was not added to the culture medium. The concentrations were chosen based on the published effective physiological doses [5, 15-17, 25-27], plasma hormone concentrations [14, 28-30], and our preliminary studies. These salmonid hormones have approximately 60% amino-acid identities to the medaka counterparts (NCBI accession no. or Ensemble medaka genomic database browser ID: medaka growth hormone: ENSORLP00000024332, prolactin: AAP33052, somatolactin: AAT58046; [1, 13]) and have high specificities for their respective receptors in fish, unlike mammalian hormones which bind equally to other hormone receptors in fish [13, 31, 32]. The use of these salmonid hormones to study the specific physiological roles in many teleost species has been well established [25, 27, 29, 33, 34]. All the culture medium was replaced with freshly prepared medium daily. Although explants were occasionally found to adhere to the bottom of the plate well, they typically remained unattached during culture. The tissue culture maintained structural integrity for 8 days based on the presence of intact nuclei and cell-to-cell borders [23]. The cultured esophageal explants were fixed in 4% paraformaldehyde in phosphate-buffered saline (PBS) at 4°C for 4 h for histological analysis (N = 3-5) or snap frozen in liquid nitrogen for quantification of apoptosis.

2.3. Cell proliferation assay

At given time points, cultured explants were pulsed with an oxidation-reduction indicator WST-1 (10% vol/vol, Roche, Tokyo, Japan) for 4 h and color development ($A_{450\ nm}$-$A_{600\ nm}$) was quantified to measure the activity of mitochondrial dehydrogenases. This activity is proportional to the number of viable cultured cells and is expressed as the cell proliferating index [35]. The result after pre-incubation (on day 0) was used to correct for differences in initial tissue content per esophageal slice, and also for quantification of apoptosis.

2.4. Quantification of apoptosis

DNA internucleosomal fragmentation in the esophagus was assessed using a cell death detection ELISA kit (Roche, Tokyo, Japan) according to the manufacturer's instructions. This kit uses a quantitative sandwich ELISA that specifically measures the histone region (H1, H2A, H2B, H3, and H4) of mono- and oligonucleosomes [36] in teleosts [37] that are released during apoptosis, but not during necrosis [38]. After a 10-minute reaction, color development (A_{405} nm-A_{492} nm) was quantified using an MTP-300 microplate reader (Corona, Ibaragi, Japan).

2.5. Proliferating cell nuclear antigen (PCNA) immunohistochemistry

To label proliferating cells in the esophagus, we used a mouse monoclonal antibody (clone PC10; Sigma, Tokyo, Japan) against proliferating cell nuclear antigen (PCNA), as described previously for teleosts [14, 19, 33]. In our previous study on the teleost esophagus [19], the level of PCNA immunoreactivity was in agreement with the uptake of [^{3}H]-thymidine. Slides were immersed in 0.3% H_2O_2 in methanol at 20°C for 30 min to inactivate endogenous peroxidase activity. After washing in PBS, the sections were placed in 5% normal goat serum in PBS at room temperature for 1 h to block non-specific binding. Sections were subsequently incubated at 4°C overnight with the primary antibody diluted 1:100 in a solution containing 0.5% Triton X-100 and 1% BSA (Sigma, Tokyo, Japan) in PBS. Sections were then washed 3 times in PBS, incubated with peroxidase-labeled goat anti-mouse secondary antibody (Sigma, Tokyo, Japan) diluted 1:70 in PBS containing 0.5% Triton X-100 and 1% BSA at room temperature for 1 h, and then developed for 5 min with DAB substrate solution (Roche, Tokyo, Japan). Controls omitting the PCNA primary antibody were performed and yielded no immunoreactivity.

2.6. *In situ* 3'-end labeling of DNA (TUNEL)

Nuclei of apoptotic cells were detected by the TUNEL method [39] using an *in situ* cell death detection kit (Roche, Tokyo, Japan; [14, 19, 33]). The TUNEL procedure produces results that are similar to those obtained with analysis of internucleosomal DNA fragmentation in the esophagus using gel electrophoresis, and appears to discriminate apoptosis from necrosis [19]. Fixed tissue samples were dehydrated through graded alcohol concentrations and embedded in Paraplast. Sections were cut at 5 μm and attached to 3-aminopropyltriethoxysilane-coated slides. The sections were then treated with 20 μg/ml proteinase K (Roche, Tokyo, Japan) at 20°C for 30 min, washed in PBS for 15 min, and immersed in 0.3% H_2O_2 in methanol at 20°C for 30 min to inactivate endogenous peroxidase activity. After washing in PBS, the sections were incubated with TdT and fluorescein-labeled dUTP at 37°C for 1 h in a humidified chamber. The reaction was terminated by transferring the slides to PBS for 15 min. The sections were then incubated with peroxidase-labeled anti-fluorescein antibody at 37°C for 30 min and then for 5 min with DAB substrate solution (Roche, Tokyo, Japan). Omission of TdT gave completely negative results.

2.7. Statistical analysis

The significance of differences between the means for cell proliferation were analyzed using two-way repeated measures analysis of variance (ANOVA), with time within groups (after application of treatment) as one factor and treatment among or between groups as the other factor. Since there was a significant interaction between treatment and time, each time was analyzed separately to identify differences among the treatments using the appropriate post-hoc test. The significance of differences among means for concentration-response relationships for apoptosis was also tested using ANOVA followed by a post-hoc test. All data were checked for normality and equal variances. Where assumptions of normality or equal variances were not satisfied, equivalent non-parametric tests were used. Results were considered significant for $P < 0.05$.

3. Results

The effects of growth hormone, prolactin and somatolactin (1, 10 and 100 ng/ml) on esophageal cell proliferation for 8 days in culture are shown in Figures 1 and 2. Addition of prolactin at 10 ng/ml to the culture medium significantly ($P < 0.001$) enhanced cell proliferation after 4 and 8 days (Figs. 1A and 2). Significant ($P < 0.05$) induction of cell proliferation was also observed at 1 day after treatment with 10 ng/ml growth hormone. In contrast, the esophagus did not respond significantly ($P > 0.05$) to treatment with somatolactin at any concentration. Similar results were obtained from six separate trials. Based on the highly significant results for prolactin treatment in the cell proliferation assays, the localization of the proliferating cells was examined in esophagi cultured for 8 days with or without 10 ng/ml prolactin (Fig. 1B). In control esophagi, labeling with an antibody against PCNA revealed few proliferating cell nuclei in the epithelium. In contrast, esophagi treated with prolactin had many PCNA-labeled nuclei in the epithelium and mucus cells in the epithelium were seemed to be more abundant than those in control tissue. No obvious longitudinal regionalization of the epithelial structure, including localization of proliferating cells, was observed.

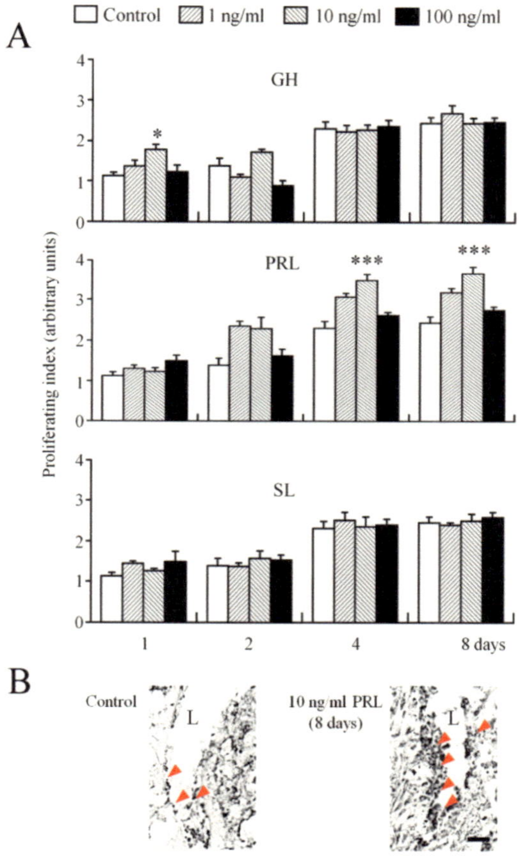

Figure 1. Effects of 1-100 ng/ml growth hormone (GH), prolactin (PRL) and somatolactin (SL) on cell proliferation of esophageal explants cultured for 1-8 days (A). Values are means ± SEM ($N = 4$-6) and are expressed in arbitrary units normalized to the results on day 0 (initial tissue content). * $P < 0.05$, *** $P < 0.001$ vs. the control on the same day. Proliferating cell (dark muclei, arrowheads) based on labeling by PCNA immunocytochemistry in the esophageal epithelium after 8 days in culture (B). A few PCNA-positive nuclei were detected in the epithelium in control esophagi, whereas many labeled nuclei appeared in the epithelium in esophagi treated with 10 ng/ml prolactin. *L*: lumen. Representative results are shown. Scale bar = 50 μm.

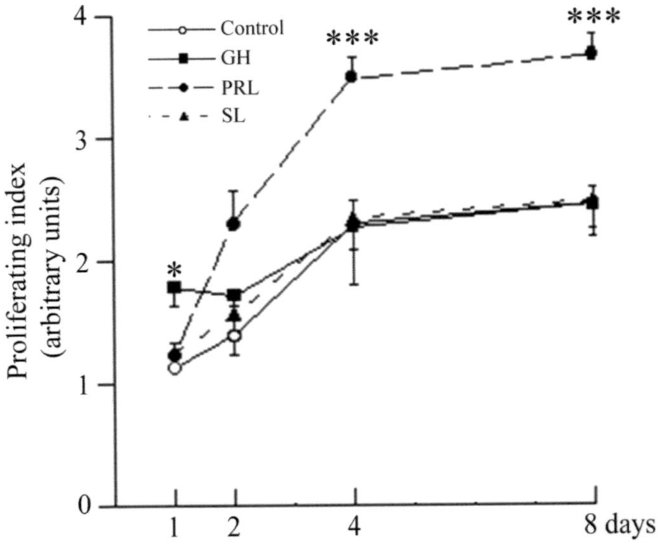

Figure 2. Effects of 10 ng/ml growth hormone (GH), prolactin (PRL) and somatolactin (SL) on cell proliferation of esophageal explants cultured for 1-8 days (redrawn from Fig. 1). Values are means ± SEM ($N = 4\text{-}6$) and are expressed in arbitrary units normalized to the results on day 0 (initial tissue content). * $P < 0.05$, *** $P < 0.001$ vs. the control on the same day.

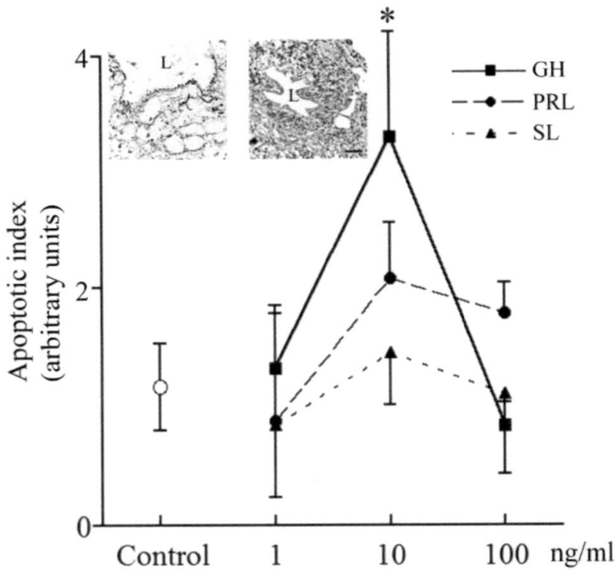

Figure 3. Effects of growth hormone (GH), prolactin (PRL) and somatolactin (SL) on esophageal apoptosis after 8 days of culture. Values are means ± SEM ($N = 4\text{-}5$) and are expressed in arbitrary units normalized to the initial tissue content. * $P < 0.05$ vs. control. Apoptosis in the esophageal epithelium detected in a TUNEL assay after 8 days in culture (left and right insets). A few TUNEL-positive nuclei were observed in the epithelium in control esophagi (left inset), whereas numerous labeled nuclei appeared in the epithelium of esophagi treated with 10 ng/ml growth hormone (right inset). L: lumen. Representative results are shown. Scale bar = 50 μm.

We examined the effects of growth hormone, prolactin and somatolactin (1, 10 and 100 ng/ml) on esophageal apoptosis after 8 days of culture, since esophageal apoptosis has been shown to be induced significantly 5-10 days after salinity acclimation and hormonal treatment of fish [14, 19, 33]. Addition of growth hormone (10 ng/ml) to the culture medium significantly induced esophageal apoptosis ($P < 0.05$), whereas prolactin and somatolactin showed no significant effects at any doses (Fig. 3). Similar results were obtained from three separate trials. Based on these results, the localization of apoptotic cells was examined in esophagi cultured for 8 days with or without 10 ng/ml growth hormone. In control esophagi cultures, there were few apoptotic cells based on TUNEL staining of DNA fragments (Fig. 3, left inset), whereas a large number of apoptotic cells were observed in esophageal epithelia treated with 10 ng/ml growth hormone for 8 days (Fig. 3, right inset). No obvious longitudinal regionalization of apoptotic cells was observed.

4. Discussion

Prolactin is an important hormone for freshwater adaptation in teleost species, whereas growth hormone is involved in seawater adaptation in several euryhaline fishes [3]. In accord with the greater permeability of the esophagus in seawater-acclimated euryhaline fish than in freshwater-acclimated fish [20], we have previously shown that apoptosis throughout the esophageal epithelium occurs for the simple columnar epithelium in seawater and that cell proliferation is induced for the stratified epithelium, which is composed of numerous mucus cells, in fresh water [14, 19]. We have also shown that injection of prolactin stimulates cell proliferation in the esophageal epithelium [33], but neither the mode nor specificity of the action of prolactin is clear. The present study shows that the esophagus of medaka is responsive to prolactin and growth hormone after several days in culture, with induction of cell proliferation and apoptosis, respectively. This is the first demonstration of opposite *in-vitro* effects of prolactin and growth hormone on the teleost osmoregulatory organ. The 10-ng/ml concentrations of prolactin and growth hormone required for these specific responses were similar to the physiologically increased levels observed in the plasma of several teleost fishes during acclimation to different salinities [14, 29, 30]. The time course is also similar to those for esophageal cell proliferation and apoptosis as well as for plasma prolactin and growth hormone in euryhaline fishes during salinity acclimation and after *in-vivo* hormonal treatment [14, 19, 33]. The *in-vitro* response to prolactin in the esophagus is consistent with the localization of prolactin receptors in proliferating cells of esophageal epithelia found in our previous study [14]. The growth hormone receptor is also expressed in the gastrointestinal tracts of fishes, which accounts for the ability of growth hormone to act on these organs [8, 11, 40-42]. Taken together, these results suggest that the osmoregulatory esophagus is one of the primary targets for the actions of prolactin and growth hormone during acclimation of euryhaline fishes to fresh water and seawater, respectively.

The *in-vitro* effects of prolactin on the permeability of trout gill epithelia [16, 43] may also be associated with direct stimulation of cell proliferation by prolactin, as proposed above for the medaka esophagus. Prolactin has also been shown to induce cell proliferation in jejunal explants from fetal rat [44], and several studies have shown direct effects of prolactin on cell proliferation throughout vertebrates [21]. In teleosts, prolactin induces proliferative responses in cultured salmonid leukocytes [25, 26], and promotes osteoblastic activities in goldfish scales *in vitro* [27]. However, the epithelium appears to be the major target, as in human keratinocytes and prostate epithelial cells [3, 45, 46], and it is likely that a primary function of prolactin in teleost osmoregulation is direct stimulation of cell proliferation in osmoregulatory epithelia. On the other hand, prolactin has also been shown to stimulate apoptosis in newt spermatogonia and rat luteal tissues [47, 48]. In addition, we suggested that the inhibitory effect of prolactin on osteoclastic activity in goldfish scales is mediated in part through osteoclast apoptosis [27]. Further studies of intracellular signaling pathway will elucidate how prolactin regulates these cell turnover. At any rate, one of prolactin's primary functions may be control of cell proliferation/apoptosis. Indeed, the prolactin receptors belong to the large superfamily of class 1 "cytokine" receptors.

There are few reports on the *in vitro* actions of growth hormone on teleost osmoregulatory organs, although growth hormone appears to be an important hormone for seawater adaptation. Direct regulatory roles of growth hormone on the gill Na^+,K^+-ATPase and heat-shock protein 70 in climbing perch and silver sea bream have been described [15, 17, 18]. Our experiment reveals direct effects of growth hormone on esophageal cell turnover. Induction of cell proliferation was observed 1 day after addition of 10 ng/ml growth hormone, whereas epithelial apoptosis was stimulated after 8 days. The direct action of growth hormone on cell proliferation may occur through locally produced insulin-like growth factor I (IGF-I), since IGF-I has been suggested to mediate the direct proliferative effects of growth hormone in mammalian gastrointestinal tracts [49, 50]. On the other hand, the stimulation of apoptosis by long-term growth hormone exposure is at variance with the commonly reported protective role of the growth hormone /IGF-I axis against cell death [51]. However, increases in myocyte apoptosis are associated with high levels of growth hormone in patients with acromegaly [52] and in 9-month-old transgenic mice overexpressing growth hormone [53]. Furthermore, coho salmon implanted with growth hormone for 2 weeks showed stimulated Na-dependent proline absorption in the intestine [4], which may reflect increased permeability of the apoptotic intestinal epithelia in seawater.

At 100 ng/ml prolactin or growth hormone, the above significant effects on esophageal cell turnover were disappeared. Very high doses of these hormones may also activate receptors for the other hormones even in homologous systems. It is reported that prolactin can bind to growth hormone receptor in tilapia (*Oreochromis mossambicus*) [54], and that growth hormone has an ability to bind to somatolactin receptor in salmon (*Oncorhynchus masou*) [13]. In addition, our results may also be related to the functional distinction of multiple prolactin receptor isoforms in teleost fish [55]. These receptors have different sensitivities to prolactin and may have the distinct physiological functions as described above [27, 49, 50, 55-57].

In our previous study using this esophagus culture system, low levels of cortisol stimulate epithelial apoptosis through glucocorticoid receptors in seawater, whereas high levels of cortisol induce epithelial cell proliferation also via glucocorticoid receptors in freshwater [23]. Interactions of prolactin/growth hormone with glucocorticoid may play an important role in the cell turnover in osmoregulatory esophageal epithelia during acclimation to different salinities. In the gill, cortisol is suggested to promote the differentiation of the ion-secretory chloride cell (seawater-form) with growth hormone, and also expedite the differentiation of ion-uptake chloride cell (freshwater-form) by interacting with prolactin [3, 58]. In the amphibian metamorphosis, on the other hand, thyroid hormones with glucocorticoid signaling induce apoptosis in the regression of tadpole tail, whereas prolactin prevents this apoptosis [22](Fig. 4B). Although apoptosis by glucocorticoid appear to be conserved throughout the vertebrates, thyroid hormone has no significant effect on esophageal cell proliferation or apoptosis in euryhaline fish [33]. Therefore, we hypothesize that thyroid hormones are involved only in irreversible metamorphosis and/or developmental processes.

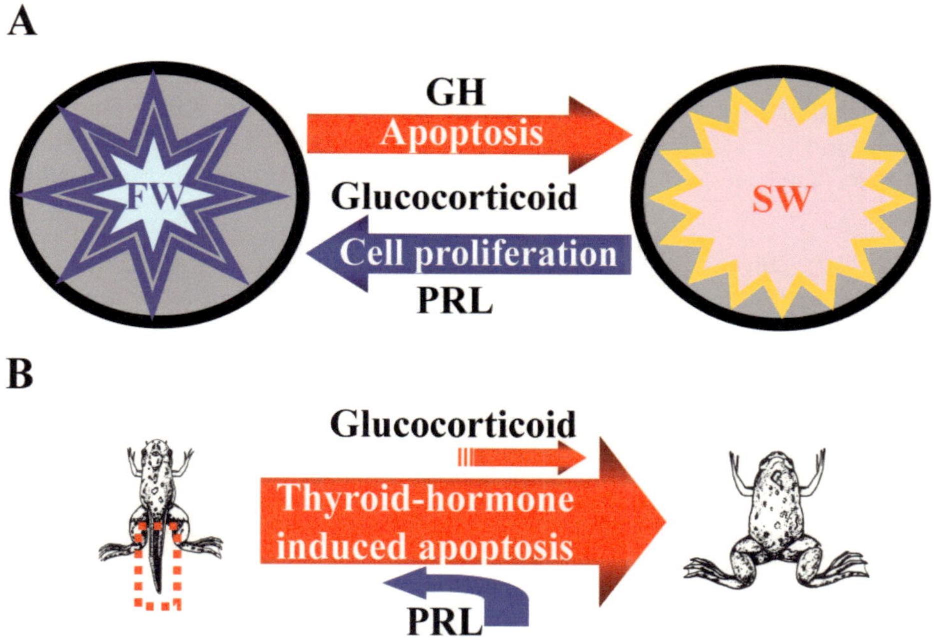

Figure 4. The summary representation of the epithelial differentiation in the esophagus of an euryhaline teleost during adaptation to different salinities. During freshwater (FW) adaptation, glucocorticoid signaling (cortisol-glucocorticoid receptor) and prolactin (PRL) stimulate epithelial cell proliferation for the stratified epithelium, resulting in the low permeability. During seawater (SW) adaptation, growth hormone (GH) and glucocorticoid signaling induce epithelial apoptosis for the simple epithelium with the high permeability (A). In the amphibian metamorphosis, thyroid hormones with glucocorticoid signaling induce apoptosis in tadpole tail whereas prolactin inhibits the apoptosis induced by thyroid hormones in regression of tadpole tail (B).

5. Conclusions

Our *in vitro* study in medaka esophagi indicates that prolactin directly induces the epithelial cell proliferation for the stratified epithelium and this response appears to be important in the freshwater adaptive process. Furthermore, growth hormone directly stimulates the apoptosis for the simple epithelium and seems to be a key factor in seawater acclimation (Fig. 4A). To clarify the mechanism of prolactin/growth hormone actions in osmoregulation, future investigations using molecular tools are required to examine the relationship among the esophageal proliferating/apoptotic cells and important gene/protein expression patterns (e.g. prolactin/ growth hormone receptors, IGF-I and IGF-I receptor as well as transporters/pumps and intercellular junctions such as Na^+,K^+,ATPase, Na^+,K^+,$2Cl^-$ cotransporter, aquaporins., tight junctions, gap junctions and claudins. A further study is also required determine if the apoptosis induced by growth hormone in medaka esophagus is also characteristic of other species.

Author details

Hideya Takahashi*
Ushimado Marine Institute, Faculty of Science, Okayama University, Ushimado, Setouchi, Japan
Graduate School of Natural Science and Technology, Okayama University, Kitaku Tsushimanaka, Okayama, Japan
Department of Environmental Science, Faculty of Science, Niigata University, Ikarashi, Niigata, Japan

Hiroki Kudose, Chiyo Takagi and Tatsuya Sakamoto
Ushimado Marine Institute, Faculty of Science, Okayama University, Ushimado, Setouchi, Japan
Graduate School of Natural Science and Technology, Okayama University, Kitaku Tsushimanaka, Okayama , Japan

Shunsuke Moriyama
School of Marine Biosciences, Kitasato University, Ofunato, Iwate, Japan

Acknowledgement

This study was supported in part by grants to T.S (Grants-in-Aid for Scientific Research (C) Nos. 17570049, 19570057 and from JSPS) and to H.T (JSPS Research Fellowships for Young Scientists Nos. 192156 and 214892).

6. References

[1] Rand-Weaver M, Kawauchi H, Ono M. Evolution of the Structure of the Growth Hormone and Prolactin Family. Schreibman MP, Scanes CG, Pang PKT. (eds.) The Endocrinology of Growth, Development, and Metabolism in Vertebrates. Academic Press: San Diego; 1993. p13-42.

[2] Kaneko T. Cell Biology of Somatolactin. International Review of Cytology 1996; 169:1-24.

* Corresponding Author

[3] Sakamoto T, McCormick S. Prolactin and Growth Hormone in Fish Osmoregulation. General and Comparative Endocrinology 2006; 147(1):24-30.

[4] Collie NL, Stevens JJ. Hormonal Effects on L-Proline Transport in Coho Salmon (*Oncorhynchus Kisutch*) Intestine. General and Comparative Endocrinology 1985; 59(3):399-409.

[5] Lu M, Swanson P, Renfro JL. Effect of Somatolactin and Related Hormones on Phosphate Transport by Flounder Renal Tubule Primary Cultures. American Journal of Physiology 1995; 268(3):R577-582.

[6] Goss GG, Perry SF, Fryer JN, Laurent P. Gill Morphology and Acid-Base Regulation in Freshwater Fishes. Comparative Biochemistry and Physiology-Part A: Molecular & Integrative Physiology 1998; 119(1):107-115.

[7] Furukawa F, Watanabe S, Inokuchi M, Kaneko T. Responses of Gill Mitochondria-Rich Cells in Mozambique Tilapia Exposed to Acidic Environments (Ph 4.0) in Combination with Different Salinities. Comparative Biochemistry and Physiology-Part A: Molecular & Integrative Physiology 2011; 158(4):468-476.

[8] Sakamoto T, Hirano T. Growth Hormone Receptors in the Liver and Osmoregulatory Organs of Rainbow Trout: Characterization and Dynamics During Adaptation to Seawater. Journal of Endocrinology 1991; 130(3):425-433.

[9] Auperin B, Rentier-Delrue F, Martial JA, Prunet P. Characterization of a Single Prolactin (Prl) Receptor in Tilapia (*Oreochromis Niloticus*) Which Binds Both Prli and Prlii. Journal of Molecular Endocrinology 1994; 13(3):241-251.

[10] Sandra O, Le Rouzic P, Cauty C, Edery M, Prunet P. Expression of the Prolactin Receptor (Tiprl-R) Gene in Tilapia Oreochromis Niloticus: Tissue Distribution and Cellular Localization in Osmoregulatory Organs. Journal of Molecular Endocrinology 2000; 24(2):215-224.

[11] Lee LT, Nong G, Chan YH, Tse DL, Cheng CH. Molecular Cloning of a Teleost Growth Hormone Receptor and Its Functional Interaction with Human Growth Hormone. Gene 2001; 270(1-2):121-129.

[12] Kajimura S, Kawaguchi N, Kaneko T, Kawazoe I, Hirano T, Visitacion N, et al. dentification of the Growth Hormone Receptor in an Advanced Teleost, the Tilapia *Oreochromis Mossambicus*) with Special Reference to Its Distinct Expression Pattern in he Ovary. Journal of Endocrinology 2004; 181(1):65-76.

[13] Fukada H, Ozaki Y, Pierce AL, Adachi S, Yamauchi K, Hara A, et al. Identification of the Salmon Somatolactin Receptor, a New Member of the Cytokine Receptor Family. Endocrinology 2005; 146(5):2354-2361.

[14] Takahashi H, Prunet P, Kitahashi T, Kajimura S, Hirano T, Grau E, et al. Prolactin Receptor and Proliferating/Apoptotic Cells in Esophagus of the Mozambique Tilapia *Oreochromis Mossambicus*) in Fresh Water and in Seawater. General and Comparative Endocrinology 2007; 152(2-3):326-331.

[15] Leena S, Oommen O. Hormonal Control on Enzymes of Osmoregulation in a Teleost, *Anabas Testudineus* (Bloch): An in Vivo and in Vitro Study. Endocrine Research 2000; 26(2):169-187.

[16] Kelly SP, Wood CM. Prolactin Effects on Cultured Pavement Cell Epithelia and Pavement Cell Plus Mitochondria-Rich Cell Epithelia from Freshwater Rainbow Trout Gills. General and Comparative Endocrinology 2002; 128(1):44-56.

[17] Deane EE, Woo NY. Growth Hormone Attenuates Branchial Hsp70 Expression in Silver Sea Bream. Fish Physiology and Biochemistry 2010; 36(2):135-140.

[18] Deane EE, Woo N. Growth Hormone Increases Hsc70/Hsp70 Expression and Protects against Apoptosis in Whole Blood Preparations from Silver Sea Bream. Annals of the New York Academy of Sciences 2005; 1040:288-292.

[19] Takahashi H, Sakamoto T, Narita K. Cell Proliferation and Apoptosis in the Anterior ntestine of an Amphibious, Euryhaline Mudskipper (*Periophthalmus Modestus*). Journal of Comparative Physiology B 2006; 176(5):463-468.

[20] Grosell M. The Role of the Gastrointestinal Tract in Salt and Water Balance. In: Grosell M, Farrell, A., Brauner C. (eds.) The Multifunctional Gut of Fish. San Diego: Academic Press; 2012. p136-156.

[21] Sakamoto T, Oda A, Narita K, Takahashi H, Oda T, Fujiwara J, et al. Prolactin: Fishy Tales of Its Primary Regulator and Function. Annals of the New York Academy of Sciences 2005; 1040:184-188.

[22] Tata JR. Amphibian Metamorphosis as a Model for the Developmental Actions of Thyroid Hormone. Molecular and Cellular Endocrinology 2006; 246(1-2):10-20.

[23] Takagi C, Takahashi H, Kudose H, Kato K, Sakamoto T. Dual in Vitro Effects of Cortisol on Cell Turnover in the Medaka Esophagus Via the Glucocorticoid Receptor. Life Sciences 2011; 88(5-6):239-245.

[24] Sakamoto T, Kozaka T, Takahashi A, Kawauchi H, Ando M. Medaka (*Oryzias Latipes*) as a Model for Hypoosmoregulation of Euryhaline Fishes. Aquaculture 2001; 193(3-4):347-354.

[25] Sakai M, Kobayashi M, Kawauchi H. In Vitro Activation of Fish Phagocytic Cells by Gh, Prolactin and Somatolactin. Journal of Endocrinology 1996; 151(1):113-118.

[26] Yada T, Muto K, Azuma T, Ikuta K. Effects of Prolactin and Growth Hormone on Plasma Levels of Lysozyme and Ceruloplasmin in Rainbow Trout. Comp Biochem Physiol C Toxicol Pharmacol 2004; 139(1-3):57-63.

[27] Takahashi H, Suzuki N, Takagi C, Ikegame M, Yamamoto T, Takahashi A, et al. Prolactin Inhibits Osteoclastic Activity in the Goldfish Scale: A Novel Direct Action of Prolactin in Teleosts. Zoolog Science 2008; 25(7):739-745.

[28] Kaneko T, Hirano T. Role of Prolactin and Somatolactin in Calcium Regulation in Fish. ournal of Experimental Biology 1993; 184(2):31-45.

[29] Sakamoto T, Hirano T. Expression of Insulin-Like Growth Factor I Gene in Osmoregulatory Organs During Seawater Adaptation of the Salmonid Fish: Possible Mode of Osmoregulatory Action of Growth Hormone. Proceedings of the National Academy of Sciences of the United States of America 1993; 90(5):1912.

[30] Breves JP, Hirano T, Grau EG. Ionoregulatory and Endocrine Responses to Disturbed Salt and Water Balance in Mozambique Tilapia Exposed to Confinement and Handling Stress. Comparative Biochemistry and Physiology-Part A: Molecular & Integrative Physiology 2010; 155(3):294-300.

[31] Fukada H, Ozaki Y, Pierce AL, Adachi S, Yamauchi K, Hara A, et al. Salmon Growth Hormone Receptor: Molecular Cloning, Ligand Specificity, and Response to Fasting. General and Comparative Endocrinology 2004; 139(1):61-71.

[32] Prunet P, Auperin B. Prolactin Receptors. In: Sher-wood NM and Hew CL. (eds) Molecular Endocrinology of Fish. San Diego: Academic Press; 1994. p 367-391.

[33] Takahashi H, Takahashi A, Sakamoto T. In Vivo Effects of Thyroid Hormone, Corticosteroids and Prolactin on Cell Proliferation and Apoptosis in the Anterior ntestine of the Euryhaline Mudskipper (*Periophthalmus Modestus*). Life Sciences 2006; 79(19):1873-1880.

[34] Planas JV, Swanson P, Rand-Weaver M, Dickhoff WW. Somatolactin Stimulates in Vitro Gonadal Steroidogenesis in Coho Salmon, Oncorhynchus Kisutch. General and Comparative Endocrinology 1992; 87(1):1-5.

[35] Sakamoto T, Ojima N, Yamashita M. Induction of Mrnas in Response to Acclimation of Trout Cells to Different Osmolalities. Fish Physiology and Biochemistry 2000; 22(3):255-262.

[36] Chin AC, Lee WD, Murrin KA, Morck DW, Merrill JK, Dick P, et al. Tilmicosin Induces Apoptosis in Bovine Peripheral Neutrophils in the Presence or in the Absence of Pasteurella Haemolytica and Promotes Neutrophil Phagocytosis by Macrophages. Antimicrob Agents Chemother 2000; 44(9):2465-2470.

[37] Andreu-Vieyra CV, Buret AG, Habibi HR. Gonadotropin-Releasing Hormone Induction of Apoptosis in the Testes of Goldfish (*Carassius Auratus*). Endocrinology 2005; 146(3):1588-1596.

[38] Bassing CH, Alt FW. The Cellular Response to General and Programmed DNA Double Strand Breaks. DNA Repair (Amst) 2004; 3(8-9):781-796.

[39] Gavrieli Y, Sherman Y, Ben-Sasson SA. Identification of Programmed Cell Death in Situ Via Specific Labeling of Nuclear DNA Fragmentation. Journal of Cell Biology 1992; 119(3):493-501.

[40] Filby AL, Tyler CR. Cloning and Characterization of Cdnas for Hormones and/or Receptors of Growth Hormone, Insulin-Like Growth Factor-I, Thyroid Hormone, and Corticosteroid and the Gender-, Tissue-, and Developmental-Specific Expression of Their Mrna Transcripts in Fathead Minnow (*Pimephales Promelas*). General and Comparative Endocrinology 2007; 150(1):151-163.

[41] Pierce AL, Fox BK, Davis LK, Visitacion N, Kitahashi T, Hirano T, et al. Prolactin Receptor, Growth Hormone Receptor, and Putative Somatolactin Receptor in Mozambique Tilapia: Tissue Specific Expression and Differential Regulation by Salinity and Fasting. General and Comparative Endocrinology 2007; 154(1-3):31-40.

[42] Tomy S, Chang YM, Chen YH, Cao JC, Wang TP, Chang CF. Salinity Effects on the Expression of Osmoregulatory Genes in the Euryhaline Black Porgy Acanthopagrus Schlegeli. General and Comparative Endocrinology 2009; 161(1):123-132.

[43] Zhou B, Kelly SP, Wood CM. Response of Developing Cultured Freshwater Gill Epithelia to Gradual Apical Media Dilution and Hormone Supplementation. Journal of Experimental Zoology Part A: Comparative Experimental Biology 2004; 301(11):867-881.

[44] Bujanover Y, Wollman Y, Reif S, Golander A. A Possible Role of Prolactin on Growth and Maturation of the Gut During Development in the Rat. Journal of Pediatric Endocrinology & Metabolism 2002; 15(6):789-794.

[45] Girolomoni G, Phillips JT, Bergstresser PR. Prolactin Stimulates Proliferation of Cultured Human Keratinocytes. Journal of Investigative Dermatology 1993; 101(3):275-279.

[46] Crepin A, Bidaux G, Vanden-Abeele F, Dewailly E, Goffin V, Prevarskaya N, et al. Prolactin Stimulates Prostate Cell Proliferation by Increasing Endoplasmic Reticulum Content Due to Serca 2b over-Expression. Biochemical Journal 2007; 401:49-55.

[47] Abe S. Hormonal Control of Meiosis Initiation in the Testis from Japanese Newt, Cynops Pyrrhogaster. Zoological Science 2004; 21(1):691-704.

[48] Kiya T, Endo T, Goto T, Yamamoto H, Ito E, Kudo R, et al. Apoptosis and Pcna Expression Induced by Prolactin in Structural Involution of the Rat Corpus Luteum. ournal of Endocrinological Investigation 1998; 21(5):276-283.

[49] Wheeler EE, Challacombe DN. The Trophic Action of Growth Hormone, Insulin-Like Growth Factor-I, and Insulin on Human Duodenal Mucosa Cultured in Vitro. Gut 1997; 40(1):57-60.

[50] Ersoy B, Ozbilgin K, Kasirga E, Inan S, Coskun S, Tuglu I. Effect of Growth Hormone on Small Intestinal Homeostasis Relation to Cellular Mediators Igf-I and Igfbp-3. World ournal of Gastroenterology 2009; 15(43):5418-5424.

[51] Vincent AM, Feldman EL. Control of Cell Survival by Igf Signaling Pathways. Growth Hormone & IGF Research 2002; 12(4):193-197.

[52] Frustaci A, Chimenti C, Setoguchi M, Guerra S, Corsello S, Crea F, et al. Cell Death in Acromegalic Cardiomyopathy. Circulation 1999; 99:1426-1434.

[53] Bogazzi F, Russo D, Raggi F, Ultimieri F, Urbani C, Gasperi M, et al. Transgenic Mice Overexpressing Growth Hormone (Gh) Have Reduced or Increased Cardiac Apoptosis hrough Activation of Multiple Gh-Dependent or -Independent Cell Death Pathways. Endocrinology 2008; 149(11):5758-5769.

[54] Shepherd BS, Sakamoto T, Nishioka RS, Richman NH, 3rd, Mori I, Madsen SS, et al. Somatotropic Actions of the Homologous Growth Hormone and Prolactins in the Euryhaline Teleost, the Tilapia, *Oreochromis Mossambicus*. Proc Natl Acad Sci U S A 1997; 94(5):2068-2072.

[55] Huang X, Jiao B, Fung CK, Zhang Y, Ho WK, Chan CB, et al. The Presence of Two Distinct Prolactin Receptors in Seabream with Different Tissue Distribution Patterns, Signal Transduction Pathways and Regulation of Gene Expression by Steroid Hormones. Journal of Endocrinology 2007; 194(2):373-392.

[56] Breves JP, Seale AP, Helms RE, Tipsmark CK, Hirano T, Grau EG. Dynamic Gene Expression of Gh/Prl-Family Hormone Receptors in Gill and Kidney During Freshwater-Acclimation of Mozambique Tilapia. Comparative Biochemistry and Physiology Part A: Molecular & Integrative Physiology 2011; 158(2):194-200.

[57] Kline JB, Roehrs H, Clevenger CV. Functional Characterization of the Intermediate soform of the Human Prolactin Receptor. Journal of Biological Chemistry 1999; 274(50):35461-35468.

[58] McCormick SD. Endocrine Control of Osmoregulation in Teleost Fish. American Zoologist 2001; 41(4):781-794.

Use of the Bovine Prolactin Gene (*bPRL*) for Estimating Genetic Variation and Milk Production in Aboriginal Russian Breeds of *Bos taurus* L.

I.V. Lazebnaya, O.E. Lazebny, S.R. Khatami and G.E. Sulimova

Additional information is available at the end of the chapter

http://dx.doi.org/10.5772/54756

1. Introduction

Prolactin is a protein hormone mainly, but not exclusively produced by lactotroph cells of the anterior pituitary. Its role in lactogenesis and galactopoiesis (maintenance of milk secretion) is well demonstrated [1, 2]. Therefore, the gene encoding it (*PRL*) is considered to be one of the key links in the gene network constituting the hereditary component of milk productivity. Test systems for cattle breeding have been developed based on the associations of the *PRL* gene polymorphism with milk yield and quality.

Inbreeding, which decreases the genetic variation and viability of animals, is a well-known negative consequence of artificial selection. Its impact is further aggravated by the recent trend towards globalization of some cattle breeds [3]. Therefore, conservation of aboriginal breeds adapted to local conditions (which are not infrequently extreme) is necessary in countries with wide zonal climatic variations.

This is especially important when a breed in question has pronounced adaptive characteristics and its population is small. Yakut cattle represent one of such breeds (Figure 1a); it is unique among Russian breeds in terms of ecological plasticity. These cattle live in the northernmost part of the *Bos taurus* species range, a hardly accessible region of the subarctic zone of the Republic of Sakha (Yakutia), Russia, surrounded with mountain ridges. The morphological and physiological characteristics of Yakut cattle and their biochemical and behavioral adaptations allow free grazing almost round the year despite a severe continental climate, with the mean air temperatures usually varying from –43°C in winter to +25°C in summer (the lowest and highest temperatures on record are –65°C and +38°C, respectively). These animals can live on rough foods. Their body, including the udder, is covered with long, thick hair protecting them from cold and gnats. The color of aboriginal Yakut cattle varies from black and red to a leopard pattern with white spots on the head and lower trunk. This breed is exceptionally resistant to tuberculosis, leukemia, and brucellosis. Yakut cattle are small, with the shoulder height shorter than 1 m and the live weights of bulls and cows of 500–550 and 350–400 kg, respectively. The milk yield is low (2100–2350 kg in the breeding stock), but the fat content of milk is as high as 7.3% [4]. Yakut cattle have long been providing local residents (mostly Yakuts) with beef and dairy products. Cattle leather is widely used in Yakut ethnic handicrafts; Yakuts traditionally make comfortable, durable, beautiful leather clothes. Excavations in the Olekminsk district of Yakutia have revealed remnants of nomad camps containing fossil bones of domestic cattle, which suggests an ancient origin of this breed [5].

Bestuzhev and Kostroma cattle are dual-purpose breeds. Bestuzhev cattle selected for both beef and milk production were bred from local cattle in Samara province, Russia, in the late 18th century (Figure 1b). English Shorthorn cattle were used for its improvement, the offspring being crossed with the Holland, Shorthorn, Simmental, and some other breeds. The breed was completely formed by the mid-19th century. Bestuzhev cattle are well adapted to the continental climate of the Volga basin. The animals are red; the color intensity varies from light-red to dark-red or cherry-red. Some animals have white spots, mostly on the lower trunk, udder, and head. The mean milk yield of Bestuzhev cattle is 5502–8250 kg; the mean fat content of milk is 3.82–4.0% (the maximum content is 5.5%) [4]. Bestuzhev cattle are especially valuable because they are almost free of hereditary diseases and abnormalities and are resistant to tuberculosis and leukemia.

Kostroma cattle are classified with the group of brown cattle (Figure 1c). The breed was registered in 1944. These cattle are characterized by a high growing capacity, strong constitution, and steady inheritance of commercially valuable traits, including a good milk quality. The Kostroma breed is regarded as one of the most productive dual-purpose breeds. The live weights of Kostroma bulls and cows are 800–900 and 550–650 kg, respectively; the fat and protein contents of milk are as high as 3.9 and 3.6%, respectively. The milk yield varies from 6000–8000 to 10,500 kg [4]. The Kostroma breed is characterized by a high total frequency of the *BoLA–DRB3* gene alleles determining the leukemia resistance (on average, 35.9%) [6].

Yaroslavl cattle, formed as a native cattle breed in the 16th century, have the highest milk yield and the best milk composition among all native Russian breeds (Figure 1d). Their milk contains, on average, 4.37% of fat (maximum content, 5.0%) and 3.4–3.6% of protein; the dry matter content is 13.6% (compared to 12.3–12.5% in other breeds) [4]. Yaroslavl cattle are usually black, except the white head with a black mask around the eyes and the white lower trunk. Yaroslavl cattle were first mentioned in the literature in the mid-19th century. Bestuzhev cattle were named after the original breeder; Yaroslavl, Yakut, and Kostroma cattle, after the region of origin.

The balance between the increase in the milk yield and quality of cattle breeds and preservation of diversity both within and between breeds of *B. taurus* is a complicated problem. Therefore, analysis of the variation of the gene markers that are affected by artificial selection because of their associations with milk yield and composition would be useful for breed monitoring.

The bovine prolactin gene (*bPRL*) is traditionally regarded as a good candidate gene for marker-assisted selection (MAS) [7] for milk production parameters, because it has been located to chromosome 23 at 43 cM, close to the quantitative trait loci (QTLs) (36, 41, and 42 cM) [8-11]. In addition, it is known that the binding of the *bPRL* gene product with its receptor (PRLR) initiates a signaling cascade that activates the transcription of a number of genes, including the genes of milk proteins (caseins and lactalbumin).

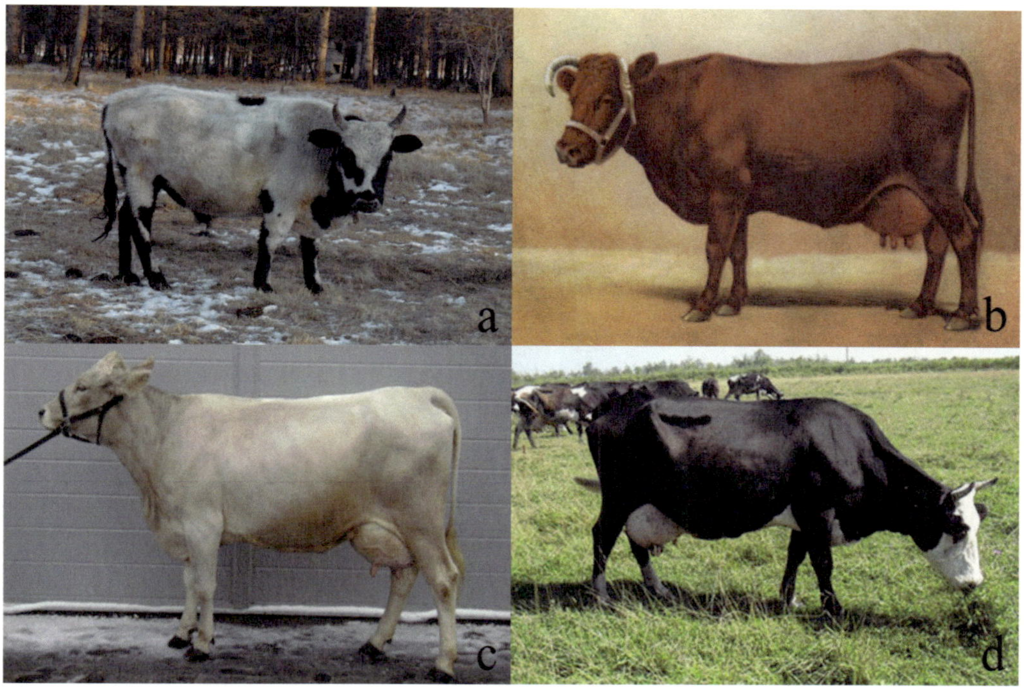

Figure 1. (a) Yakut, (b) Bestuzhev, (c) Kostroma, and (d) Yaroslavl cattle breeds [12, 13, 14, 15].

Note that this regulatory cascade involves growth hormone (Figure 2), because it is recognized not only by its own receptor (GHR), but also by PRLR [16]. The prolactin and growth hormone genes are very similar to each other, because they have resulted from duplication of a common ancestral gene. They have the same general structure (five exons and four introns) [17] and a common positive transcription factor (PITI) [18].

The specifics of the *bPRL* and *bGH* genes suggest their combined effect on milk production; however, this has been paid little attention until now. Most studies on the polymorphism of milk production genes deal with isolated effects of individual genes. Many data on the polymorphisms of both *bPRL* and *bGH* genes and their relationship with the milk yield and composition have been accumulated. For example, a synonymous A–G transition has been found in the codon of amino acid residue 103 of bPRL in the third exon of its gene; this mutation results in an *Rsa*I polymorphic site [19]. The *AA* and *AB* genotypes have been shown to be associated with the milk yield and protein content in Polish Black & White, Holstein Friesian, and Brown Swiss cattle [19-21]. Other associations have been found in Russian Red Pied cattle [22]. The C–G transversion in the third exon of the *bGH* gene (nucleotide position 2141) is known to be related to milk production traits. This SNP entails the disappearance of an *Alu*I restriction site and the substitution of valine for leucine (Leu → Val) at position 127 of the bGH amino acid sequence. There is evidence for a stronger dependence of the milk yield on the *LL* genotype than the *LV* genotype in Black Pied and Holstein Friesian cattle [23, 24]. However, Mitra *et al.* [25] and Dybus *et al.* [20] note a positive dependence of the milk yield and both fat and protein contents on the *V* allele in Holstein and Polish Black & White cattle. Study of the combined effect of the *bPRL* and *bGH* genes might explain some contradictions about the associations of individual markers of these genes. Although associations of the *bPRL*(*Rsa*I) and *bGH*(*Alu*I) polymorphisms with milk yield and quality have been extensively studied, the combined effect of SNPs of these genes has been hardly considered at all.

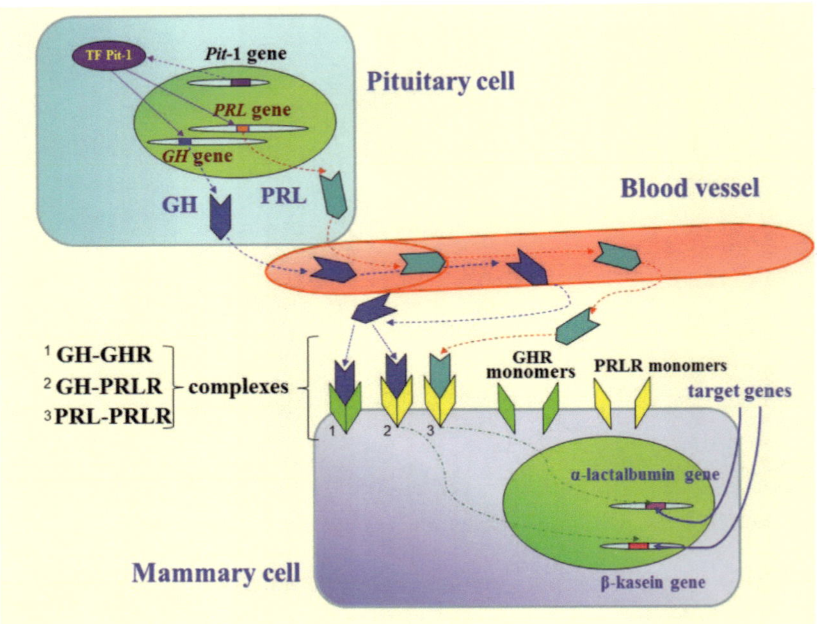

Top: an anterior pituitary cell. Chromosomes carrying the transcription factor (*Pit*-1), growth hormone (*GH*), and prolactin (*PRL*) genes are shown in the nucleus (a green oval). The product of *Pit*-1 (TF Pit-1) activates the transcription of the prolactin and growth hormone genes. The corresponding hormones (GH and PRL, shown in dark blue and light blue, respectively) enter the bloodstream and reach mammary cells, where they are recognized by transmembrane receptors (GHR and PRLR, respectively). This initiates regulatory cascades activating the transcription of the milk protein (β-casein and α-lactalbumin) genes. The prolactin and growth hormone receptors are shown in yellow and green, respectively. The growth hormone competes with prolactin for the prolactin receptor.

Figure 2. Schematic representation of the regulatory cascade involving the prolactin gene.

The goal of this study was twofold. First, we compared the Kostroma, Bestuzhev, Yakut, and Yaroslavl breeds both with one another and with some other Russian and foreign breeds (literature data) with respect to genetic variation as estimated from the *Rsa*I polymorphism of the prolactin gene. Second, we estimated the effect of the *Rsa*I polymorphism of the *bPRL* gene, as well as the effect of its combination with the *Alu*I polymorphism of the *bGH* gene, on milk production in Yaroslavl cattle.

2. Materials and methods

We used PCR–RFLP analysis to study the *Rsa*I polymorphism of the *bPRL* gene in Yakut cattle (n = 41) in the Republic of Sakha (Yakutia), Bestuzhev cattle (n = 57) in Samara region, Kostroma cattle (n =124) in Kostroma region, and Yaroslavl cattle (n = 113) in Yaroslavl region of Russia. The possible effects of the *bPRL*(*Rsa*I) polymorphism and its combination with the *bGH*(*Alu*I) polymorphism on milk production in Yaroslavl cattle were estimated.

DNA was isolated from 200-μl samples of whole blood using a Diatom™ DNA Prep kit (IsoGeneLab., Russia). Fragments of *bPRL* (156 bp) and *bGH* (223 bp) [25] were amplified in a Tertsik thermal cycler by the standard methods using a GenePak™PCR Core kit (IsoGene Lab., Russia). The DNA digestion with the *Rsa*I and *Alu*I restriction endonucleases was performed as recommended by the manufacturer (MBI Fermentas, Lithuania). The oligonucleotides F_{PRL} (5'-CGAGTCCTTATGAGCTTGATTCTT-3') and R_{PRL} (5'-GCCTTCCAGAAGTCGTTTGTTTTC-3') served as primers for the *bPRL* gene fragments; F_{GH} (5'-GCTGCTCCTGAGGGCCCTTCG-3') and R_{GH} (5'-GCGGCGGCACTTCATGACCCT-3'), for the *bGH* gene fragments. The following amplification profiles were used: for the *bPRL* gene fragments, one cycle of 94°C for 4 min; 35 cycles of 94°C for 30 s, 58°C for 30 s, and 72°C for 30 s; and one cycle of 72°C for 10 min; for the *bGH* gene fragments, one cycle of 94°C for 4 min; 35 cycles of 94°C for 45 s, 67°C for 45 s, and 72°C for 45 s; and one cycle of 72°C for 10 min. The amplification products were detected by means of 2% agarose gel electrophoresis (0.5 μg/ml ethidium bromide in 1X TBE buffer). The restriction products were visualized in 2% agarose gel (the *bGH* gene) or 6% polyacrylamide gel (the *bPRL* gene) (0.5 μg/ml ethidium bromide in 1X TBE buffer). The results of electrophoresis were recorded by means of a UVT-1 transilluminator (312 nm) and a ViTran-1 photodocumentation system (Biokom, Russia). The alleles were identified as follows: *Rsa*I(–) and *Rsa*I(+) corresponded to the *A* and *B* alleles of the *bPRL* gene, respectively; *Alu*I(–) and *Alu*I(+), to the *V* and *L* alleles of the *bGH* gene, respectively.

The PopGene [26] and STATISTICA 8.0 [25] software packages were used for statistical treatment of the results. Pairwise comparisons of the allele and heterozygote frequencies (observed heterozygosity, H_{obs}) in the group of breeds studied were performed using the Fisher exact test. For similar comparisons using published data on other Russian and foreign breeds, we additionally calculated the expected heterozygosity (H_{exp}) where its values were not presented. The G^2 test was used for pairwise comparisons of the breeds with respect to the genotype frequencies and H_{exp}. The fit of the observed frequencies of heterozygous genotypes to those expected from the Hardy–Weinberg equilibrium was tested using the PopGene software. The dependence of the milk yield (in kilograms) and fat and protein contents (in percent) on the *bPRL* and *bGH* genotypes in Yaroslavl cattle was estimated by one-way and two-way ANOVA with the use of the STATISTICA 8.0 software.

3. Results and discussion

3.1. Genetic structure

The genotype and allele frequencies of the *bPRL* gene studied in four Russian cattle breeds are shown in Table 1.

Breed		*bPRL*(*Rsa*I) genotypes			*Rsa*I alleles of the *bPRL* gene	
Yakut	(*n*)	*AA* (23)	*AB* (14)	*BB* (4)	*A* (60)	*B* (22)
(*n* = 41)	*p*±*s.e.*	0.561±0.078	0.341±0.074	0.098±0.046	0.732±0.098	0.268±0.098
		H_{exp}± s.e.	0.393±0.120			
Yaroslavl	(*n*)	*AA* (48)	*AB* (50)	*BB* (15)	*A* (146)	*B* (80)
(*n* = 113)	*p*±s.e.	0.425±0.047	0.442±0.047	0.133±0.032	0.646±0.064	0.354±0.064
		H_{exp}± s.e.	0.461±0.066			
Bestuzhev	(*n*)	*AA* (27)	*AB* (24)	*BB* (6)	*A* (78)	*B* (36)
(*n* = 57)	*p*±s.e.	0.474±0.066	0.421±0.065	0.105±0.041	0.684±0.087	0.316±0.087
		H_{exp}± s.e.	0.432±0.085			
Kostroma	(*n*)	*AA* (69)	*AB* (48)	*BB* (7)	*A* (186)	*B* (62)
(*n* = 124)	*p*±s.e.	0.556±0.045	0.387±0.044	0.056±0.021	0.750±0.055	0.250±0.055
		H_{exp}± s.e.	0.375±0.133			

Notes: *p*± s.e. is the genotype (allele) frequency and its standard error; the number of animals with the given genotype is indicated in parentheses; *n* is the sample size; H_{exp} ± s.e. is the expected heterozygosity and its standard error.

Table 1. The frequencies of the *Rsa*I restriction genotypes and alleles of the *bPRL* gene in four Russian cattle breeds

The G^2 test did not show significant differences between the breeds studied with respect to the genotype or allele frequencies for the *bPRL* gene. The genotype frequency distributions in the breeds studied fit the Hardy–Weinberg equilibrium. The *A* allele was prevailing in all breeds studied; its frequency was two to three times higher than the *B* allele frequency. Thus, these breeds had similar genetic structures in terms of the given SNP despite their different origins and directions of artificial selection.

The distribution of the *Rsa*I alleles of the *bPRL* gene is characterized by a higher frequency of the *A* allele in most breeds studied (Figure 3). In Indian Jersey cattle [28], the frequencies of the two alleles were approximately equal. The *A* allele frequency was lower in Polish Jersey cattle [29], which deserves special attention. These differences in allele frequencies may have resulted from different histories of selection for milk yield in different breeds. The breeds of *B. taurus* exhibit a considerable genotypic variation with respect to the *bPRL* gene marker used in this study. This can be seen in the diagram of the genotype frequency distribution (Figure 4). The group of four Russian cattle breeds studied here significantly differed in the genotype frequency distribution from Russian Black & White [31] and Russian Red Pied [22], but not Lithuanian Black & White [30]; ($p < 0.006$ with the Bonferroni correction).

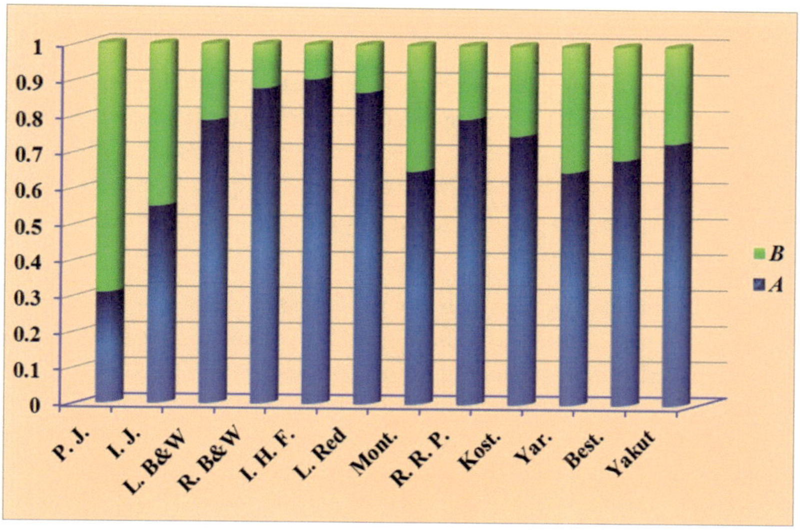

Designations: *A* and *B*, alleles of the *bPRL* gene; P, Polish; J, Jersey; I, Indian; L, Lithuanian; B&W, Black and White; R, Russian; Holstein Friesian; Mont, Montebeliard; R.R.P., Russian Red Pied; Kostr, Kostroma; Yar, Yaroslavl; Best, Bestuzhev.

The diagram is based on published data on Polish Jersey [29], Indian Jersey, Indian Holstein Friesian [28], Lithuanian Black & White, Lithuanian Red [30], Russian Black & White [31], Montebeliard [32], and Russian Red Pied [22] cattle.

Figure 3. Distribution of *bPRL*(*Rsa*I) allele frequencies in the four breeds studied and in other Russian and foreign breeds. The abscissa shows the breeds; the ordinate shows the allele frequencies (in fractions of unity).

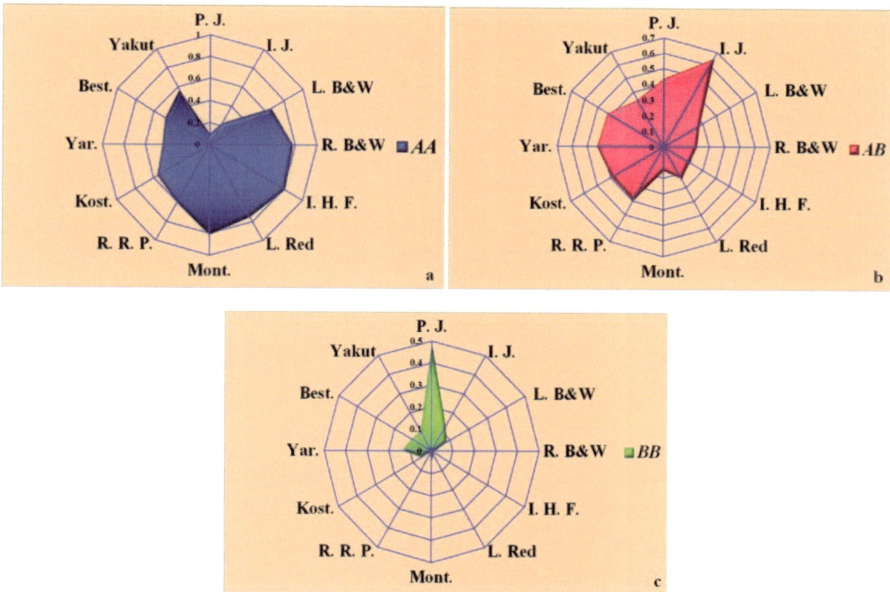

Designations: *AA*, *AB*, and *BB*, *bPRL* genotypes. For designations of the breeds, see Figure 2.

Figure 4. Distribution of *bPRL* genotype frequencies in the four breeds studied and in other Russian and foreign breeds. The radial axes show the breeds and the corresponding genotype frequencies.

3.2. Genetic variation

The observed (H_{obs}) and expected (H_{exp}) heterozygosities (Table 1) for the *bPRL* gene did not differ significantly from each other in any breed studied; nor did any two breeds differ in these parameters. This was unexpected, considering the substantial differences between these breeds in the *HinfI* site of the *bPit-1* transcription factor gene (exon 6) and the *AluI* site of the *bGH* growth hormone gene (exon 5) (our unpublished data), which are also associated with milk productivity.

In order to compare the genetic diversity in the Russian cattle breeds studied here with those in other Russian and foreign breeds (Figure 5), we calculated the H_{exp} for all breeds analyzed. The observed and expected heterozygosities for the *bPRL* gene did not differ significantly in most breeds (Figure 5). The Indian Jersey breed was an exception ($\chi^2 = 13.77$, $\nu = 1$, $p = 0.00021$); the excess of heterozygotes in these cattle apparently resulted from artificial selection.

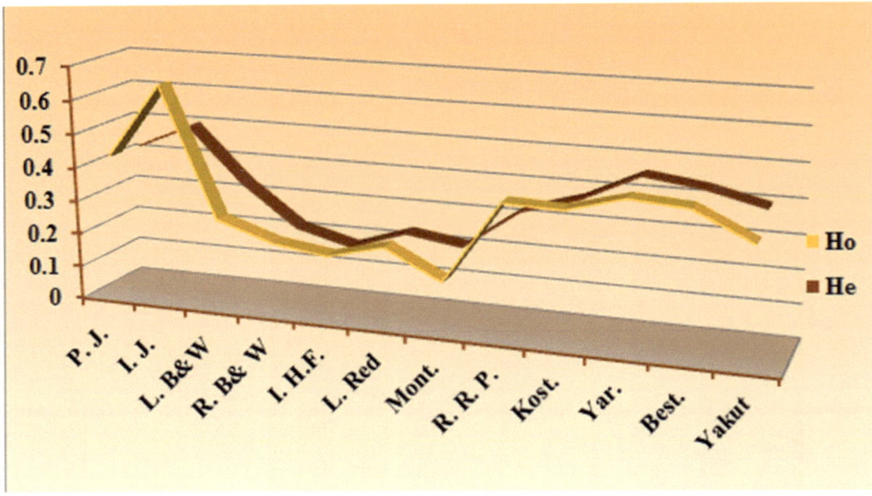

Designations: H_{obs} and H_{exp}, the observed and expected heterozygosities, respectively. For designations of the breeds, see Figure 2. The diagram is based on the expected heterozygosity levels calculated from published data on Montebeliard [32], Russian Red Pied [22], Polish Jersey [29], Lithuanian Black & White, Lithuanian Red [30], Indian Jersey, and Indian Holstein Friesian [28] cattle.

Figure 5. The observed and expected heterozygosities for the *bPRL* gene markers in Russian and foreign cattle breeds. The abscissa shows the breeds; the ordinate shows the heterozygosity coefficients (in fractions of unity).

Four Russian breeds studied did not differ from one another in the genetic variation (H_{exp}). At the same time, as can be seen in Figure 5, this group had significantly higher H_{exp} values compared to Russian Red Pied [22] Indian Holstein Friesian [28], and Montebeliard [32], cattle ($G^2 = 36.13$, $\nu = 4$, $p = 3.0 \cdot 10^{-7}$; $G^2 = 39.19$, $\nu = 4$, $p = 1.0 \cdot 10^{-7}$; $G^2 = 16.72$, $\nu = 4$, $p = 0.0022$; and $G^2 = 19.41$, $\nu = 4$, $p = 0.0007$, respectively; after the Bonferroni correction).

Thus, the heterozygosity levels in the Kostroma, Bestuzhev, Yakut, and Yaroslavl breeds are significantly higher than in the breeds used for comparison. This indicates a stable state of the breeds studied. However, since artificial selection alters genetic variation, regular monitoring of cattle breeds for the given *Rsa*I genetic marker is advisable.

3.3. Search for associations of SNPs of the prolactin and somatotropin genes with milk production traits in Yaroslavl cattle

Advances in molecular genetic analysis based on PCR have given rise to novel marker systems for direct genotyping at the DNA level that are independent of the animal's sex and age. This makes the procedures less time-consuming and more accurate.

The *Rsa*I polymorphism of the *bPRL* gene (Table 1), as well as the *Alu*I polymorphism in exon 5 of the *bGH* gene, was used to search for associations of these genes with milk production traits, including the milk yield and milk fat and protein contents, in Yaroslavl cattle. We found the following frequency distribution of genotypes: *LL* ($n = 32$), 0.283 ± 0.042; *LV* ($n = 63$), 0.558 ± 0.047; *VV* ($n = 18$), 0.159 ± 0.034. The genotype frequency distribution in these breeds fit the Hardy–Weinberg equilibrium. Table 1 shows the frequency distribution of *bPRL* genotypes. *AAVL* ($n = 29$) and *ABVL* ($n = 27$) are the most frequent combined genotypes of these genes; the *AALL* and *ABLL* genotypes are somewhat rarer ($n = 12$ and $n = 16$, respectively).

We used ANOVA to estimate the isolated effect of the *bPRL* gene and the combined effect of the *bPRL* and *bGH* genes on milk production traits (the milk yield in kilograms and the percentage fat and protein contents for the first three lactations) in Yaroslavl cattle. Table 3 shows the dependence of these parameters for the third lactation on the *bPRL*(*Rsa*I) polymorphism as estimated by one-way ANOVA. The *bPRL* gene was found to affect the fat content of milk ($F_{(2;63)} = 3.18$, $p = 0.048$) but not the milk yield or protein content.

	Lactation 3								
		Milk Yield (kg)				Fat (%)			
Factor	D. F.	SS	MS	F	P	SS	MS	F	P
PRL(*Rsa*1)	2	0.03	0.015	0.5	0.629	0.002	0.001	3.19	**0.0478**
Error	63	2.021	0.032			0.0232	0.0004		
		Protein (%)							
		SS	MS	F	P				
*Rsa*1(*PRL*)	2	0.0005	0.0003	2.34	0.104				
Error	63	0.0073	0.0001						

Designations: d.f., number of degrees of freedom; SS, sum of squares; MS, mean sum of squares, *F*, Fisher's test; *p*, probability; Error, residual variance.

Table 2. Results of one-way ANOVA showing the dependence of milk production traits for the third lactation on the *PRL*(*Rsa*I) polymorphism in Yaroslavl cattle

Figures 6a–6c show the dependences of three milk production traits on the *bPRL* genotypes in Yaroslavl cattle. As can be seen in Figure 6a, cows with the *AA* genotype exhibited a significantly higher fat content of milk compared to *BB* cows ($p = 0.037$).

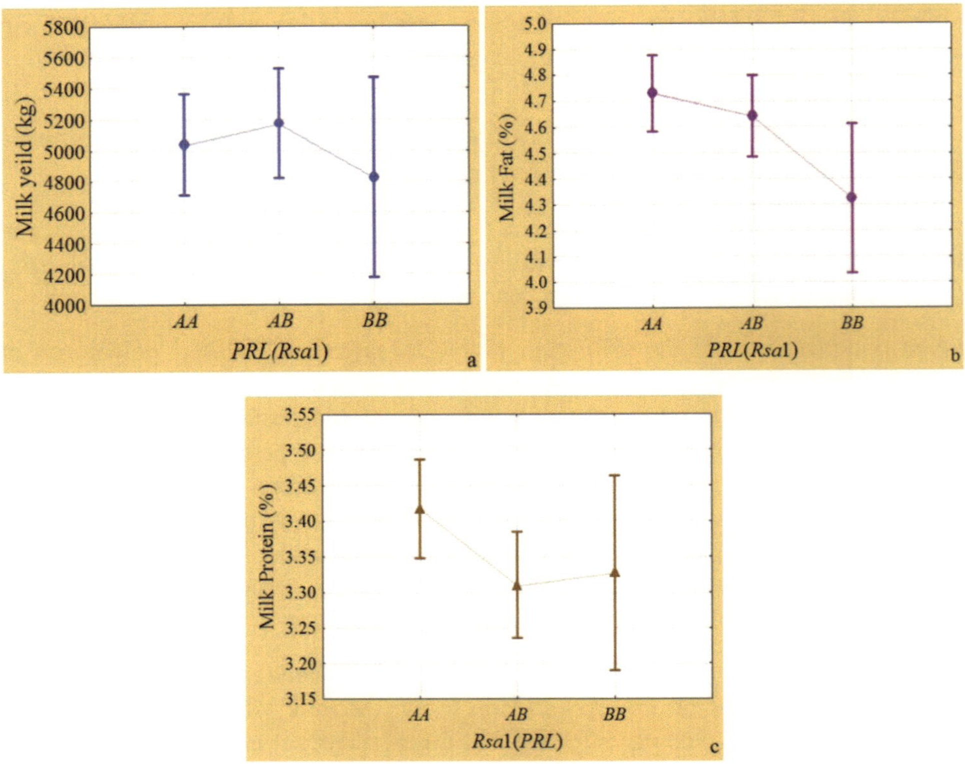

Figure 6. Dependence of (a) the milk yield (in kilograms), (b) the fat content, and (c) the protein content of milk of the third lactation on the *bPRL* genotypes in Yaroslavl cattle. The abscissas show the *bPRL* genotypes; the ordinates show the mean values of the traits; vertical bars are 0.95 confidence intervals.

Considering that quantitative traits, including milk production traits, are each determined by a number of genes, we also estimated the possible combined effect of two factors, the *bPRL* and *bGH* genes, on the milk production traits using two-way ANOVA. The analysis did not reveal a significant isolated effect of any one-locus genotype for any lactation. Still it showed that the *bPRL* genotype tended to affect the third-lactation milk fat content (p = 0.064), which was in contrast to the results of one-way ANOVA showing its significant effect (Table 2). Like one-way ANOVA, the two-way analysis demonstrated that *AA* cows were characterized by a higher fat content of milk than *BB* cows. However, the main result concerning the relationship between the *bPRL* and *bGH* gene polymorphisms and milk production was that we found combined effects of these two genes on the fat and protein contents of first-lactation milk in Yaroslavl cattle ($F_{(4;104)} = 2.59$, $p = 0.041$ and $F_{(4;104)} = 2.93$, $p = 0.024$, respectively) (Table 3).

In order to identify the genotypes whose carriers significantly differed in the mean percentage fat and protein contents of milk, we performed post-hoc pairwise comparisons of these traits in cows with different combined genotypes of the *bPRL* and *bGH* genes. Table 4 shows the results of this analysis. In terms of the milk fat content, cows with the *ABLL* genotype significantly differed from those with the *AAVL, AALL, ABVV,* and *BBVL* genotypes; and cows with the *BBVV* genotype significantly differed from those with the *ABVV* and *BBVL* genotypes. In terms of the milk protein content, *AALL* cows significantly differed from *AAVV, ABVL, ABLL,* and *BBLL* cows; and *BBVV* cows, from *BBLL* ones.

Effect	Lactation 1								
	Trait	Milk Yield				Fat (%)			
	D.f.	SS	MS	F	P	SS	MS	F	P
PRL(*Rsa*I)	2	0.006	0.003	0.2	0.858	4.0E-05	2.0E-05	0.060	0.939
GH(*Alu*I)	2	0.084	0.042	2.1	0.123	0.001	2.6E-04	0.920	0.401
PRL(*Rsa*I) **GH*(*Alu*I)	4	0.064	0.016	0.8	0.520	0.003	0.001	2.590	**0.041**
Error	104	2.049	0.020			0.029	2.8E-04		

	Lactation 1				
	Trait	Protein (%)			
Effect	D.f.	SS	MS	F	P
PRL(*Rsa*I)	2	2.4E-05	1.2E-05	0.100	0.908
GH(*Alu*I)	2	2.3E-04	1.1E-04	0.890	0.412
PRL(*Rsa*I) **GH*(*Alu*I)	4	0.001	3.7E-04	2.930	**0.024**
Error	104	0.013	1.3E-04		

Designations are the same as in Table 2.

Table 3. Results of two-way ANOVA showing the dependence of the milk production parameters on the *bPRL* and *bGH* genes and their interaction in Yaroslavl cattle

Figure 7 graphically shows the combined effects of the *bPRL* and *bGH* genes. The milk yield (in kilograms) and the fat and protein contents of milk of the first lactation in Yaroslavl cows are plotted in Figures 7a, 7b, and 7c, respectively, against the *bPRL* genotypes (*AA, AB,* and *BB*). The *bGH* genotypes are indicated by dots of different colors. The points corresponding to the same *bGH* genotype but different *bPRL* genotypes are connected by dotted lines. As evident from Figure 7, there was no consistent dependence of the fat or protein content on the dose of any allele of any gene. Let us consider how the mean milk fat content depended on the *bPRL* genotypes in combination with different *bGH* genotypes (Figure 7b). The combinations of the *AA* genotype of the *bPRL* gene with different *bGH* genotypes did not differ significantly from one another, and neither did the combinations of the *BB* genotype of the *bPRL* gene with different *bGH* genotypes. In contrast, the mean percentage fat content of milk of *AB* cows was significantly lower if they had the *LL* genotype of the *bGH* gene than if they had the *VV* genotype. This indicates gene interaction, which should be taken into account because otherwise the effects of individual genes on the formation of these traits would be incorrectly estimated. Note that, among the combined genotypes of the *bPRL* and *bGH* genes shown in Figure 7, the *AALL, AAVL, ABVV,* and *BBVL* genotypes were characterized by a significantly higher milk fat content of milk compared to the *ABLL* gene (Figure 7b).

Combined *bPRL* and *bGH* genotypes (*bPRL*(*Rsa*I)–*bGH*(*Alu*I))									
	AAVV	*AAVL*	*AALL*	*ABVV*	*ABVL*	*ABLL*	*BBVV*	*BBVL*	*BBLL*
AAVV		0.933	0.725	0.243	0.945	0.182	0.272	0.267	0.968
AAVL	0.102		0.701	0.163	0.809	**0.041**	0.175	0.186	0.984
AALL	**0.038**	0.378		0.336	0.572	**0.044**	0.139	0.369	0.806
ABVV	0.067	0.484	0.986		0.125	**0.008**	**0.038**	0.955	0.339
ABVL	0.432	0.181	**0.058**	0.125		0.069	0.218	0.143	0.919
ABLL	0.733	0.086	**0.029**	0.068	0.570		0.882	**0.009**	0.259
BBVV	0.058	0.343	0.725	0.736	0.108	0.064		**0.042**	0.312
BBVL	0.559	0.368	0.153	0.208	0.960	0.727	0.159		0.36
BBLL	0.713	0.086	**0.036**	0.054	0.293	0.491	**0.045**	0.387	

Table 4. Results of post-hoc comparisons of the mean first-lactation fat (above the diagonal) and protein (below the diagonal) contents of milk of Yaroslavl cows with different combined *bPRL–bGH* genotypes

Regarding the dependence of the mean protein content of milk in Yaroslavl cattle on the *bPRL* genotypes combined with different *bGH* genotypes (Figure 7c), the combined *AALL* genotype differs from *AAVV*, and *BBVV* differed from *BBLL*. In contrast, no combination of the *AB* genotype of *bPRL* with a *bGH* genotype differed from its combination with any other *bGH* genotype in this respect. Note that, in the given sample of Yaroslavl cattle, the *AAVV, ABLL,* and *BBLL* genotypes were preferable over the *AALL* genotype in terms of the percentage protein content of milk, as was the *BBLL* genotype over the *BBVV* genotype.

Thus, in Yaroslavl cattle, the *AA* genotype of the *bPRL* gene was characterized by a significantly higher percentage fat content of milk than the *BB* genotype, in contrast to Russian Red Pied cattle, where *AB* cows had a higher milk fat content than *AA* and *BB* cows ($p < 0.05$) [22]. Our study has been the first to demonstrate the combined effect of the *bPRL* and *bGH* genes (i.e., their combined genotypes) on the milk fat and protein contents. A number of other authors have also studied the relationship of milk production with combined genotypes of SNPs in the same or different genes; however, the possibility of their combined effect has almost never been considered. One exception is the study on the effects of the combined genotypes of the *Alu*I and *Msp*I polymorphic sites in exon 5 and intron 3, respectively, of the growth hormone gene in Polish Black & White cattle [20]. However, these authors studied combined *bGH* genotypes as a single factor; hence, they did not consider the effect of interaction between individual SNPs on the traits studied. In addition, the marker system used by them was hardly suitable for revealing the interaction of these SNPs because they were located in the same gene.

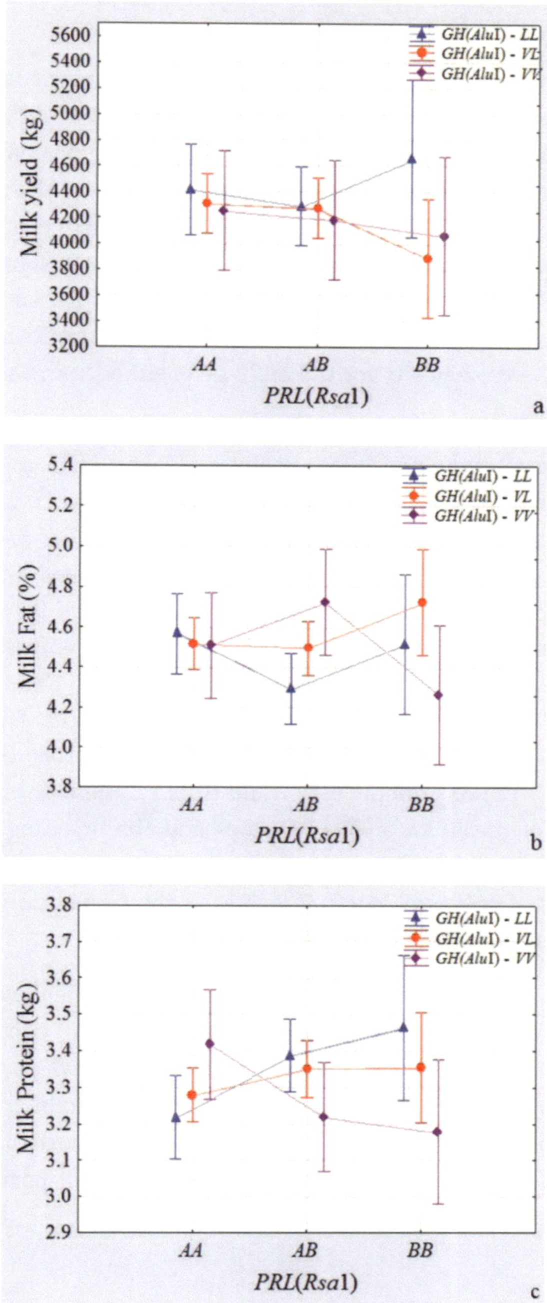

Figure 7. Dependence of (a) the milk yield (in kilograms), (b) the fat content, and (c) the protein content of milk of the first lactation on combined genotypes of the *bPRL* and *bGH* genes in Yaroslavl cattle. The abscissas show the *bPRL* genotypes (*AA, AB,* and *BB*); the ordinates show the mean values of the traits; vertical bars are 0.95 confidence intervals. Different *bGH* genotypes are denoted by dots of different colors; the points corresponding to the same *bGH* genotype but different *bPRL* genotypes are connected by dotted lines.

4. Conclusion

We have found that four Russian cattle breeds, Yakut, Bestuzhev, Kostroma, and Yaroslavl cattle, are similar in genetic structure. All of them are characterized by a low frequency of the *BB* genotype of the *Rsa*I polymorphic site in the *bPRL* gene (from 0.056 ± 0.021 to 0.133 ± 0.031) and high frequencies of heterozygotes and homozygotes for the *A* allele. The breeds of *B. taurus* exhibit a considerable genotypic variation with respect to the *bPRL* gene marker used in this study. The group of these four Russian cattle breeds significantly differs in the genotype frequency distribution from other breeds, such as Russian Black & White and Russian Red Pied. At the same time, these four breeds do not differ significantly in the observed or expected heterozygosity for the *bPRL* gene either from each other or from other breeds used for comparison.

We have demonstrated a combined effect of the *bPRL* and *bGH* genes on the percentage protein and fat contents of milk. Each trait has been found to be significantly positively associated with some of the combined genotypes. No genotype has been found to positively affect both traits. At the same time, some genotypes are associated positively with one trait and negatively with the other one: *ABVV* cows are characterized by a high fat content and low protein content of milk, while this is the other way round with *ABLL* cows. This could be used for selecting cattle for high individual productivity traits. Note that only one combined genotype (*BBVV*) is unfavorable in terms of both traits. However, being doubly homozygous, it may serve as a reserve for obtaining genotypes that are valuable in terms of either fat (*ABVV* and *BBVL*) or protein (*AAVV* and *BBLL*) content of milk. Thus, the study of the combined effects of the *bPRL* and *bGH* genes and the breeding practice taking these effects into account allow the cattle productive potential to be analyzed in more detail. In addition, involvement of epistatic gene interaction in the formation of selectively valuable quantitative traits has been further confirmed.

We believe that data on the *bPRL*(*Rsa*I) SNP marker and the heterozygosity estimates calculated from its allele frequencies may be used in programs for conservation of aboriginal breeds while maintaining the optimal balance between the goals of artificial selection and preservation of the genetic diversity, which is necessary for sustained reproduction of cattle breeds with all their unique characters. This is especially important because of the rapid decrease in the stocks of cattle breeds and the related threat of partial loss of the genetic resources for stockbreeding on a global scale. [33].

Author details

I.V. Lazebnaya and G.E. Sulimova
Department of Comparative Genetics of Animals,
Vavilov Institute of General Genetics, Russian Academy of Sciences, Moscow,
Russian Federation

O.E. Lazebny
Department of Genetics, Koltsov Institute of Developmental Biology, Russian Academy of Sciences, Moscow, Russian Federation

S.R. Khatami
Department of Genetics, Faculty of Science,
Shahid Chamran University of Ahvaz, Ahvaz, Iran
Department of Comparative Genetics of Animals,
Vavilov Institute of General Genetics, Russian Academy of Sciences, Moscow, Russian Federation

Acknowledgement

This study was supported by the Subprogram of the Presidium of the Russian Academy of Sciences "Gene Pools and Gene Diversity," State Contract no. 14.740.11.0164 in the framework of the Federal Target Program "Science and Education Professionals of Innovative Russia," and the Russian Foundation for Basic Research (grant no. 12-04-92214 Mong_a).

5. References

[1] Bernichtein S., Touraine P., Goffin V. REVIEW New concepts in prolactin biology. Journal of Endocrinology 2010;206(1) 1–11.

[2] Horseman N.D., Zhao W., Montecino-Rodriguez E., Tanaka M., Nakashima K., Engle S.J., Smith F., Markoff E., Dorshkind K. Defective mammopoiesis, but normal hematopoiesis, in mice with a targeted disruption of the prolactin gene. EMBO Journal 1997;16(23) 6926–6935.

[3] Rischkowsky B., Pilling D., editors. The State of the World's Animal Genetic Resources for Food and Agriculture Food and Agriculture Organization of the United Nations. FAO. Rome. 2007. ISBN 978-92-5-105762-9

[4] Ernst L.K., Dmitriev N.G., Paronyan I.A., editors. Geneticheskie resursy selskokhozyaistvennykh zhivotnykh v Rossii i sopredel'nykh stranakh (Genetic Resources of Farm Animals in Russia and Neighboring Countries). St. Petersburg, Russia: VNIIGRZh; 1994.

[5] Korotov G.P. Krupnyi Rogatyi Skot Yakutskoi FSSZ i Metody Ego Uluchsheniya (Yakut Cattle and Breeding Methods of Its Improvement). Yakutsk, USSR: Yakutknigoizdat; 1983.

[6] Sulimova G.E., Lazebnaja I.V., Perchun A.V., Voronkova V.N., Ruzina M.N., Badin G.A. Uniqueness of Kostroma breed of cattle from a position of molecular genetics. Advances in science and technology of Agro-Industrial Complex 2011;9 52-54.

[7] Weller J.I. Quantitative Trait Loci Analysis in Animals. London: CABI Publishing; 2001.

[8] Bennewitz J., Reinsch N., Guiard V., Fritz S., Thomsen H., Looft C., Kühn C., Schwerin M., Weimann C., Erhardt G., Reinhardt F., Reents R., Boichard D., Kalm E. Multiple quantitative trait loci mapping with cofactors and application of alternative variants of the false discovery rate in an enlarged granddaughter design. Genetics 2004;168(2) 1019-1027.

[9] Ashwell M.S., Rexroad Jr. C.E., Miller R.H., Van Raden P.M., Da Y. Detection of loci affecting milk production and health traits in an elite US Holstein population using microsatellite markers. Animal Genetics 1997;28(3) 216-222.

[10] Zhang Q., Boichard D., Hoeschele I., Ernst C., Eggen A., Murkv B., Pfistergenskow M., Witte L.A., Grignola F.E., Uimari P., Thaller G., Bishop M.D. Mapping quantitative trait loci for milk production and health of dairy cattle in a large outbred pedigree. Genetics 1998;149(4) 1959-1973.

[11] Plante Y., Gibson J.P., Nadesalingam J., Mehrabani-Yeganeh H., Lefebvre S., Vandervoort G., Jansen G.B. Detection of quantitative trait loci affecting milk production traits on 10 chromosomes in Holstein cattle. J. Dairy Sci. 2001;84(6) 1516-1524.

[12] http://fermer.ru/files/blog/2012/03/137153/yak4.jpg

[13] http://agrolib.ru/rastenievodstvo/item/f00/s00/e0000992/index.shtml

[14] http://agrobk.ru/kostromskaya

[15] http://frunze37.ru/zhivotnovodstvo/

[16] Svensson L.A., Bondensgaard K., Nørskov-Lauritsen L., Christensen L., Becker P., Andersen M.D., Maltesen M.J., Rand K.D., Breinholt J. Crystal Structure of a Prolactin Receptor Antagonist Bound to the Extracellular Domain of the Prolactin Receptor. The Journal of Biological Chemistry 2008;283(27) 19085–19094.

[17] Camper S.A., Luck D.N., Yao, Y., Woychik R.P., Goodwin R.G., Lyons R.H., Rottman F.M. Characterization of the bovine prolactin gene. DNA 1984;3(3) 237-249.

[18] Inoue K., Goda H., Mogi Ch., Tomida M., Tsurugano Sh.. Chapter 6. The Role of Glucocorticoids and Retinoic Acid in the Pituitary Endocrine Cell Differentiation. In: Handa R.J., Hayashi Sh., Terasawa E., Kawata M. (eds.) Neuroplasticity, Development, and Steroid Hormone Action. Boca Raton, FL: CRC Press; 2001. p73-80.

[19] Chung E.R. Chung E.R., Rhim T.J., Han SK. Associations between PCR-RFLP markers of growth hormone and prolactin genes and production traits in dairy cattle. Korean J. Anim. Sci. 1996;38(X) 321-336.

[20] Dybus A., Grzesiak W., Szatkowska I., Błaszczyk P. Association between the growth hormone combined genotypes and dairy traits in Polish Black-and-White cows. Animal Science Papers and Reports 2004;22(2) 185-194.

[21] Chrenek P., Huba J., Oravcova M., Hetenyi L., Peskovieova D., Bulla J. Genotypes of *bGH* and *bPRL* genes in relationships to milk production. 50th Annual Meeting: Book of Abstracts, 1999, Eaap, Zurich. 1999.

[22] Alipanah M., Kalashnikova L., Rodionov G. Association of prolactin gene variants with milk production traits in Russian Red Pied cattle. Iranian Journal of Biotechnology 2007;5(3) 158-161.

[23] Sabour M.P., Lin C.Y., Smith C. Association of genetic variants of bovine growth hormone with milk production traits in Holstein cattle. Journal of Animal Breeding and Genetics 1997;114(X) 435-442.

[24] Zwierzchowski L., Krzyzewski J., Strzalkowska N., Dymnicki E. Effect of polymorphism of growth hormon (*GH*), *Pit*-1, and leptin (*LEP*) genes,cow's age, lactation stage and somatic cell count on milk yield and composition of Polish Black-and-White cows. Animal Science Papers and Reports 2002;20(4) 213.

[25] Mitra A., Schlee P., Balakrishman C.R., Pirchner F. Polymorphisms at Growth-Hormone and Prolactin Loci in Indian Cattle and Buffalo. Journal of Animal Breeding and Genetics 112, 71-74. 1995

[26] Yeh F.C., Yang R.-C., Boyle T.B.J., Ye Z-H., Mao J.X. PopGene, the User-Friendly Shareware For Population Genetic Analysis. Molecular Biology and Biotechnology Centre, University of Alberta, Canada. 1997.

[27] StatSoft, Inc. STATISTICA (Data Analysis Software System), version 8.0. 2008, www.statsoft.com.

[28] Kumari R., Singh K.M., Soni K.J., Patel R.K., Chauhan J.B., Sambasiva-Rao K.R.S. Genotyping of the Polymorphism Within Exon 3 of Prolactin Gene in Various Dairy Breeds by PCR RFLP (Brief report). Archiv Tierzucht / Archives Animal Breeding 2008;51(3) 298-299.

[29] Dybus A., Grzesiak W., Kamieniecki H., Szatkowska I., Sobek Z., Blaszczyk P., Czerniawska- Piatkowska, E. Zych S., Muszynska M. Association of Genetic Variants of Bovine Prolactin With Milk Production Traits of Black-and-White and Jersey Cattle. Archiv Tierzucht / Archives Animal Breeding 2005;48(2) 149-156.

[30] Skinkytė R., Zwierzchowski L., Riaubaitė L., Baltrėnaitė L., Miceikienė I. Distribution of Allele Frequencies Important to Milk Production Traits in Lithuanian Black and White and Lithuanian Red Cattle. Veterinary Medicine and Zootechnics (Veterinarija ir Zootechnika) 2005;31(53) 93-96.

[31] Goryacheva T.S., Goncharenko G.M. Polymorphism in κ-Casein and Prolactin Genes and Their Influence on Dairy Productivity of Cows of the Black-and-White Breed. Agricultural biology 2010;4 51-54.

[32] Ghasemi N., Zadehrahmani M., Rahimi G., Hafezian S.H. Associations Between Prolactin Gene Polymorphism and Milk Production in Montebeliard Cows. International Journal of Genetics and Molecular Biology 2009;1(3) 48.

[33] FAO. 2007. The State of the World's Animal Genetic Resources for Food and Agriculture, edited by Barbara Rischkowsky & Dafydd Pilling. Rome.

Chapter 4

Prolactin in the Immune System

Lorenza Díaz, Mauricio Díaz-Muñoz, Leticia González,
Saúl Lira-Albarrán, Fernando Larrea and Isabel Méndez

Additional information is available at the end of the chapter

http://dx.doi.org/10.5772/53538

1. Introduction

Prolactin (PRL) is a protein hormone, as well as a cytokine, which is synthesized and secreted from specialized cells of the anterior pituitary gland, named lactotrophs. More than 300 functions exerted by PRL in vertebrates have been recognized; and they reflect the ubiquitous distribution of its receptors, as well as the fact that PRL is synthesized in many extrapituitary tissues. Among these sites of PRL synthesis are cells of the immune system, such as macrophages, natural killer cells, and T- and B-lymphocytes. Regulation of PRL synthesis is organ specific, which confers additional complexity to the spectrum of PRL actions. In the physiology of the immune system, PRL acts by stimulating the secretion of other cytokines and the expression of cytokine receptors, and also as a growth and survival factor. In pathological conditions, increased levels of PRL could cause deterioration of the subject's condition. In this review, we integrate the information on regulation of PRL synthesis with that concerning its physiological and pathological actions in extrapituitary tissues, highlighting those in the immune system.

2. Regulation of prolactin expression and secretion in the pituitary and at extrapituitary sites

PRL was originally identified as a neuroendocrine hormone of pituitary origin; however, its synthesis is not limited to the hypophysis since numerous extrapituitary tissues also express this protein, including the placenta, ovary, testis, mammary gland, skin, adipose tissue, endothelial cells, and immune cells [1]. This wide-spread PRL expression might explain its involvement in very different processes such as reproduction, metabolism, immunology, and behavior.

PRL expression and secretion are regulated by different stimuli provided by the environment and the internal milieu. Although pituitary PRL secretion is under a tonic and predominantly inhibitory control exerted by dopamine of hypothalamic origin, other factors within the brain, pituitary gland, and peripheral organs have been shown to inhibit or stimulate PRL secretion as well [2-5]. Therefore, pituitary PRL expression depends on the balance between inhibitory and stimulatory molecules such as hormones, cytokines, and other factors that orchestrate the cascade of intracellular events involving numerous signaling pathways. Prominent among these signaling cascades are the cAMP/protein kinase A (PKA), the phosphatidylinositol/Ca^{++}/protein kinase C (PKC), and the mitogen-activated protein kinase (MAPK) pathways. In addition, the PRL gene seems to follow a pulsatile transcription dynamic with refractive phases in the transcription cycles [4]. In the pituitary, a direct relation between transcribed mRNA and released protein cannot be easily established, since different, post-transcriptional processes may alter the final protein production; these include mRNA degradation, protein storage, and regulation of secretion. Pituitary PRL secretion depends on the action of secretagogues which act on the cell membrane of lactotrophs, rapidly releasing stored PRL by means of calcium-dependent exocytosis. In contrast, extrapituitary cells seem to have little storage capacity and consequently, PRL is released after synthesis [2, 5]. Therefore, extrapituitary PRL is basically

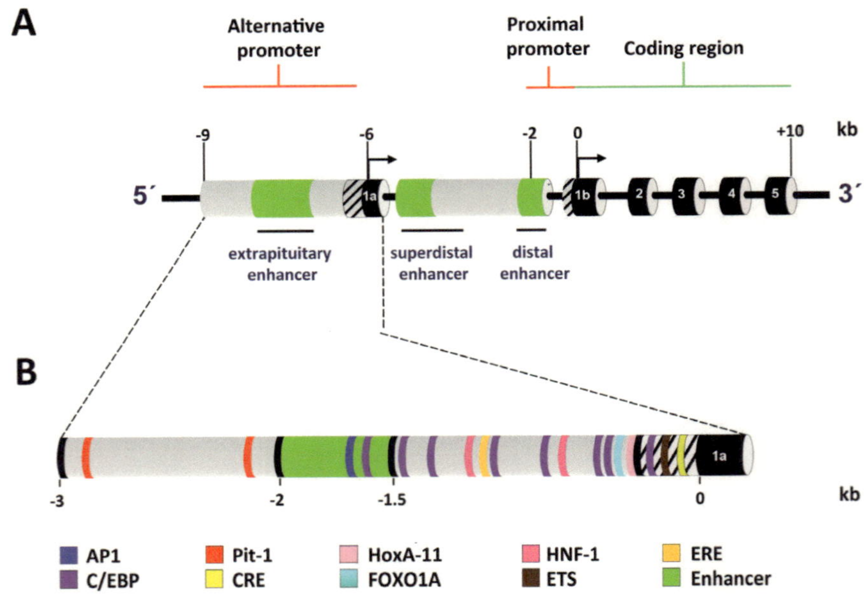

Figure 1. Schematic representation of the human PRL gene. A) The alternative and proximal promoters, as well as the coding region are depicted. Exons are represented by black boxes with corresponding exon numbers (1a, 1b, 2-5). Exon 1a, located 5.8 kb upstream of the proximal start site, drives extrapituitary PRL expression. B) Extended diagram of human PRL alternative promoter showing the location of predicted transcription factor binding sites. The superdistal promoter is about 3.0 kb in length. Consensus sequences for transcription factors are depicted and shown in different colors. The figure is not drawn to scale. AP1: activator protein 1; C/EBP: CCAAT/enhancer binding protein; Pit-1: pituitary-specific transcription factor 1; CRE: cyclic-AMP response element; HoxA-11: homeobox A11; FOXO1A: forkhead box protein O1A; HNF-1: hepatocyte nuclear factor 1; ETS: E-twenty six; ERE: estrogen response element. Enhancer regions are represented in green.

regulated at the level of transcription. The regulation of PRL gene expression is quite complex, due to the presence of several enhancer and silencer domains as well as the formation of chromatin loops with consequences for transcription dynamics. Two independent promoters with differential responses to regulatory mediators direct PRL transcription in a cell-type specific manner [4].

The human PRL locus consists of a single gene containing 5 coding exons transcribed directly from a pituitary-specific promoter (proximal promoter) and a non-coding exon (1a) transcribed from an alternative promoter (also known as the decidual or superdistal promoter) with a transcriptional start site located 5.8 kb upstream of exon 1b (Figure 1). This alternative promoter drives expression in extrapituitary tissues [4, 5] and seems to have evolved from a long terminal repeat transposable element, previously described as primate specific [6]. The differential promoter usage produces different sized gene products, which may vary in a cell-specific manner depending on the functional elements used within the particular promoter. In general, extrapituitary PRL mRNA is ~150 bp longer than pituitary PRL mRNA; however, mRNA identical to that in the pituitary gland has been found in normal and tumoral breast tissues, breast cell lines, and prostate [7, 8]. Therefore, the dichotomy of promoter usage in pituitary versus extrapituitary sites is not absolute [9].

As a consequence of the distal transcription start site, the alternative promoter does not respond to the same regulators of gene expression that operate with the proximal promoter, such as the pituitary transcriptional factor-1 (Pit-1), which is paramount for the activation of pituitary PRL transcription. An exception to this generalization is the hormonal form of vitamin D, calcitriol, which stimulates PRL expression in pituitary cells as well as in decidua and resting lymphocytes. Other cell-specific cases will be further discussed below.

2.1. Regulation of PRL in the immune system

In the immune system, PRL is thought to act as a locally produced cytokine with relevance for immune regulation and modulation of T- and B-cell function. Nevertheless, the molecular mechanisms regulating PRL expression in the immune system and the factors implicated are still not fully understood. Within the immune system, PRL is produced by T- and B-lymphocytes, macrophages, thymocytes, mononuclear and natural killer cells. However, in peripheral blood-mononuclear cells (PBMC), PRL production is mainly associated with the T-lymphocyte fraction [2, 10]. Because it uses the alternative promoter, lymphocyte PRL expression is independent of Pit-1, progesterone, estrogen, thyrotropin-releasing hormone (TRH), dihydrotestosterone, and insulin, among other classical modulators of PRL in the hypophysis. In contrast, PRL expression in T-lymphocytes is stimulated by cAMP, retinoic acid, and calcitriol, while it is inhibited by dexamethasone and some interleukins [10-15].

2.1.1. cAMP and modulators of the cAMP/CREB pathway

Consistent evidence, including studies in different leukemic cell lines as well as PBMC from normal patients, has shown that PRL gene expression is significantly stimulated by cAMP, its analogues and first messengers that signal through the cAMP/PKA pathway [12, 13, 16]. The second messenger cAMP induces PRL gene expression by activating PKA, which migrates to the nucleus and phosphorylates target proteins such as the cAMP response element binding protein (CREB). However, in the eosinophilic leukemia cell line EoL-1, it seems that cAMP induces PRL expression by two different signaling cascades: the classic PKA-dependent pathway leading to the phosphorylation of CREB, and a PKA-independent pathway leading to the phosphorylation of p38 [12]. Known first messengers that activate the cAMP/PKA pathway are prostaglandin-E_2 and terbutaline, a β_2-adrenergic agonist that enhances PRL expression in PBMC and some leukemic cell lines either alone or in combination with PMA or ionomycin [17]. These observations are most likely explained by the cAMP response element (CRE) located -25 bp upstream of the PRL alternative promoter (Figure 1). Furthermore, this CRE encourage additional studies of the regulation of PRL by other physiological modulators of the immune system that operate through cAMP as a second messenger. This would be especially relevant in pathological conditions associated with increased PRL levels such as autoimmune diseases and cancer, where alterations in extrapituitary PRL promoter regulation might play a role in the pathophysiology of these disorders.

2.1.2. Dopamine and cell-activating factors

Quite interestingly, the nervous and the immune systems use a common chemical language for intra- and inter-system communication. Indeed, both systems produce a common set of neurotransmitters and cytokines that act on a shared repertoire of receptors [18]. Regarding dopamine, which is the primary neuroendocrine inhibitor of PRL secretion in the anterior pituitary gland, some evidence supports the involvement of this neurotransmitter in the regulation of lymphocyte PRL production and release [3]. Indeed, differential expression of all dopamine receptor subtypes has been detected by flow cytometry in human immune cells [19]. Specifically in lymphocytes, pharmacological studies indicate expression of the dopamine receptors D_2, D_3, D_4, and D_5 [3, 20, 21]. In the secondary lymphoid tissues, D_3 is the predominant dopamine receptor and it is highly and selectively expressed in naive $CD8^+$T cells of both humans and mice [22]. The differential expression of dopamine receptor subtypes in the lymphocyte subsets as well as the alterations in dopamine-mediated effects under conditions of stress [23]; need to be taken into consideration when studying regulatory mechanisms involved in cell activation/suppression processes. Indeed, since D_1 and D_5 couple with $G_{\alpha s}$ proteins increasing cAMP, while D_2, D_3, and D_4 couple with $G_{\alpha i}$ proteins, inhibiting the production of cAMP, a different cell response is to be expected depending on the receptor subtype that is expressed, as seen in activated T cells [24].

In addition, some immune cells such as lymphocytes produce endogenous dopamine, which may induce autocrine/paracrine actions. The effects of dopamine in the immune system are highly dependent on the context and dopamine concentration [25]; moreover, its effects on immune cells also depend on their activation state, which, at the same time, is modulated by dopamine itself [25, 26]. Indeed, dopamine interacts directly with dopaminergic receptors on normal human T-cells, triggering characteristic features of activated lymphocytes [26].

These data are in agreement with unpublished observations from our group which indicated that dopamine regulates prolactin expression in PBMC, as well as expression of its own receptor [27]. Moreover, our results showed that activation of PBMC with phytohemagglutinin (PHA), concanavalin-A (Con-A), or phorbol myristate acetate (PMA) significantly reduced PRL mRNA in all cases. Notably, the inhibitory effect of Con-A upon PRL mRNA expression persisted in the presence of a cAMP analogue (Figure 2), suggesting that cell activation with this lectin disrupts the cAMP/PKA signaling pathway, which is involved in PRL upregulation in lymphocytes as previously mentioned. In accordance with our results, Gerlo *et al* showed that PMA and ionomycin inhibited PRL gene expression in normal PBMC, but elicited differential effects in several leukemic cell lines [17]. Altogether, these observations suggest that under an *in vivo* scenario, modification of the lymphocytes activation status by dopamine might alter their PRL expression, an idea which warrants further investigation. *In vitro*, even if PRL gene expression is decreased by cell activation, the final PRL concentration in the culture media might be elevated due to the larger number of PRL-producing cells. This agrees with several other studies showing that mitogen stimulation is not required for PRL mRNA expression and exerts no appreciable effect on the level of PRL transcripts [10].

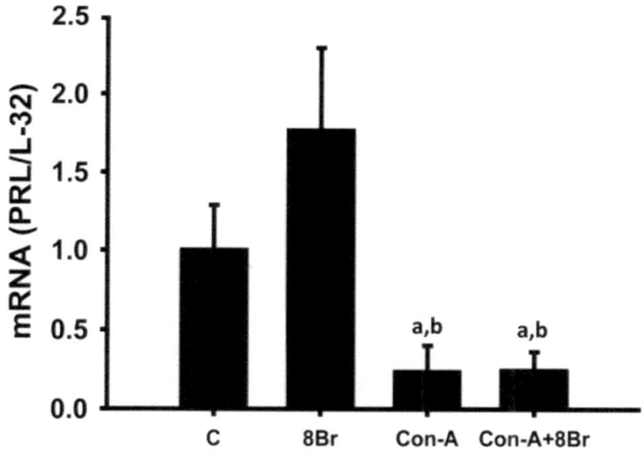

Figure 2. Effect of lymphocyte activators on PRL mRNA levels. PBMC from 3 pregnant women were incubated for 24 h in the presence of 8-Bromo-cAMP (8Br, 1 mM), concanavalin-A (Con-A, 1 mg/mL), or both. PRL mRNA expression was evaluated after normalization against L-32 mRNA by real time PCR. a = $P < 0.05$ vs control (C); b = $P < 0.05$ vs 8Br. An arbitrary value of 1 was given to control data.

2.1.3. Calcitriol

Previous findings in human lymphocytes suggested that calcitriol effects were exerted only after cell activation, which is necessary for the induction of the 50-kDa classic vitamin D receptor (VDR). Nevertheless, recent findings from our group clearly showed VDR-mediated effects in resting lymphocytes. We also described a constitutive, 75-kDa VDR species that might participate in calcitriol-dependent PRL upregulation in these cells.

Indeed, as in the case of decidua and the pituitary, calcitriol stimulated both, PRL mRNA expression and protein production in resting PBMC through a VDR-mediated mechanism [15]. Interestingly, this effect was only seen in quiescent lymphocytes and was not detected in Jurkat T-lymphoma cells. Genomic effects of calcitriol upon the alternative PRL promoter are likely to occur in lymphocytes, in view of previous results in decidua [28] together with the fact that the decidual form of the PRL transcript is expressed in human blood lymphocytes [10, 29]. Nevertheless, further studies are required to clarify the specific interaction of the VDR with the PRL promoter region in lymphocytes, since it is known that the pituitary promoter contains functional sequences that confer VDR responsiveness. Indeed, calcitriol stimulated PRL promoter activity in cultured pituitary GH3 cells [30, 31], an effect that was further corroborated *in vivo* [32]. The fact that calcitriol regulates PRL in immune cells might be relevant in specific physiological contexts, considering the immunomodulatory actions of this secosteroid. Certainly, calcitriol effects in the immune system appear to occur at the level of T-helper (Th) cells, where it acts as an immunosuppressive factor. Calcitriol inhibits mainly Th1 cytokines [33], as confirmed by its abilities to prevent or ameliorate autoimmune diseases and to inhibit allograft rejection responses [34, 35]. The upregulation of lymphocyte-derived PRL by calcitriol could help explain the condition of hyperprolactinemia reported in some granulomatous disorders such as sarcoidosis, a disease associated with increased calcitriol production by macrophages, and characterized by abnormal accumulation of inflammatory cells such as T-lymphocytes [36, 37]. Indeed, calcitriol is synthesized by macrophages, dendritic cells, and both T- and B-cells by means of expressing the enzyme CYP27B1, which catalyzes the synthesis of the secosteroid from its inactive precursor, calcidiol [38]. Thus, in immune cells, PRL secretion might be regulated by locally produced calcitriol providing, at this level, paracrine and or autocrine immunomodulatory effects.

2.1.4. Cytokines

Structural analyses of PRL and its receptors have revealed their relation to the cytokine/hematopoietin family. Standing as a leukocyte-derived cytokine in the immune system, PRL is regulated by other cytokines in an autocrine and paracrine manner. In T-lymphocytes, interleukin (IL)-2, IL-1β, and IL-4 reduced PRL mRNA, while IL-10 and interferon-γ had no effect [11]. On the other hand, in myeloid leukemic cells, the PRL alternative promoter was activated by the proinflammatory cytokine tumor necrosis factor alpha (TNF-α). A TNF-α-responsive region was located between -1842 and -1662 of the extrapituitary PRL promoter. Interestingly, the stimulatory effect of TNF-α upon PRL was blocked by a protein kinase C (PKC) inhibitor [14]. Since TNF-α is a master proinflammatory cytokine, its involvement in PRL stimulation might have clinical relevance in view of several studies indicating that leukocyte-derived PRL is involved in autoimmune and hematological disorders [39-41]. Indeed, hyperprolactinemia and increased secretion of lymphocyte PRL have been reported in systemic lupus erythematosus (SLE) [42], which is an autoimmune disease characterized by abnormal production of autoantibodies and proinflammatory cytokines [43]. Moreover, hyperprolactinemia has been associated with SLE disease activity [41, 42, 44, 45].

2.2. Regulation of PRL in the placenta and endometrium

PRL functions in reproduction vary within species. For example, while in rodents the presence of PRL is mandatory to achieve a normal estrous cycle, support the corpus luteum for progesterone production and maintenance of gestation, in humans the role of PRL is more likely relevant during lactation, since it does not support the corpus luteum nor significantly participates in the menstrual cycle [5]. The decidua develops from the uterine lining throughout the late luteal phase of the menstrual cycle, and during pregnancy the decidua constitutes the maternal component of the placenta. Considered a marker of decidualization, PRL is one of the most dramatically induced genes in decidualized endometrial cells. The placental decidua secretes very large amounts of PRL that accumulates in the amniotic fluid, peaking between 16 and 22 weeks of gestation (~5000 ng/mL) and falling to ~500 ng/mL at term [46]. Regarding PRL regulation, activation of the cAMP/PKA pathway is known to induce the activity of the alternative PRL promoter in human decidual cells through the transcription factors CREB and CCAAT/enhancer-binding protein (C/EBP) [47, 48]. In this regard, eight C/EBP binding sites have been described in the decidual PRL promoter (Figure 1). Decidualization is mainly triggered and supported by progesterone. Accordingly, upregulation of PRL gene expression steadily increases due to high progesterone levels during pregnancy. Indeed, progesterone potently stimulates decidual PRL production [49, 50], which is achieved in part by cross-talk with the cAMP/PKA signaling pathway [51], and is synergized by a number of factors such as prostaglandin E, corticotropin releasing factor, and the free α-subunit of gonadotropin [52-54]. Furthermore, in human endometrium explants and endometrial stromal (ES) cells, progesterone and relaxin induced stromal differentiation (decidualization) and PRL secretion [50, 55]. Interestingly, in primary ES cell cultures, cAMP activated the alternative PRL promoter in a biphasic manner, with an initial, weak induction during the first 12 hours, followed by a more intense induction afterwards. It was concluded that the early response depended upon the CRE located at approximately -12 bp upstream of the PRL alternative promoter, whereas the major activation depended upon a region between positions -332 and -270 bp, which kinetics differed from classic CRE-mediated responses [55].

In addition to the decidualized endometrium of the late luteal phase and of pregnancy, the human myometrium, which is the muscle layer of the uterus, is considered to be a secondary source of PRL. Nevertheless, the regulation of myometrial PRL differs significantly from that of the decidua. Indeed, myometrial PRL expression seems to be under inhibitory control *in vivo,* as concluded from experimental findings showing that myometrial PRL release increased with time in culture. Moreover, in myometrial explant cultures, medroxyprogesterone acetate inhibited PRL production [2, 56]. This observation, together with the fact that PRL circulating levels are unchanged throughout the human menstrual cycle, suggests that further studies are needed to completely clarify the mechanistic details of PRL regulation by progesterone in the human myometrium.

Besides progesterone, other stimulators of decidual PRL synthesis and release are insulin, insulin-like growth factor-1, and calcitriol [28, 57, 58]. Since the human decidua is able to synthesize calcitriol and express the VDR, PRL regulation by this secosteroid is more likely autocrine in nature. However, considering that inflammatory cytokines such as TNF-α, IL-1α, IL-1β, IL-2, IL-8, and transforming growth factor-β (TGF-β1) inhibit decidual PRL expression [59, 60], and that calcitriol is a potent inhibitor of placental inflammatory cytokine production [61, 62], calcitriol might also be acting as a paracrine upregulator of decidual PRL. In addition, IL-4 decreased both the level of PRL mRNA and its release from myometrial tissue, whereas IL-6 exerted no effect [63]. Recently, the transcriptional regulators HoxA-10, HoxA-11, and FOXO1A, which are essential for decidualization, have been shown to interact physically and functionally to upregulate the expression of a gene battery in differentiating endometrium. In particular, this core set of transcription factors cooperatively upregulate PRL in differentiating ES cells by binding to an enhancer region located between positions −395 and −148 of the decidual prolactin promoter (Figure 1) [64].

2.3. Regulation of PRL in the breast and adipose tissue

In addition to uptake of PRL from the blood, mammary epithelial cells synthesize PRL during pregnancy and lactation. It has been suggested that the production of mammary PRL requires a systemic trophic factor, because PRL mRNA declined with time in cultured rat mammary gland explants [65]; however, this proposal requires further investigation since PRL regulation is thought to differ between species. Interestingly, the number of PRL variants in human milk exceeds that found in serum, indicating that the breast may be a post-transcriptional processing site [66]. In support of this possibility, incubation of mammary slices in the presence of PRL resulted in the formation of fragments of PRL [67]. Although there are two Pit-1 consensus sequences located at -2186 and -2800 bp within the alternative promoter (Figure 1), the expression of extrapituitary PRL is thought to be independent of Pit-1. However, Pit-1 expression in normal and cancerous human breast tissue has been reported [68]. Moreover, the experimental over-expression of Pit-I in MCF-7 cells significantly increased expression of PRL mRNA, while PRL protein expression was significantly reduced after Pit-I knockdown, suggesting that in this cell line, PRL transcription is driven by the proximal pituitary promoter and is due to Pit-I binding to this region [69]. Alternatively, distal upstream Pit-1 consensus sequences could also be participating.

As in the case of the pituitary, studies performed in the human mammary cell line T47D showed that estrogen directly induces PRL gene expression [70]. A functional, non-canonical, estrogen responsive element (ERE) and an AP1 site have been located in the PRL distal promoter (Figure 1). Moreover, both estrogen receptors α and β bind directly to this ERE, which suggests that estrogens regulating autocrine PRL in the human breast may contribute to breast development and cancer progression.

It is noteworthy that most local PRL production in the breast occurs in adipose rather than in glandular tissue [71]. Whereas PRL release from glandular explants was suppressed by progesterone, neither estrogen nor progesterone altered PRL expression in adipose explants [71]. This dissimilar regulation of PRL in adjacent tissues is not unusual, and was also observed in decidua and myometrium. Therefore, the interactions between stromal, glandular, and adipose tissue should be taken into consideration for PRL regulation studies in the mammary gland. Even if the main source of PRL in breast adipose tissue seems to be the mature adipocyte, both the subcutaneous and visceral adipose depots also produce PRL [72]. As in other locations, the regulation of PRL release from primary human breast preadipocytes is stimulated by activators of the cAMP/PKA pathway. Indeed, recent studies have shown that, similar to its action in the pituitary, dopamine suppresses PRL gene expression and release in adipocytes through inhibition of cAMP, followed by the suppression of PKA activity [73]. Moreover, in primary human breast preadipocytes, isoproterenol, a β-adrenergic receptor agonist, and the pituitary adenylate cyclase activating peptide, increased PRL mRNA expression and release. This effect was suppressed by several protein kinase inhibitors, suggesting involvement of multiple signaling cascades [74].

Another interesting issue to be addressed is whether regulators of metabolic and endocrine activities of adipocytes such as insulin and cytokines affect PRL secretion in these cells. This question is particularly relevant in conditions such as obesity and inflammation. Contrary to results obtained in cultured rat mammary gland explants [65], PRL release from human adipose explants and mature adipocytes increased with time, indicating removal from inhibition [72]. Interestingly, insulin suppressed PRL expression and release from differentiated adipocytes but moderately stimulated PRL release from non-differentiated cells. Nevertheless, considering that preadipocytes represent only a small fraction of the total cell population within adipose tissue, the overall effect of insulin on PRL is likely inhibitory [72].

3. Prolactin in the physiology of the immune system

PRL is a highly versatile hormone/cytokine that displays a wide spectrum of effects in a variety of tissues. In fact, more than 300 actions by PRL have been described in vertebrates. In pancreatic beta cells, pancreas, liver, and T-lymphocytes, PRL can regulate proliferation [75, 76] while in prostate, pancreatic beta cells, lymphocytes, ovarian carcinoma cells, breast cancer cells, and others, PRL acts as an antiapoptotic factor. [77-81]. These effects are mediated by its receptors, which are members of the class I hematopoietin/cytokine receptor family [76]. In the immune system, PRL receptors expression have been detected in several cells such as splenocytes, thymocytes, bone marrow cells, PBMC, lymphocytes, and monocytes [76]. Both PRL and the PRL receptor are constitutively expressed by resting T-cells [29], which indicates that PRL may influence the immune system even during steady-state conditions.

PRL has a wide range of effects on the regulation of the immune system. Administration of PRL to hypophysectomised rats provokes weight gain of two lymphoid tissues, spleen and thymus [82]. In lymphocytes, PRL reverses anemia, leukopenia, and thrombocytopenia induced by hypophysectomy [83], and it increases antibody production [84]. PRL has also been reported to increase receptor levels for interleukin (IL)-2 and PRL [76]. Using PRL receptor knockdown, autocrine PRL actions could be elucidated. In T- lymphocytes in which the PRL receptor was silenced, proliferation induced by phytohemagglutinin (PHA) was significantly reduced. Moreover, the expression of certain co-stimulatory molecules (CD137, CD154) and the secretion of cytokines (IL-2 and IL-4) induced by PHA activation were suppressed in these cells [85]. Although PRL has been observed to act in a cooperative fashion with IL-2 to influence proliferation in the immune system, there is evidence indicating that PRL can act as a T-cell growth factor, independently of IL-2 [86-88]. In addition to stimulating proliferation, PRL has been shown to inhibit apoptosis of lymphocytes [79, 89, 90]. In BALB/c mice expressing a transgene for the heavy chain of a pathogenic anti-DNA antibody, inducing moderate hyperprolactinemia (a 2-fold increase in the serum PRL concentration) increases the number of autoreactive B-cells with the follicular phenotype and leads to their activation, with subsequent anti-DNA antibody production as well as IgG deposition in the kidneys [91]. The induction of hyperprolactinemia promotes autoreactivity inasmuch as it breaks B-cell tolerance, acting on the mechanisms of B-cell tolerance induction at three levels: B cells receptor-mediated deletion, receptor editing, and anergy [91].

Despite evidence of an immunomodulatory role of PRL, it has been shown that the development of the immune system was unaffected in both PRL and PRL-receptor knockout mice [92]. The effects due to the lack of PRL action were probably compensated by redundancy of the cytokine network. Data support the immunomodulatory role of PRL in normal murine and human cells and in *in vivo* models after procedures such as hypophysectomy and ovariectomy. More studies are needed to determine the involvement of PRL in physiological and/or pathological conditions, and to explore its therapeutic potential in diseases of the immune system.

4. Prolactin in the pathology of the immune system.

4.1. Prolactin and autoimmunity

The interrelationship between PRL and the immune system has been elucidated over the last 2 decades, opening important new horizons in the field of immunoendocrinology [93]. The autoimmune diseases are more common in females, and sex hormones could have an important role in this gender bias. Estrogens and PRL modify the immune phenotype and functions; furthermore, they are able to modulate both the innate and adaptive immunological response. PRL exerts an immunostimulatory effect and might promote the development of autoimmune diseases by different mechanisms, such as impairing the negative selection of auto reactive B-lymphocytes occurring during B-cell maturation into fully functional B-cells [94]. Moreover, PRL induces an anti-apoptotic effect, enhances the proliferative response to antigens and mitogens, and increases the production of immunoglobulin, cytokines, and autoantibodies. In murine models of some autoimmune diseases there is a clear association between hyperprolactinemia and disease progression. Indeed, moderate hyperprolactinemia has been found in a cohort of patients with autoimmune diseases like SLE, rheumatoid arthritis (RA), Sjogren´s syndrome (SS), Hashimoto´s thyroiditis (HT), and multiple sclerosis (MS) [95-98]. These data are controversial, since some studies have not found a consistent correlation between PRL levels and disease activity in humans [99]. These discrepancies could be explained by genetic, environmental, and hormonal factors related to susceptibility; these factors might influence the progression of autoimmune disorders, might alter PRL circadian rhythm thereby contributing to disease by modifying the immune response [100], and could even change PRL isoforms and anti-PRL antibodies that reduce the biological activity of PRL [101]. The PRL molecule undergoes posttranslational modifications generating several molecular species. In contrast to high molecular weight PRL species (>100 kDa), monomeric PRL (23 kDa) is associated with SLE clinical activity [102]. An association of PRL levels with anti-dsDNA antibodies and with anti-Ro and anti-La antibodies has been reported [94].

The physiology of the immune system involves a balance between the two arms of the cellular immune response. T-helper cells type 1 (Th1) and type 2 (Th2) elicit cell- and humoral-mediated responses, respectively. PRL is involved in regulating both Th1 and Th2 responses, particularly the former. Altered PRL levels associated with either Th1 or Th2 dominance often characterize autoimmune diseases [103]. Evidence observed in animal models and human disorders suggest that Th1 cytokines (IFN-γ, IL-2 and TNF-α) are involved in the genesis of organ-specific autoimmune diseases, such as RA, MS, insulin-dependent diabetes mellitus (IDDM), and thyroid autoimmunity. In contrast, Th2 responses tend to dominate in circumstances such as SLE, and in systemic and allergic conditions, such as HT (Figure 3) [103].

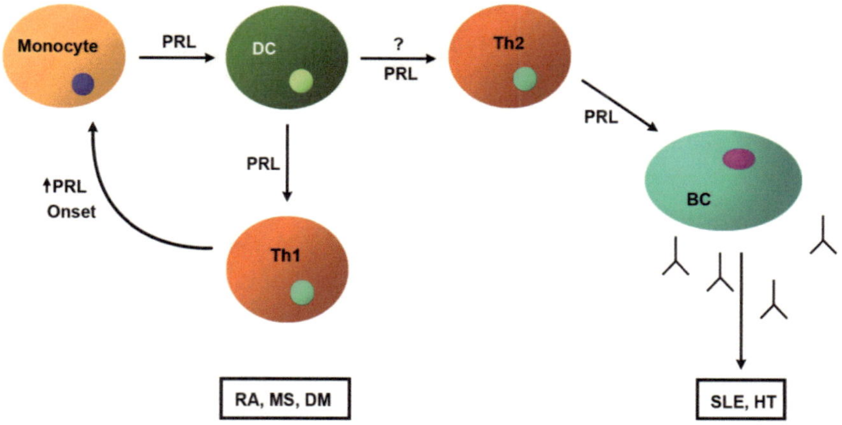

Figure 3. The role of PRL in autoimmune diseases. PRL induces monocytes maturation to dendritic cells (DC) through increasing major histocompatibility complex and co-stimulatory molecules. Furthermore, PRL induces T-cell activation and production of pro-inflammatory cytokines. Imbalances between Th1 and Th2 result in different autoimmune diseases. BC, B-cells; SLE, systemic lupus erythematosus; RA, rheumatoid arthritis; MS, multiple sclerosis; DM, diabetes mellitus; HT, Hashimoto's thyroiditis.

4.1.1. Systemic lupus erythematosus

SLE is an autoimmune disease nine times more common in young women of reproductive age than in men. The expected rate of hyperprolactinemia is 0.4% in healthy adults [104, 105], whereas mild to moderate hyperprolactinemia occurs in 15-33% of SLE patients of both genders [102, 106]. Furthermore, elevated lymphocyte PRL gene expression has been identified in a cohort of female SLE subjects [42, 44]. In the majority of SLE - hyperprolactinemia patients the cause of the enhanced PRL levels is unknown, which suggests impaired regulation of PRL synthesis in SLE. In this regard, observations from our group showed an increased central dopaminergic tone in SLE and normoprolactinemic female patients, but with enhanced levels of PRL from lymphocytes; this finding suggests that lymphocyte-derived PRL might contribute to altering the functional activity of the hypothalamic dopaminergic system in order to maintain serum PRL within a physiological range in SLE [42]. In this study, after metoclopramide administration, mRNA expression and secretion of lymphocyte-derived PRL increased only in PBMC from control women and not in those from SLE patients. These observations indicate that dopamine could have a direct effect on PRL synthesis in normal lymphocytes that is absent in SLE lymphocytes.

Murine SLE encompasses several strains of inbred mice and hybrids (NZB, NZB x NZW F1, MRL lpr/lpr, BXSB) that variably manifest autoimmune disturbances such as accelerated hypergammaglobulinemia, immune complex glomerulonephritis and mortality, increased anti-DNA antibody levels and immune complex formation, as well as suppression of lymphoproliferation, symptoms that closely resemble those of human SLE [107]. In this model, induced hyperprolactinemia exacerbates disease activity, which leads to premature death regardless of the gender. Interestingly, in non-lupus prone BALB/c mice, treatment with high or physiological doses of PRL favours the development of an SLE-like phenotype, because this hormone breaks down the B-cell tolerance [91]. In addition, administration of bromocriptine, a dopamine receptor agonist that blocks prolactin secretion by the anterior pituitary ameliorates disease progression in murine SLE models [108, 109], indicating a potential role of PRL in the pathogenesis of SLE. Furthermore, clinical trials treating SLE with bromocriptine, have suggested a beneficial effect in patients with mild and moderate disease activity. Bromocriptine suppresses the levels of immunoglobulins, autoantibodies, and immune complexes in lupus glomerulonephritis, both in animal models and SLE patients [103, 107]. This drug is also associated with lower cytokine secretion and proliferation of T- cells. Furthermore, a clinical trial using bromocriptine in pregnant SLE patients suggests that it may help prevent maternal-fetal complications secondary to this disease [110, 111].

4.1.2. Rheumatoid arthritis

Clinical observations in humans and experimental data in animal models have also implicated PRL in other autoimmune diseases such as RA. This common autoimmune condition is an inflammatory disease that presents a diurnal rhythm of disease activity. An imbalance in favor of proinflamatory hormones like PRL, as opposed to levels of anti-inflammatory hormones, could be responsible for this diurnal rhythm of disease [112]. In both genders, however, associations between RA and PRL have been inconsistent [98, 100, 113-118]. A recent study shows an increase of PRL in serum and synovial fluid from subjects affected with RA perhaps indicating that this cytokine acts as a proinflammatory factor to increase disease severity and joint damage in RA [119]. However, further studies are still needed in this area.

4.1.3. Multiple Sclerosis

Patients with MS, a Th1-dominated autoimmune disease, have slightly, but significantly higher PRL levels than normal subjects, and an association between this biomarker and the course of the disease course should be considered [120]. One-third of MS subjects exhibit hyperprolactinemia, which is claimed to be a sensitive indicator for hypothalamic lesions [97]. In experimental animal models of MS, treatment with bromocriptine decreases both PRL secretion and disease severity [121]. These data support the idea that PRL is involved in the pathogenesis of MS.

4.1.4. Hashimoto thyroiditis

In HT, an endocrine autoimmune disease, hyperprolactinemia and low serum cortisol levels have been found [122]. In addition, the high prevalence of anti-thyroid antibodies in the presence of hyperprolactinemia in HT suggests a role for PRL in this autoimmune disease, particularly since hyperprolactinemia correlates with HT only in subjects with hypothyroidism, suggesting a role of PRL in this autoimmune disease. Furthermore, another association between PRL and endocrine autoimmune diseases has been noted in subjects with a combined deficiency of pituitary hormones (GH; PRL; TSH) due to antibodies against Pit-1 [123].

4.1.5. Prolactin and diabetes

Diabetes mellitus (DM) is a complex disease characterized by hyperglycemia, dyslipidemia and disorders of protein metabolism. High levels of glucose in serum are a consequence of defects in insulin secretion, insulin action, or both. Indeed, DM is classified as type 1 (DM1) with an autoimmune etiology that causes a total absence of insulin secretion, or as type 2 (DM2) caused by a combination of resistance to insulin action and an inadequate compensatory insulin secretion response [124, 125].

Studies in human and murine experimental models have demonstrated a stimulatory effect of PRL and other structurally related hormones (placental lactogen and growth hormone) on both insulin secretion and proliferation of β-cells [126, 127]. Furthermore, studies in PRL receptor-deficient mice highlight the importance of these hormones in pancreatic islet development. PRLR-deficient mice had a 26-42% lower islet-cell density ($P < 0.01$), and beta-cell mass and insulin mRNA levels in pancreatic cells were 20-30% lower compared with wild-type mice [75]. Furthermore, insulin secretion in response to glucose was blunted in PRLR-deficient males in vivo. The precise mechanism by which PRL induces insulin gene transcription is still unclear since PRL binding induces low promoter activation of STAT5b, indicating that other pathways might be involved. The effects of many of the insulin signaling inhibitors occur downstream of PRL signaling pathways; however, the mechanism by which PRL impairs insulin signaling remains to be elucidated [128].

The effects of PRL have been studied in subjects with DM. For example, hyperprolactinemia has been identified in patients with DM1; however, the precise role of PRL in the progression of this disease is unclear. In contrast, PRL is one factor that can modify the clinical course of diabetic retinopathy (DR), one of the main complications of DM2 and a leading cause of blindness in working-age adults. The DR is associated with an excessive retinal vasopermeability and this could be inhibited by intraocular vasoinhibins, a family of peptides derived from proteolysis of PRL. Indeed, in a case-controlled study of diabetic patients, decreased serum PRL levels contributed to the development and progression of DR [129]. Furthermore, in a pharmacologically induced murine model of DM, hyperprolactinemia led to vasoinhibins accumulation within the retina, which reduced retinal vasopermeability induced by the vascular endothelial growth factor (VEGF) or streptozotocin, and this phenomenon is reversed by bromocriptine [130]. Therefore, circulating PRL influences the progression of DR after its intraocular conversion to vasoinhibins [130]. This important observation may provide a novel approach to protect DM subjects against the development of DR [131] , which was recently demonstrated in a murine model using gene therapy [132]. In summary, *in vitro* experiments and *in vivo* studies revealed that vasoinhibins are potent inhibitors of angiogenesis in the retina by several mechanisms, inhibiting proangiogenic effects of VEGF.

5. Effects of prolactin, circadian rhythms, and sleep on immune function

5.1. Background

Circadian rhythms are defined as ~24-h fluctuations in a variety of behavioral, physiological, and metabolic parameters driven by biological pacemakers and oscillators. The rhythmic changes are endogenous, meaning they are independent of environmental clues. At the same time, circadian rhythms are entrained by external inputs that are classified as photic (light–darkness alternation) and non-photic (food availability, pheromones, social interactions). Although they have been described across the entire phylogenetic scale (from prokaryotes to vertebrates), the various mechanisms that underlie circadian rhythms are better understood in mammals. In this group the principal pacemaker is the suprachiasmatic nucleus (SCN), which is a hypothalamic structure situated above the optic chiasm and close to the third ventricle. The SCN is synchronized by means of the conduction of photic stimuli from the melanopsin-enriched ganglionar retinal cells directly to the dorsal section of the SCN. Experiments done *in vitro* with isolated SCN preparations have demonstrated that this oscillator can show 24-h rhythmicity in electrical and metabolic activity for several weeks. The capacity for self-sustained oscillatory activity is based on the cyclic expression of a set of specialized genes and proteins that form the core of the molecular clock. The set of "clock" gene proteins interact in a network of positive and negative feedback loops, ultimately giving the SCN the ability to measure ~24-h time periods. The circadian rhythmicity elicited by the SCN is eventually communicated to other tissues and organs through several output pathways that enable the circadian variations in endocrine patterns, physiological responses, metabolic activities, and behavior [133].

The circadian system is hierarchical; it is formed by the SCN as principal pacemaker, but also includes a set of peripheral oscillators which are dependent on SCN activity to accomplish a coordinated and harmonized overall day-to-day response. These peripheral oscillators are present, not only in thoracic and abdominal organs (heart, lungs, liver, pancreas, and others), but also in cerebral regions different from the SCN (amigdala, hippocampus, other hypothalamic nuclei, etc). Many of these peripheral oscillators are endocrine glands and biological targets for the secreted hormones. The coordination between SCN and peripheral oscillators is lost in some circumstances, such as restricted feeding schedules [134]. It has been proposed that a state of good fitness involves the appropriate coordination between the SCN (as a master pacemaker) and the other oscillators (slave clocks). Hence, a lack of communication among oscillators could promote adverse symptoms such as jet-lag and maladies associated with shift work [135].

Many biological functions are under the command of the circadian system. In the end, the evolutive explanation considers the 24-h rhythmic fluctuations as adaptations that allow biological tasks to be performed at a most appropriate time for the organisms, according to their diurnal or nocturnal profile. Some examples illustrating this concept are: 1) cortisol in humans is secreted a short time before awakening as a response to the fasting condition and in preparation for wakefulness; 2) growth hormone is released during the non-REM stage of sleep; 3) for predators, the search for food occurs when prey are most likely available and is coordinated with the time for rest and sleep.

Sleep is a complex process that is modulated by both circadian and homeostatic regulation. This dual control is evident in situations of sleep deprivation. In this circumstance, the animal will compensate for the lack of sleep regardless of the time of day, and the subject will fall sleep as a function of the amount of previous time awake. Not very much is known about the brain structures and neurotransmitters involved in the coordination and interplay between the circadian and homeostatic control of the sleep activity. The functions that have been attributed to sleep are diverse, but some of the principal ones are: energy restoration, memory processing, and neural plasticity [136].

In mammals and some birds, sleep is divided into 2 principal phases: sleep without rapid eye movement (NREM) and sleep with rapid eye movement (REM). These 2 stages are characterized mainly by polysomnographic criteria: for example, NREM sleep shows brain waves of high amplitude and low frequency and a clear muscular tone. In contrast, during REM sleep the brain waves become desynchronized, have low voltage, and the muscular tone is lost. Interestingly, the muscles that allow the ocular movements are the only ones that can become active. In humans, 75-80% of sleep time is dedicated to NREM and the rest to REM sleep, with the episodes of REM sleep becoming more frequent at the end of the night [137]. Because some characteristics of REM sleep and the wakeful state are similar, REM has been called paradoxical sleep.

Multiple factors have been invoked as having some role in the control of circadian rhythmicity, including the physiological adaptations in the sleeping activity. This section will be focused on the role of PRL in modulating both processes, acting as an endocrine signal and as an immunological mediator.

5.2. Circadian profile of prolactin in physiological and pathological conditions

PRL displays ultradian and circadian variations in humans [138]. On average, PRL is significantly higher at night, with a clear acrophase or peak close to midnight. However, between 6 and 8 peaks of PRL are also observed during the 24-h period, indicating a concurrent ultradian pattern [139]. The amplitude of the PRL diurnal rhythm is reduced during aging [140]. Hypothalamic PRL secretion is highly dependent on the suppression of the inhibitory input of dopamine. In rats, it has been shown that dopamine control of PRL release is modulated by circadian action from the SCN. In experimental animals, circulating PRL was reported to show complex rhythmicity under the regulation of several hypothalamic factors, including that is exerted by the vasoactive intestinal peptide (VIP) secreted by the SCN [141]. Levels of PRL produced by the lactotrophs of the anterior pituitary gland increase in the afternoon, but this PRL peak is abolished when VIP is not released from the SCN, indicating a circadian contribution to the temporal PRL profile. PRL secretion is also regulated by sexual activity, mainly in female rats. Mating promotes the release of oxytocin, which favors PRL synthesis and release. Hence, circadian modulation of blood PRL is coordinated with ultradian events and also with sporadic physiological responses. Most of the genes that show circadian rhythmicity contain a specific response element known as the E-box. However, PRL is an exception, since the circadian fluctuations involve daily chromatin remodeling carried out by the factors NONO (Non-POU domain-containing octamer-binding protein) and SFPQ (splicing factor proline-glutamine rich) [142]. PRL has also been implicated in circannual rhythmicity in rams. In this context, the role of PRL in reproductive physiology, which fluctuates according to the photoperiodic regulation during the year, is dependent mainly on the pineal gland, and it persists after the hypothalamo-pituitary connection is severed [143].

In patients with Parkinson´s disease, the rhythmic pattern of PRL secretion is not altered [139], but schizophrenic patients under treatment with atypical antipsychotic drugs such as perospirone show larger daily fluctuations of PRL [144]. However, loss of PRL rhythmicity during hyperprolactinemia episodes has been associated with obesity. One of the apparent causes of increased adipose tissue reservoirs is inhibition of the lipolytic enzyme lipoprotein lipase by PRL [145]. Hyperprolactinemia also affects daily changes of GABA and taurine concentrations in various hypothalamic areas, with potential consequences for eating and drinking behaviors [146]. Hypersecretion of PRL has been associated with the Carney complex (a syndrome of spotty skin pigmentation, myxomas, endocrine overactivity, and schwannomas), which is a multiple neoplasia condition with various endocrine abnormalities [147]. Elevation of PRL at night has also been associated with the worsening of a pathological condition known as SUNCT (recurrent short-lasting unilateral neuralgiform headache attacks with conjunctival injection and tearing) [148]. High PRL concentrations are involved in the pathogenesis of SLE in human beings and experimental animals by an unknown mechanism [149]. A hypothesis related to the onset of winter depression in women has postulated a defect of neural pathways afferent to the paraventricular nucleus that promote a reduction of serum PRL concentration. In this perspective, winter depression would also under the influence of estrogen responses [150]. Reduced PRL at night has also been associated with women suffering from fibromyalgia, a medical disorder characterized by chronic, widespread pain, and allodynia (pain due to a stimulus which does not normally provoke painful response) [151].

5.3. Prolactin and sleep

PRL concentrations are elevated during sleep, even if sleep is delayed [152], and short periods of sleep deprivation in humans are associated with lower nocturnal PRL levels in comparison to normal sleep [153]. PRL has been shown to be a hypnogenic factor, acting as a promoter of REM sleep: systemic or intracerebroventricular injection of PRL in rats and rabbits increased REM episodes, but in rats, only during the light period [154]. Supporting this observation, it was reported that antiserum against PRL and genetically PRL-deficient rodents showed reduced frequency of REM sleep [155]. It has been suggested that PRL may enhance a REM-promoting mechanism rather than initiate REM episodes. A putative mechanism by which PRL enhances REM sleep is the activation of the mitochondrial enzyme pyruvate dehydrogenase, which catalyzes the synthesis of acetyl-coenzyme A. This metabolic intermediate may favor the generation of acetylcholine in cholinergic terminals of brain areas that are involved in promoting REM sleep [156].

Besides its action in REM episodes, PRL has been postulated to be a modulator of NREM sleep in lactating women [157]. The predominant underlying hormonal alteration occurring in lactation is a marked increase in circulating PRL. Because the PRL concentration is elevated for several months in women that breastfeed, the increase in NREM sleep in this situation has been explained as a result of chronic hyperprolactinemia [158].

5.4. The circadian system and the sleep–wake cycle as modulators of the immune function. Role of prolactin

The immunological network is influenced by the physiological timing organization, but at the same time, the circadian rhythmicity is regulated by factors elicited by the immune system. This reciprocal modulation has been documented in physiological and pathological conditions in humans, and some related molecular and cellular mechanisms have been explored in experimental animals. It has been reported that the number and properties of cellular components of the immune system show circadian variations, for example: 1) IgE-dependent activation by mast cells [159], 2) cell-adhesion molecule expression by human leukocytes [160], 3) activation of natural killer cells [161], 4) deterioration of clinical symptoms associated with rheumatoid arthritis in the morning following the diurnal rhythm of the pro-inflammatory cytokine IL-6 [162].

The timing regulation of the immunological function is also influenced by the numerous changes that occur during the sleep period. Sleep promotes a striking increase in the number of myeloid dendritic cell precursors producing IL-12, which implies an induction of the Th1 responses. In addition, sleep reduces plasmacytoid dendritic cells and T-cell counts without affecting the production of IFNα. Sleep also substantially decreases the number of certain subpopulations of monocytes (CD14 and CD16+), probably reflecting margination of these cells upon a sleep-related drop in catecholamine release [163]. The number of undifferentiated naïve T cells and the production of pro-inflammatory cytokines exhibit peaks during the first hours of sleep, whereas the number of circulating immune cells with immediate effector functions and the anti-inflammatory cytokine activity peak during wakefulness. Sleep also facilitates the extravasation of T-cells and their redistribution to lymph nodes. In general, sleep enhances cytokines (such as IL-12) that promote the interaction between antigen-presenting cells and T-helper cells [164].

It has been postulated that NREM sleep facilitates the transfer of antigenic information from antigen-presenting cells to antigen-specific Th cells; as a consequence, sleep after vaccination has been observed to boost immunological memory [165]. The daily profile of circulating PRL, with elevated levels during the rest periods in mammals, raises the possibility that PRL could be one of the factors involved in the enhanced immunological response associated with sleep. This role could be related in particular to the stage of NREM sleep and its accompanying pro-inflammatory endocrine milieu with the high levels of growth hormone and PRL and low concentrations of glucocorticoids and catecholamine that occur during sleep [165]. This same idea provides a rationale for the chronobiological treatment of RA. In this protocol, a low-dose, chronotherapeutic application of prednisone at night (~03:00 h) has been suggested to improve the benefits and reduce the adverse side-effects of glucocorticoid treatment in patients with RA. The low dose of prednisone during the night is as effective as a higher dose applied during the day. Again, this pharmacological scheme could be favorable because of the conjunction between PRL and other immunological supportive peptides and the proven clinical drugs [166].

6. Conclusion

The multiple actions of PRL and its diverse sites of synthesis evidence the versatility of this hormone/cytokine in the homeostasis of the organism. Besides the well-known actions of PRL on reproduction, it exerts multiple actions unrelated to the reproductive area. In the immune system PRL functions as a survival factor inasmuch as it promotes proliferation and inhibits apoptosis. This important role could help to maintain the appropriate number of immune cells in physiological conditions, and to maintain immune tolerance. Abnormal synthesis and secretion of PRL could lead to the breakdown of balance in the immune system, and consequently, could promote autorreactivity and bursting or aggravation of the clinical condition in autoimmune diseases. A deregulation in the mechanisms that control PRL synthesis could lead to enhanced PRL secretion. Nowadays, available information is limited on the biological significance of posttranslational modifications of the PRL in vivo, such as glycosylation or cleavage, which may exert different biological functions related to the immune function. In agreement with current knowledge, PRL at normal levels could be a permissive molecule, while at abnormal levels it could affect the organism homeostasis. Additional studies of PRL and its regulation, especially in the extrapituitary tissues, are needed in order to understand better the role of PRL in the physiology and pathophysiology of autoimmune diseases.

Author details

Lorenza Díaz, Leticia González, Saúl Lira-Albarrán and Fernando Larrea
Department of Reproductive Biology, Instituto Nacional de Ciencias Médicas y Nutrición Salvador Zubirán. México, D. F. México

Mauricio Díaz-Muñoz and Isabel Méndez*
Department of Cellular and Molecular Neurobiology, Instituto de Neurobiología, Universidad Nacional Autónoma de México (UNAM), Campus UNAM-Juriquilla, Querétaro, México

Acknowledgement

We thank Fernando López-Barrera for his expert technical assistance, and Dr. Dorothy Pless for critically editing the manuscript. Supported by UNAM (grant IB200311-22) and CONACyT (129511).

7. References

[1] Harvey S, Aramburo C, Sanders EJ (2012) Extrapituitary production of anterior pituitary hormones: an overview. Endocrine. 41:19-30.
[2] Ben-Jonathan N, Mershon JL, Allen DL, Steinmetz RW (1996) Extrapituitary prolactin: distribution, regulation, functions, and clinical aspects. Endocr Rev. 17:639-669.
[3] Freeman ME, Kanyicska B, Lerant A, Nagy G (2000) Prolactin: structure, function, and regulation of secretion. Physiol Rev. 80:1523-1631.
[4] Featherstone K, White MR, Davis JRE (2012) The Prolactin Gene: A Paradigm of Tissue Specific Gene Regulation with Complex Temporal Transcription Dynamics. J Neuroendocrinol.
[5] Ben-Jonathan N, LaPensee CR, LaPensee EW (2008) What can we learn from rodents about prolactin in humans? Endocr Rev. 29:1-41.
[6] Gerlo S, Davis JR, Mager DL, Kooijman R (2006) Prolactin in man: a tale of two promoters. Bioessays. 28:1051-1055.
[7] Shaw-Bruha CM, Pirrucello SJ, Shull JD (1997) Expression of the prolactin gene in normal and neoplastic human breast tissues and human mammary cell lines: promoter usage and alternative mRNA splicing. Breast Cancer Res Treat. 44:243-253.

* Corresponding Author

[8] Dagvadorj A, Collins S, Jomain JB, Abdulghani J, Karras J, Zellweger T, et al. (2007) Autocrine prolactin promotes prostate cancer cell growth via Janus kinase-2-signal transducer and activator of transcription-5a/b signaling pathway. Endocrinology. 148:3089-3101.

[9] Bernichtein S, Touraine P, Goffin V (2010) New concepts in prolactin biology. J Endocrinol. 206:1-11.

[10] Montgomery DW (2001) Prolactin production by immune cells. Lupus. 10:665-675.

[11] Gerlo S, Verdood P, Hooghe-Peters EL, Kooijman R (2005) Modulation of prolactin expression in human T lymphocytes by cytokines. J Neuroimmunol. 162:190-193.

[12] Gerlo S, Verdood P, Hooghe-Peters EL, Kooijman R (2005) Multiple, PKA-dependent and PKA-independent, signals are involved in cAMP-induced PRL expression in the eosinophilic cell line Eol-1. Cell Signal. 17:901-909.

[13] Gerlo S, Verdood P, Hooghe-Peters EL, Kooijman R (2006) Multiple cAMP-induced signaling cascades regulate prolactin expression in T cells. Cell Mol Life Sci. 63:92-99.

[14] Gerlo S, Verdood P, Kooijman R (2006) Tumor necrosis factor-alpha activates the extrapituitary PRL promoter in myeloid leukemic cells. J Neuroimmunol. 172:206-210.

[15] Diaz L, Martinez-Reza I, Garcia-Becerra R, Gonzalez L, Larrea F, Mendez I (2011) Calcitriol stimulates prolactin expression in non-activated human peripheral blood mononuclear cells: breaking paradigms. Cytokine. 55:188-194.

[16] Reem GH, Ray DW, Davis JR (1999) The human prolactin gene upstream promoter is regulated in lymphoid cells by activators of T-cells and by cAMP. J Mol Endocrinol. 22:285-292.

[17] Gerlo S, Vanden Berghe W, Verdood P, Hooghe-Peters EL, Kooijman R (2003) Regulation of prolactin expression in leukemic cell lines and peripheral blood mononuclear cells. J Neuroimmunol. 135:107-116.

[18] Blalock JE (2005) The immune system as the sixth sense. J Intern Med. 257:126-138.

[19] McKenna F, McLaughlin PJ, Lewis BJ, Sibbring GC, Cummerson JA, Bowen-Jones D, et al. (2002) Dopamine receptor expression on human T- and B-lymphocytes, monocytes, neutrophils, eosinophils and NK cells: a flow cytometric study. J Neuroimmunol. 132:34-40.

[20] Bondy B, de Jonge S, Pander S, Primbs J, Ackenheil M (1996) Identification of dopamine D4 receptor mRNA in circulating human lymphocytes using nested polymerase chain reaction. J Neuroimmunol. 71:139-144.

[21] Ricci A, Amenta F (1994) Dopamine D5 receptors in human peripheral blood lymphocytes: a radioligand binding study. J Neuroimmunol. 53:1-7.

[22] Watanabe Y, Nakayama T, Nagakubo D, Hieshima K, Jin Z, Katou F, et al. (2006) Dopamine selectively induces migration and homing of naive CD8+ T cells via dopamine receptor D3. J Immunol. 176:848-856.

[23] Saha B, Mondal AC, Basu S, Dasgupta PS (2001) Circulating dopamine level, in lung carcinoma patients, inhibits proliferation and cytotoxicity of CD4+ and CD8+ T cells by D1 dopamine receptors: an in vitro analysis. Int Immunopharmacol. 1:1363-1374.

[24] Ilani T, Strous RD, Fuchs S (2004) Dopaminergic regulation of immune cells via D3 dopamine receptor: a pathway mediated by activated T cells. FASEB J. 18:1600-1602.

[25] Levite M (2012) Dopamine in the Immune System: Dopamine receptors in immune cells, potent effects, endogenous production and involvement in immune and neuropsychiatric diseases. In: Mia L, editor. Nerve-Driven Immunity: Neurotransmitters and Neuropeptides in the Immune System: Springer-Verlag/Wien; pp. 1-46.

[26] Levite M, Chowers Y, Ganor Y, Besser M, Hershkovits R, Cahalon L (2001) Dopamine interacts directly with its D3 and D2 receptors on normal human T cells, and activates beta1 integrin function. Eur J Immunol. 31:3504-3512.

[27] Mendez I, González L., Martínez I., Larrea F. Dopamine Inhibits Prolactin Expression and Enhances DRD2 Expression in Peripheral Mononuclear Cells. The Endocrine Society's 91st Annual Meeting; 2009; Washington, DC., USA.

[28] Delvin EE, Gagnon L, Arabian A, Gibb W (1990) Influence of calcitriol on prolactin and prostaglandin production by human decidua. Mol Cell Endocrinol. 71:177-183.

[29] Pellegrini I, Lebrun JJ, Ali S, Kelly PA (1992) Expression of prolactin and its receptor in human lymphoid cells. Mol Endocrinol. 6:1023-1031.

[30] Haug E, Bjoro T, Gautvik KM (1987) A permissive role for extracellular Ca2+ in regulation of prolactin production by 1,25-dihydroxyvitamin D3 in GH3 pituitary cells. J Steroid Biochem. 28:385-391.

[31] Castillo AI, Jimenez-Lara AM, Tolon RM, Aranda A (1999) Synergistic activation of the prolactin promoter by vitamin D receptor and GHF-1: role of the coactivators, CREB-binding protein and steroid hormone receptor coactivator-1 (SRC-1). Mol Endocrinol. 13:1141-1154.

[32] Tornquist K (1987) Effect of 1,25-dihydroxyvitamin D3 on rat pituitary prolactin release. Acta Endocrinol (Copenh). 116:459-464.

[33] Baeke F, Takiishi T, Korf H, Gysemans C, Mathieu C (2010) Vitamin D: modulator of the immune system. Curr Opin Pharmacol. 10:482-496.

[34] Adorini L, Amuchastegui S, Daniel KC (2005) Prevention of chronic allograft rejection by Vitamin D receptor agonists. Immunol Lett. 100:34-41.

[35] Adorini L, Penna G (2008) Control of autoimmune diseases by the vitamin D endocrine system. Nat Clin Pract Rheumatol. 4:404-412.

[36] Sharma OP (2000) Hypercalcemia in granulomatous disorders: a clinical review. Curr Opin Pulm Med. 6:442-447.

[37] Turkington RW, MacIndoe JH (1972) Hyperprolactinemia in sarcoidosis. Ann Intern Med. 76:545-549.

[38] Hewison M (2010) Vitamin D and the immune system: new perspectives on an old theme. Endocrinol Metab Clin North Am. 39:365-379, table of contents.

[39] Stevens A, Ray DW, Worthington J, Davis JR (2001) Polymorphisms of the human prolactin gene--implications for production of lymphocyte prolactin and systemic lupus erythematosus. Lupus. 10:676-683.

[40] Nagafuchi H, Suzuki N, Kaneko A, Asai T, Sakane T (1999) Prolactin locally produced by synovium infiltrating T lymphocytes induces excessive synovial cell functions in patients with rheumatoid arthritis. J Rheumatol. 26:1890-1900.

[41] Hatfill SJ, Kirby R, Hanley M, Rybicki E, Bohm L (1990) Hyperprolactinemia in acute myeloid leukemia and indication of ectopic expression of human prolactin in blast cells of a patient of subtype M4. Leuk Res. 14:57-62.

[42] Mendez I, Alcocer-Varela J, Parra A, Lava-Zavala A, de la Cruz DA, Alarcon-Segovia D, et al. (2004) Neuroendocrine dopaminergic regulation of prolactin release in systemic lupus erythematosus: a possible role of lymphocyte-derived prolactin. Lupus. 13:45-53.

[43] Aringer M, Smolen JS (2004) Tumour necrosis factor and other proinflammatory cytokines in systemic lupus erythematosus: a rationale for therapeutic intervention. Lupus. 13:344-347.

[44] Larrea F, Martinez-Castillo A, Cabrera V, Alcocer-Varela J, Queipo G, Carino C, et al. (1997) A bioactive 60-kilodalton prolactin species is preferentially secreted in cultures of mitogen-stimulated and nonstimulated peripheral blood mononuclear cells from subjects with systemic lupus erythematosus. J Clin Endocrinol Metab. 82:3664-3669.

[45] Jara LJ, Gomez-Sanchez C, Silveira LH, Martinez-Osuna P, Vasey FB, Espinoza LR (1992) Hyperprolactinemia in systemic lupus erythematosus: association with disease activity. Am J Med Sci. 303:222-226.

[46] Ben-Jonathan N, Munsick RA (1980) Dopamine and prolactin in human pregnancy. J Clin Endocrinol Metab. 51:1019-1025.

[47] Telgmann R, Maronde E, Tasken K, Gellersen B (1997) Activated protein kinase A is required for differentiation-dependent transcription of the decidual prolactin gene in human endometrial stromal cells. Endocrinology. 138:929-937.

[48] Pohnke Y, Kempf R, Gellersen B (1999) CCAAT/enhancer-binding proteins are mediators in the protein kinase A-dependent activation of the decidual prolactin promoter. J Biol Chem. 274:24808-24818.

[49] Brosens JJ, Hayashi N, White JO (1999) Progesterone receptor regulates decidual prolactin expression in differentiating human endometrial stromal cells. Endocrinology. 140:4809-4820.

[50] Maslar IA, Ansbacher R (1986) Effects of progesterone on decidual prolactin production by organ cultures of human endometrium. Endocrinology. 118:2102-2108.

[51] Gellersen B, Brosens J (2003) Cyclic AMP and progesterone receptor cross-talk in human endometrium: a decidualizing affair. J Endocrinol. 178:357-372.

[52] Frank GR, Brar AK, Cedars MI, Handwerger S (1994) Prostaglandin E2 enhances human endometrial stromal cell differentiation. Endocrinology. 134:258-263.

[53] Ferrari A, Petraglia F, Gurpide E (1995) Corticotropin releasing factor decidualizes human endometrial stromal cells in vitro. Interaction with progestin. J Steroid Biochem Mol Biol. 54:251-255.

[54] Nemansky M, Moy E, Lyons CD, Yu I, Blithe DL (1998) Human endometrial stromal cells generate uncombined alpha-subunit from human chorionic gonadotropin, which

can synergize with progesterone to induce decidualization. J Clin Endocrinol Metab. 83:575-581.

[55] Telgmann R, Gellersen B (1998) Marker genes of decidualization: activation of the decidual prolactin gene. Hum Reprod Update. 4:472-479.

[56] Gellersen B, Bonhoff A, Hunt N, Bohnet HG (1991) Decidual-type prolactin expression by the human myometrium. Endocrinology. 129:158-168.

[57] Thrailkill KM, Golander A, Underwood LE, Handwerger S (1988) Insulin-like growth factor I stimulates the synthesis and release of prolactin from human decidual cells. Endocrinology. 123:2930-2934.

[58] Thrailkill KM, Golander A, Underwood LE, Richards RG, Handwerger S (1989) Insulin stimulates the synthesis and release of prolactin from human decidual cells. Endocrinology. 124:3010-3014.

[59] Jikihara H, Handwerger S (1994) Tumor necrosis factor-alpha inhibits the synthesis and release of human decidual prolactin. Endocrinology. 134:353-357.

[60] Kane NM, Jones M, Brosens JJ, Kelly RW, Saunders PT, Critchley HO (2010) TGFbeta1 attenuates expression of prolactin and IGFBP-1 in decidualized endometrial stromal cells by both SMAD-dependent and SMAD-independent pathways. PLoS One. 5:e12970.

[61] Diaz L, Noyola-Martinez N, Barrera D, Hernandez G, Avila E, Halhali A, et al. (2009) Calcitriol inhibits TNF-alpha-induced inflammatory cytokines in human trophoblasts. J Reprod Immunol. 81:17-24.

[62] Evans KN, Nguyen L, Chan J, Innes BA, Bulmer JN, Kilby MD, et al. (2006) Effects of 25-hydroxyvitamin D3 and 1,25-dihydroxyvitamin D3 on cytokine production by human decidual cells. Biol Reprod. 75:816-822.

[63] Bonhoff A, Gellersen B (1994) Modulation of prolactin secretion in human myometrium by cytokines. Eur J Obstet Gynecol Reprod Biol. 54:55-62.

[64] Lynch VJ, Brayer K, Gellersen B, Wagner GP (2009) HoxA-11 and FOXO1A cooperate to regulate decidual prolactin expression: towards inferring the core transcriptional regulators of decidual genes. PLoS One. 4:e6845.

[65] Kurtz A, Bristol LA, Toth BE, Lazar-Wesley E, Takacs L, Kacsoh B (1993) Mammary epithelial cells of lactating rats express prolactin messenger ribonucleic acid. Biol Reprod. 48:1095-1103.

[66] Ellis LA, Picciano MF (1995) Bioactive and immunoreactive prolactin variants in human milk. Endocrinology. 136:2711-2720.

[67] Baldocchi RA, Tan L, Nicoll CS (1992) Processing of rat prolactin by rat tissue explants and serum in vitro. Endocrinology. 130:1653-1659.

[68] Gil-Puig C, Seoane S, Blanco M, Macia M, Garcia-Caballero T, Segura C, et al. (2005) Pit-1 is expressed in normal and tumorous human breast and regulates GH secretion and cell proliferation. Eur J Endocrinol. 153:335-344.

[69] Ben-Batalla I, Seoane S, Macia M, Garcia-Caballero T, Gonzalez LO, Vizoso F, et al. (2010) The Pit-1/Pou1f1 transcription factor regulates and correlates with prolactin expression in human breast cell lines and tumors. Endocr Relat Cancer. 17:73-85.

[70] Duan R, Ginsburg E, Vonderhaar BK (2008) Estrogen stimulates transcription from the human prolactin distal promoter through AP1 and estrogen responsive elements in T47D human breast cancer cells. Mol Cell Endocrinol. 281:9-18.

[71] Zinger M, McFarland M, Ben-Jonathan N (2003) Prolactin expression and secretion by human breast glandular and adipose tissue explants. J Clin Endocrinol Metab. 88:689-696.

[72] Hugo ER, Borcherding DC, Gersin KS, Loftus J, Ben-Jonathan N (2008) Prolactin release by adipose explants, primary adipocytes, and LS14 adipocytes. J Clin Endocrinol Metab. 93:4006-4012.

[73] Borcherding DC, Hugo ER, Idelman G, De Silva A, Richtand NW, Loftus J, et al. (2011) Dopamine receptors in human adipocytes: expression and functions. PLoS One. 6:e25537.

[74] McFarland-Mancini M, Hugo E, Loftus J, Ben-Jonathan N (2006) Induction of prolactin expression and release in human preadipocytes by cAMP activating ligands. Biochem Biophys Res Commun. 344:9-16.

[75] Freemark M, Avril I, Fleenor D, Driscoll P, Petro A, Opara E, et al. (2002) Targeted deletion of the PRL receptor: effects on islet development, insulin production, and glucose tolerance. Endocrinology. 143:1378-1385.

[76] Bole-Feysot C, Goffin V, Edery M, Binart N, Kelly PA (1998) Prolactin (PRL) and its receptor: actions, signal transduction pathways and phenotypes observed in PRL receptor knockout mice. Endocr Rev. 19:225-268.

[77] Thomas LN, Morehouse TJ, Too CKL (2012) Testosterone and prolactin increase carboxypeptidase-D and nitric oxide levels to promote survival of prostate cancer cells. The Prostate. 72:450-460.

[78] Terra LF, Garay-Malpartida MH, Wailemann RA, Sogayar MC, Labriola L (2011) Recombinant human prolactin promotes human beta cell survival via inhibition of extrinsic and intrinsic apoptosis pathways. Diabetologia. 54:1388-1397.

[79] LaVoie HA, Witorsch RJ (1995) Investigation of intracellular signals mediating the anti-apoptotic action of prolactin in Nb2 lymphoma cells. Proc Soc Exp Biol Med. 209:257-269.

[80] Asai-Sato M, Nagashima Y, Miyagi E, Sato K, Ohta I, Vonderhaar BK, et al. (2005) Prolactin inhibits apoptosis of ovarian carcinoma cells induced by serum starvation or cisplatin treatment. Int J Cancer. 115:539-544.

[81] Perks CM, Keith AJ, Goodhew KL, Savage PB, Winters ZE, Holly JM (2004) Prolactin acts as a potent survival factor for human breast cancer cell lines. Br J Cancer. 91:305-311.

[82] Berczi I, Nagy E, de Toledo SM, Matusik RJ, Friesen HG (1991) Pituitary hormones regulate c-myc and DNA synthesis in lymphoid tissue. J Immunol. 146:2201-2206.

[83] Nagy E, Berczi I (1989) Pituitary dependence of bone marrow function. Br J Haematol. 71:457-462.
[84] Berczi I, Nagy E, Kovacs K, Horvath E (1981) Regulation of humoral immunity in rats by pituitary hormones. Acta Endocrinol (Copenh). 98:506-513.
[85] Xu D, Lin L, Lin X, Huang Z, Lei Z (2010) Immunoregulation of autocrine prolactin: suppressing the expression of costimulatory molecules and cytokines in T lymphocytes by prolactin receptor knockdown. Cell Immunol. 263:71-78.
[86] Matera L, Cutufia M, Geuna M, Contarini M, Buttiglieri S, Galin S, et al. (1997) Prolactin is an autocrine growth factor for the Jurkat human T-leukemic cell line. J Neuroimmunol. 79:12-21.
[87] Buckley AR (2001) Prolactin, a lymphocyte growth and survival factor. Lupus. 10:684-690.
[88] Tanaka T, Shiu RP, Gout PW, Beer CT, Noble RL, Friesen HG (1980) A new sensitive and specific bioassay for lactogenic hormones: measurement of prolactin and growth hormone in human serum. J Clin Endocrinol Metab. 51:1058-1063.
[89] Kochendoerfer SK, Krishnan N, Buckley DJ, Buckley AR (2003) Prolactin regulation of Bcl-2 family members: increased expression of bcl-xL but not mcl-1 or bad in Nb2-T cells. J Endocrinol. 178:265-273.
[90] Krishnan N, Thellin O, Buckley DJ, Horseman ND, Buckley AR (2003) Prolactin suppresses glucocorticoid-induced thymocyte apoptosis in vivo. Endocrinology. 144:2102-2110.
[91] Saha S, Gonzalez J, Rosenfeld G, Keiser H, Peeva E (2009) Prolactin alters the mechanisms of B cell tolerance induction. Arthritis Rheum. 60:1743-1752.
[92] Dorshkind K, Horseman ND (2000) The roles of prolactin, growth hormone, insulin-like growth factor-I, and thyroid hormones in lymphocyte development and function: insights from genetic models of hormone and hormone receptor deficiency. Endocr Rev. 21:292-312.
[93] De Bellis A, Bizzarro A, Pivonello R, Lombardi G, Bellastella A (2005) Prolactin and autoimmunity. Pituitary. 8:25-30.
[94] Peeva E, Venkatesh J, Michael D, Diamond B (2004) Prolactin as a modulator of B cell function: implications for SLE. Biomed Pharmacother. 58:310-319.
[95] Da Costa R, Szyper-Kravitz M, Szekanecz Z, Csepany T, Danko K, Shapira Y, et al. (2011) Ferritin and prolactin levels in multiple sclerosis. Isr Med Assoc J. 13:91-95.
[96] El-Garf A, Salah S, Shaarawy M, Zaki S, Anwer S (1996) Prolactin hormone in juvenile systemic lupus erythematosus: a possible relationship to disease activity and CNS manifestations. J Rheumatol. 23:374-377.
[97] Kira J, Harada M, Yamaguchi Y, Shida N, Goto I (1991) Hyperprolactinemia in multiple sclerosis. J Neurol Sci. 102:61-66.
[98] Neidhart M, Gay RE, Gay S (1999) Prolactin and prolactin-like polypeptides in rheumatoid arthritis. Biomed Pharmacother. 53:218-222.

[99] Shoenfeld Y, Tincani A, Gershwin ME (2012) Sex gender and autoimmunity. J Autoimmun.

[100] Chikanza IC, Petrou P, Chrousos G, Kingsley G, Panayi GS (1993) Excessive and dysregulated secretion of prolactin in rheumatoid arthritis: immunopathogenetic and therapeutic implications. Br J Rheumatol. 32:445-448.

[101] Li M, Keiser HD, Peeva E (2006) Prolactinoma and systemic lupus erythematosus: do serum prolactin levels matter? Clin Rheumatol. 25:602-605.

[102] Leanos-Miranda A, Cardenas-Mondragon G (2006) Serum free prolactin concentrations in patients with systemic lupus erythematosus are associated with lupus activity. Rheumatology (Oxford). 45:97-101.

[103] Orbach H, Shoenfeld Y (2007) Hyperprolactinemia and autoimmune diseases. Autoimmun Rev. 6:537-542.

[104] Biller BM, Luciano A, Crosignani PG, Molitch M, Olive D, Rebar R, et al. (1999) Guidelines for the diagnosis and treatment of hyperprolactinemia. J Reprod Med. 44:1075-1084.

[105] Miyai K, Ichihara K, Kondo K, Mori S (1986) Asymptomatic hyperprolactinaemia and prolactinoma in the general population--mass screening by paired assays of serum prolactin. Clin Endocrinol (Oxf). 25:549-554.

[106] Buskila D, Lorber M, Neumann L, Flusser D, Shoenfeld Y (1996) No correlation between prolactin levels and clinical activity in patients with systemic lupus erythematosus. J Rheumatol. 23:629-632.

[107] McMurray RW (2001) Prolactin in murine systemic lupus erythematosus. Lupus. 10:742-747.

[108] Blank M, Krause I, Buskila D, Teitelbaum D, Kopolovic J, Afek A, et al. (1995) Bromocriptine immunomodulation of experimental SLE and primary antiphospholipid syndrome via induction of nonspecific T suppressor cells. Cell Immunol. 162:114-122.

[109] Elbourne KB, Keisler D, McMurray RW (1998) Differential effects of estrogen and prolactin on autoimmune disease in the NZB/NZW F1 mouse model of systemic lupus erythematosus. Lupus. 7:420-427.

[110] McMurray RW, Weidensaul D, Allen SH, Walker SE (1995) Efficacy of bromocriptine in an open label therapeutic trial for systemic lupus erythematosus. J Rheumatol. 22:2084-2091.

[111] Jara LJ, Cruz-Cruz P, Saavedra MA, Medina G, Garcia-Flores A, Angeles U, et al. (2007) Bromocriptine during pregnancy in systemic lupus erythematosus: a pilot clinical trial. Ann N Y Acad Sci. 1110:297-304.

[112] Zoli A, Lizzio MM, Ferlisi EM, Massafra V, Mirone L, Barini A, et al. (2002) ACTH, cortisol and prolactin in active rheumatoid arthritis. Clin Rheumatol. 21:289-293.

[113] Fojtikova M, Tomasova Studynkova J, Filkova M, Lacinova Z, Gatterova J, Pavelka K, et al. Elevated prolactin levels in patients with rheumatoid arthritis: association with disease activity and structural damage. Clin Exp Rheumatol. 28:849-854.

[114] Brennan P, Ollier B, Worthington J, Hajeer A, Silman A (1996) Are both genetic and reproductive associations with rheumatoid arthritis linked to prolactin? Lancet. 348:106-109.

[115] Folomeev M, Nasonov EL, Prokaeva TV, Masenko VP, Ovtrakht NV (1990) [The serum prolactin levels of men with systemic lupus erythematosus and rheumatoid arthritis]. Ter Arkh. 62:62-63.

[116] Mateo L, Nolla JM, Bonnin MR, Navarro MA, Roig-Escofet D (1998) High serum prolactin levels in men with rheumatoid arthritis. J Rheumatol. 25:2077-2082.

[117] Nagy E, Chalmers IM, Baragar FD, Friesen HG, Berczi I (1991) Prolactin deficiency in rheumatoid arthritis. J Rheumatol. 18:1662-1668.

[118] Zoli A, Ferlisi EM, Lizzio M, Altomonte L, Mirone L, Barini A, et al. (2002) Prolactin/cortisol ratio in rheumatoid arthritis. Ann N Y Acad Sci. 966:508-512.

[119] Fojtikova M, Tomasova Studynkova J, Filkova M, Lacinova Z, Gatterova J, Pavelka K, et al. (2010) Elevated prolactin levels in patients with rheumatoid arthritis: association with disease activity and structural damage. Clin Exp Rheumatol. 28:849-854.

[120] Da Costa R, Szyper-Kravitz M, Szekanecz Z, Csepany T, Danko K, Shapira Y, et al. Ferritin and prolactin levels in multiple sclerosis. Isr Med Assoc J. 13:91-95.

[121] Riskind PN, Massacesi L, Doolittle TH, Hauser SL (1991) The role of prolactin in autoimmune demyelination: suppression of experimental allergic encephalomyelitis by bromocriptine. Ann Neurol. 29:542-547.

[122] Legakis I, Petroyianni V, Saramantis A, Tolis G (2001) Elevated prolactin to cortisol ratio and polyclonal autoimmune activation in Hashimoto's thyroiditis. Horm Metab Res. 33:585-589.

[123] Yamamoto M, Iguchi G, Takeno R, Okimura Y, Sano T, Takahashi M, et al. Adult combined GH, prolactin, and TSH deficiency associated with circulating PIT-1 antibody in humans. J Clin Invest. 121:113-119.

[124] Knip M, Siljander H (2008) Autoimmune mechanisms in type 1 diabetes. Autoimmun Rev. 7:550-557.

[125] Wellen KE, Hotamisligil GS (2005) Inflammation, stress, and diabetes. J Clin Invest. 115:1111-1119.

[126] Brelje TC, Scharp DW, Lacy PE, Ogren L, Talamantes F, Robertson M, et al. (1993) Effect of homologous placental lactogens, prolactins, and growth hormones on islet B-cell division and insulin secretion in rat, mouse, and human islets: implication for placental lactogen regulation of islet function during pregnancy. Endocrinology. 132:879-887.

[127] Stout LE, Svensson AM, Sorenson RL (1997) Prolactin regulation of islet-derived INS-1 cells: characteristics and immunocytochemical analysis of STAT5 translocation. Endocrinology. 138:1592-1603.

[128] Cejkova P, Fojtikova M, Cerna M (2009) Immunomodulatory role of prolactin in diabetes development. Autoimmun Rev. 9:23-27.

[129] Triebel J, Huefner M, Ramadori G (2009) Investigation of prolactin-related vasoinhibin in sera from patients with diabetic retinopathy. Eur J Endocrinol. 161:345-353.

[130] Arnold E, Rivera JC, Thebault S, Moreno-Paramo D, Quiroz-Mercado H, Quintanar-Stephano A, et al. (2010) High levels of serum prolactin protect against diabetic retinopathy by increasing ocular vasoinhibins. Diabetes. 59:3192-3197.

[131] Triebel J, Macotela Y, de la Escalera GM, Clapp C (2011) Prolactin and vasoinhibins: Endogenous players in diabetic retinopathy. IUBMB Life. 63:806-810.

[132] Ramirez M, Wu Z, Moreno-Carranza B, Jeziorski MC, Arnold E, Diaz-Lezama N, et al. Vasoinhibin gene transfer by adenoassociated virus type 2 protects against VEGF- and diabetes-induced retinal vasopermeability. Invest Ophthalmol Vis Sci. 52:8944-8950.

[133] Koukkari WL, Sothern RB (2006) Introducing biological rhythms: a primer of the temporal organization of life, with implications for health, society, reproduction and the natural environment. New York: Springer. 655 p.

[134] Aguilar-Roblero R, DÍaz-Muñoz M (2010) Chronostatic adaptations in the liver to restricted feeding: The FEO as an emergent oscillator. Sleep and Biological Rhythms. 8:9-17.

[135] Ko CH, Takahashi JS (2006) Molecular components of the mammalian circadian clock. Hum Mol Genet. 15 Spec No 2:R271-277.

[136] Saper CB, Fuller PM, Pedersen NP, Lu J, Scammell TE (2010) Sleep state switching. Neuron. 68:1023-1042.

[137] Biddle C, Oaster TR (1990) The nature of sleep. AANA J. 58:36-44.

[138] Van Cauter E (1990) Diurnal and ultradian rhythms in human endocrine function: a minireview. Horm Res. 34:45-53.

[139] Aziz NA, Pijl H, Frolich M, Roelfsema F, Roos RA (2011) Diurnal secretion profiles of growth hormone, thyrotrophin and prolactin in Parkinson's disease. J Neuroendocrinol. 23:519-524.

[140] Magri F, Locatelli M, Balza G, Molla G, Cuzzoni G, Fioravanti M, et al. (1997) Changes in endocrine circadian rhythms as markers of physiological and pathological brain aging. Chronobiol Int. 14:385-396.

[141] Egli M, Bertram R, Sellix MT, Freeman ME (2004) Rhythmic secretion of prolactin in rats: action of oxytocin coordinated by vasoactive intestinal polypeptide of suprachiasmatic nucleus origin. Endocrinology. 145:3386-3394.

[142] Guillaumond F, Boyer B, Becquet D, Guillen S, Kuhn L, Garin J, et al. (2011) Chromatin remodeling as a mechanism for circadian prolactin transcription: rhythmic NONO and SFPQ recruitment to HLTF. FASEB J. 25:2740-2756.

[143] Lincoln GA, Clarke IJ, Hut RA, Hazlerigg DG (2006) Characterizing a mammalian circannual pacemaker. Science. 314:1941-1944.

[144] Yasui-Furukori N, Furukori H, Sugawara N, Tsuchimine S, Fujii A, Inoue Y, et al. (2010) Prolactin fluctuation over the course of a day during treatments with three atypical antipsychotics in schizophrenic patients. Hum Psychopharmacol. 25:236-242.

[145] Mingrone G, Manco M, Iaconelli A, Gniuli D, Bracaglia R, Leccesi L, et al. (2008) Prolactin and insulin ultradian secretion and adipose tissue lipoprotein lipase expression in severely obese women after bariatric surgery. Obesity (Silver Spring). 16:1831-1837.

[146] Duvilanski BH, Alvarez MP, Castrillon PO, Cano P, Esquifino AI (2003) Daily changes of GABA and taurine concentrations in various hypothalamic areas are affected by chronic hyperprolactinemia. Chronobiol Int. 20:271-284.

[147] Raff SB, Carney JA, Krugman D, Doppman JL, Stratakis CA (2000) Prolactin secretion abnormalities in patients with the "syndrome of spotty skin pigmentation, myxomas, endocrine overactivity and schwannomas" (Carney complex). J Pediatr Endocrinol Metab. 13:373-379.

[148] Bosco D, Labate A, Mungari P, Vero S, Fava A (2007) SUNCT and high nocturnal prolactin levels: some new unusual characteristics. J Headache Pain. 8:114-118.

[149] Jara LJ, Vera-Lastra O, Miranda JM, Alcala M, Alvarez-Nemegyei J (2001) Prolactin in human systemic lupus erythematosus. Lupus. 10:748-756.

[150] Partonen T (1994) Prolactin in winter depression. Med Hypotheses. 43:163-164.

[151] Landis CA, Lentz MJ, Rothermel J, Riffle SC, Chapman D, Buchwald D, et al. (2001) Decreased nocturnal levels of prolactin and growth hormone in women with fibromyalgia. J Clin Endocrinol Metab. 86:1672-1678.

[152] Van Cauter E, Spiegel K (1997) Hormones and metabolism during sleep. In: Schwartz W, editor. Sleep science: integrating basic research and clinical practice. Basel: Karger; pp. 144-174.

[153] Sgoifo A, Buwalda B, Roos M, Costoli T, Merati G, Meerlo P (2006) Effects of sleep deprivation on cardiac autonomic and pituitary-adrenocortical stress reactivity in rats. Psychoneuroendocrinology. 31:197-208.

[154] Roky R, Obal F, Jr., Valatx JL, Bredow S, Fang J, Pagano LP, et al. (1995) Prolactin and rapid eye movement sleep regulation. Sleep. 18:536-542.

[155] Obal F, Jr., Garcia-Garcia F, Kacsoh B, Taishi P, Bohnet S, Horseman ND, et al. (2005) Rapid eye movement sleep is reduced in prolactin-deficient mice. J Neurosci. 25:10282-10289.

[156] Jouvet M (1994) Paradoxical sleep mechanisms. Sleep. 17:S77-83.

[157] Blyton DM, Sullivan CE, Edwards N (2002) Lactation is associated with an increase in slow-wave sleep in women. J Sleep Res. 11:297-303.

[158] Frieboes RM, Murck H, Stalla GK, Antonijevic IA, Steiger A (1998) Enhanced slow wave sleep in patients with prolactinoma. J Clin Endocrinol Metab. 83:2706-2710.

[159] Wang X, Reece SP, Van Scott MR, Brown JM (2011) A circadian clock in murine bone marrow-derived mast cells modulates IgE-dependent activation in vitro. Brain Behav Immun. 25:127-134.

[160] Niehaus GD, Ervin E, Patel A, Khanna K, Vanek VW, Fagan DL (2002) Circadian variation in cell-adhesion molecule expression by normal human leukocytes. Can J Physiol Pharmacol. 80:935-940.

[161] Masera RG, Carignola R, Sartori ML, Staurenghi AH, Angeli A (1999) Circadian abnormalities of natural killer cell activity in rheumatoid arthritis. Ann N Y Acad Sci. 876:88-90.

[162] Sierakowski S, Cutolo M (2011) Morning symptoms in rheumatoid arthritis: a defining characteristic and marker of active disease. Scand J Rheumatol Suppl. 125:1-5.

[163] Dimitrov S, Lange T, Nohroudi K, Born J (2007) Number and function of circulating human antigen presenting cells regulated by sleep. Sleep. 30:401-411.

[164] Besedovsky L, Lange T, Born J (2012) Sleep and immune function. Pflugers Arch. 463:121-137.

[165] Lange T, Dimitrov S, Bollinger T, Diekelmann S, Born J (2011) Sleep after vaccination boosts immunological memory. J Immunol. 187:283-290.

[166] Cutolo M (2012) Chronobiology and the treatment of rheumatoid arthritis. Curr Opin Rheumatol. 24:312-318.

Chapter 5

Neuregulin-1 (Nrg1): An Emerging Regulator of Prolactin (PRL) Secretion

Weijiang Zhao

Additional information is available at the end of the chapter

http://dx.doi.org/10.5772/54716

1. Introduction

1.1. Definition and structure of Neuregulin-1 (Nrg1)

Hypothalamus-derived dopamine and thyrotrophin-releasing hormone (TRH) have long been considered the main sources of prolactin (PRL) regulators in the anterior pituitary, whereas other substances also modulate PRL expression and secretion (Borrelli et al., 1992; Cai et al., 1999; Spuch et al., 2006). Recently, Vlotides for the first time observed that recombinant Nrg1 can control PRL secretion from rat RPL and growth hormone (GH) secreting lactosomatotroph GH3 cells, suggesting the emerging role of Nrg1 as a PRL regulator (Vlotides et al., 2009).

Neuregulins are homologous to epidermal growth factor (EGF) and are mainly encoded by four alternatively spliced genes: NRG-1 to -4 (Orr-Urtreger et al., 1993). Diverse splicing of the NRG-1 gene gives rise to at least six main types of Nrg1 (types I–VI) with ectodomain variation, whereas type I to III Nrg1. are the most intensively investigated. All types of Nrg1 contain an EGF-like domain, which can be classified as either α or β (Jacobsen et al., 1996; Rosnack et al., 1994). Distinct from soluble Nrg1, a membrane-tethered Nrg1 precursor has been identified that contains a transmembrane (TM) domain and an intracellular domain (ICD). The ICD can be further characterized as ICD a, b and c. The structure that links the ectodomain and the transmembrane (TM) domain is called a stalk (S), which can be further classified as S1, S2 and S4. Proteolysis of the Nrg1 precursor, a tightly regulated process, releases the soluble domains and leads to formation of autocrine/paracrine loops. However, recruitment of S3, which contains the stop codon, terminates the extension of the ectodomain into the cytoplasm and thus leads to the formation of non-membrane anchored Nrg1α/β **(See Fig 1)**.

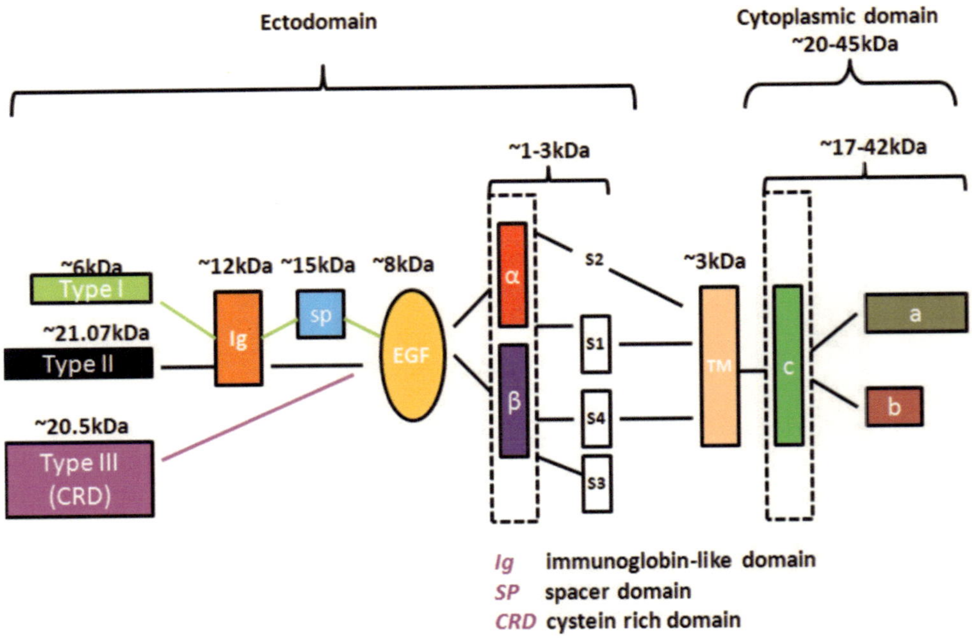

Figure 1. Schematic of type I- III Nrg1 Diverse splicing of NRG-1 gene gives rise to Type I-III Nrg1s, whose structures were schematically diagrammed. α, EGF-like domain α; β, EGF-like domain β; Ig, Ig-like domain; s, stalk domain; sp, spacer domain.

1.2. Interaction of Nrg1 with its cognate receptors and related biological functions

The bioactivity of Nrg1 is mainly mediated by homodimers comprised of their cognate receptors ErbB4 (Hahn et al., 2006) or ErbB3/ErbB2 and ErbB4/ErbB2 heterodimeric complexes (Liu et al., 2002) (See Fig 2). Nrg1 was found to specifically activate the tyrosine kinase receptor ErbB2 as a growth factor extracted from the conditioned medium of a human breast tumor cell line (Holmes et al., 1992). It exerts mitogenic activity on cultured Schwann cells as type II Nrg1 (Glial growth factor, GGF) purified from the brain and bovine pituitary anterior lobe (Lemake et al., 1984). The acetylcholine receptor-inducing activity protein (ARIA), another Nrg1 type, was shown to promote acetylcholine receptor synthesis in cultured skeletal muscle and myotubes (Jessell et al., 1979; Usdin et al., 1986). The ligand-receptor interaction initiates a complex intracellular signaling cascade in which extracellular signal-regulated kinase (ERK), serine/threonine protein kinase (AKT), mitogen-activated protein kinase (MAPK), phosphatidyl-inositol 3-kinase γ (PIK3γ), protein kinase C (PKC), and Janus kinase-signal transducers and activators of transcription (Jak-STAT) are activated. Activation of this signaling pathway leads to, among other events, tumorigenic development, cell cycle arrest, cell proliferation, differentiation, and anti-apoptotic processes (Peles et al., 1993; Liu and Kern et al., 2002; Puricelli et al., 2002). Recently, Nrgβ1 has been reported to signal mitogenesis of cortical astrocytes through ErbB1/ErbB3 heterodimeric complex (Sharif et al., 2009).

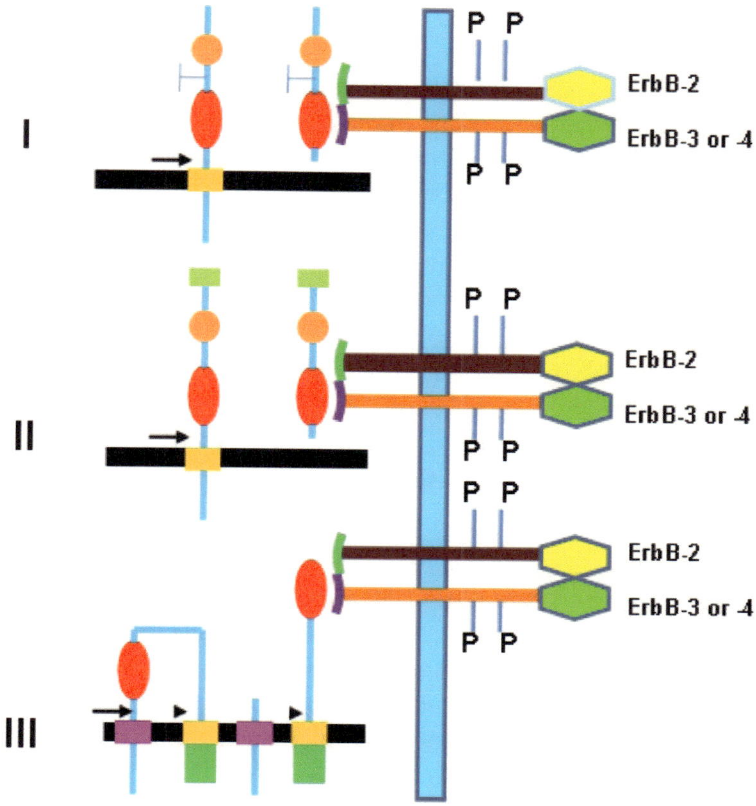

Figure 2. Schematic of type I- III Nrg1 interaction with their receptors. The initial proteolysis site was indicated by the arrow, and the site for second proteolysis was indicated by the arrow head.

2. Endogenous expression of Nrg1 in the anterior pituitary and rat lactosomatotroph GH3 cells

2.1. Expression and localization of Nrg1 and its receptor in the anterior pituitary of rat and non-human primates

The Nrg1-ErbB signaling pathway has a critical role in organ development, cell differentiation and tumorigenesis. Neuregulins have previously been described in the nervous system, especially in the cortex, spinal cord and hypothalamus. In the hypothalamus, ARIA (or Nrg1α and β) was expressed in neurons with processes projecting to the posterior pituitary gland but not in those without these projections, suggesting that hypothalamus-derived Neuregulin regulates certain functions of the pituitary (Bernstein et al., 2006; Corfas et al., 1995). Furthermore, Nrg1 receptors were reported to be expressed in hypothalamic astrocytes, where their activation as a result of paracrine Nrg1 stimulation is essential for stimulating secretion of luteinising hormone-releasing hormone (LHRH), intrapituitary gonadotrophin secretion and normal sexual puberty (Bernstein et al., 2006; Prevot et al., 2003).

Neuregulin has also been reported to be expressed in the endocrine organs, including the adrenal gland and the adult pancreas (Harari et al., 1999; Orr-Urtreger et al., 1993). Additionally, thyroid-derived cell lines and corresponding papillary carcinomas also express Nrg1 and ErbB receptors ErbB2 and ErbB4 (Fluge et al., 2000; Mincione et al., 1998). By contrast, Nrg1 expression and localization, as well as its role in the adenohypophyseal structure, have not been fully defined for a long time. Recently, exogenous Nrg1 has been reported to modulate PRL mRNA expression and PRL secretion from the rat lactosomatotroph GH3 cells, where the ErbB3 receptor was shown to correlate with malignant transformation of prolactinomas (Vlotides et al., 2009). Thus, it is essential to elucidate (i) whether the anterior pituitary gland endogenously expresses Nrg1, (ii) whether intrahypophyseal Nrg1/ErbB receptor can regulate PRL secretion and (iii) its relevance to the development of prolactinoma.

2.1.1. Multiple Nrg1 isoforms are expressed in the anterior pituitary and GH3 cells

Based on a domain RT-PCR method systematically used by Cote et al. (2005), multiple isoforms of Nrg1 were amplified. In our work, we first amplified a 392-bp band from the rat cortex and anterior pituitary cDNA, corresponding to the spacer domain (SP)-containing Ig-EGFα segment in type I Nrg1 **(Fig 3A)**. When primers spanning the Ig-like domain and the EGFβ domain were used, a band at 401 bp was amplified from the cortex, hypothalamus and anterior pituitary cDNA, representing type I Nrg1β. A 299-bp band was amplified from the cortex and hypothalamus, but not from the anterior pituitary cDNA, which represents the SP free Ig- EGFβ segment exclusively contained in type II Nrg1 **(Fig 3B)**. With primers specific to both the Ig domain and S1, S3 or S4, we found that S1 and S3 are present in type I Nrg1 in rat cortex, hypothalamus and anterior pituitary **(Fig 3C-E)**. When primers against the CRD-EGFα domain was employed, an 833-bp band was weakly amplified from the cortical cDNA and strongly amplified from the anterior pituitary and GH3 cells **(Fig 3G)**. Using primers against the CRD-EGFβ domain, an 842-bp band was amplified in all tested samples **(Fig 3H)**. With primers specific to CRD and S1, S3 or S4, we found that S1 and S3 are present in both forms of type III Nrg1 in rat cortex, hypothalamus, anterior pituitary and GH3 cells **(Fig 3I, J)**, whereas S4 was present in rat cortex and undetectable in the other samples tested **(Fig 1K)**. GAPDH signals were equal in each group, suggesting the equal loading of samples **(Fig 3F)**. To confirm the expression of membrane-anchored Nrg1, transmembrane segments were amplified by using primers specific to the different types of cytoplasmic domains. All samples tested showed two similar bands, in which the upper band represents the TM-cytoplasmic a tail segment and the lower band represents the TM-cytoplasmic b tail segment **(Fig 3L)**.

By contrast to previous studies depicting type II Nrg1 (GGF I-III) expression in the pituitary (Goodearl et al., 1993), other studies do not support this idea as a result of the absence or extremely low levels of GGF mRNA in rat pituitary with in situ hybridization (ISH) or RT-PCR (Marchionni et al., 1993). In line with the letter, the rat anterior pituitary expresses both type I Nrg1α/β and type III Nrg1α/β, whereas the GH3 cells only express type III Nrg1α/β **(Tab 1)**. This suggests that Nrg1 may have specific functions there. Furthermore, the presence of both membrane-tethered Nrg1 and soluble Nrg1 may function in an autocrine/paracrine manner.

Type	sample	α	β	S1	S3	S4	ICD-a	ICD-b	ICD-c
I	AP	+	+	+	+	-	+	+	+
	GH3	-	-	-	-	-	-	-	-
II	AP	-	-	-	-	-	-	-	-
	GH3	-	-	-	-	-	-	-	-
III	AP	+	+	+	+	-	+	+	+
	GH3	+	+	+	+	-	+	+	+

Table 1. Nrg1 domain identification in the anterior pituitary (AP) and GH3 cells (GH3) based on domain RT-PCR. α, EGF-like domain α; β, EGF-like domain β; S, stalk domain; ICD, intracellular domain.

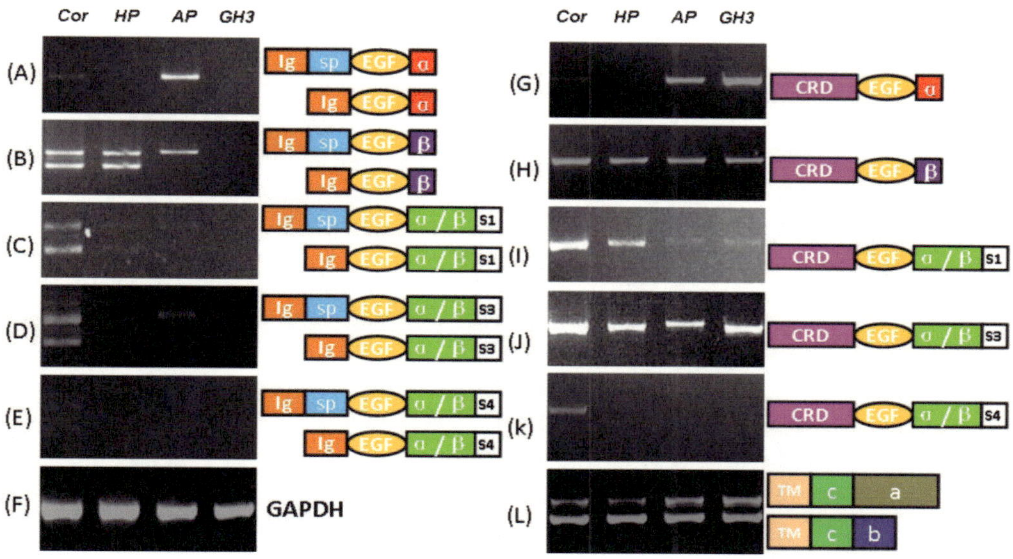

Figure 3. Domain RT-PCR for multiple Nrg1 isoforms in the rat cortex, hypothalamus, anterior pituitary and GH3 cells. Reverse transcriptase-PCR with several sets of domain specific primers amplified the expression of Nrg1 isoforms in the hypothalamus (HP) and anterior pituitary (AP) and GH3 cells (GH3). Rat cortex (Cor) serves as positive control. D-Glyceraldehyde-3-phosphate dehydrogenase (GAPDH) was used to indicate the equal loading of samples. The schematic diagrams right to the RT-PCR results indicate domains that the RT-PCR products contain. α, EGF-like domain α; β, EGF-like domain β; s, stalk domain; CRD, cysteine-rich domain; ICD, intracellular domain; TM, transmembrane domain. (Zhao et al., 2011a)

At the protein level based on Western blot, the anterior pituitary give rise to a group of bands with a wide range of molecular weights as a result of alternative splicing and post-translational modification such as hyperglycosylation. In the anterior pituitary cell lysates, bands at 140, 110, 95 and 90 kDa, representing the main Nrg1 precursors, were observed, whereas, in the hypothalamus cell lysates, a weak band at 110 kDa was observed. Soluble

Nrg1s at 36 and 30 kDa were detected in the anterior pituitary, whereas only the 36 kDa Nrg1 was detected in the hypothalamus.

In the anterior pituitary, Nrg1α/β was co-localized with Nrg1α, further confirming the domain RT-PCR and western blotting results and indicating that Nrg1α is the predominant intrapituitary Nrg1. However, Nrg1α/β was not co-localized with S-100, GH and ACTH, which serve as markers for folliculo-stellate cells, somatotrophs and corticotrophs, respectively. Notably, neighbouring localization of Nrg1 with PRL was observed, suggesting a potential interaction between lactotrophs and Nrg1 positive cells. In addition, Nrg1 was weakly detected in partial PRL positive lactotrophs. Further immunofluoresecence investigation demonstrated Nrg1α/β were co-stained with FSH or LH, both of which are markers for gonadotrophs. Significant co-localization of Nrg1α/β with either FSH or LH was noted in the transition zone between pars tuberalis and pars distalis. However, in the pars distalis, such co-localization was relatively weak. This suggests that gonadotrophs in the pars tuberalis adjacent to the pars distalis are the major source of intrapituitary Nrg1α/β (**Fig 4**) (Zhao et al., 2011a).

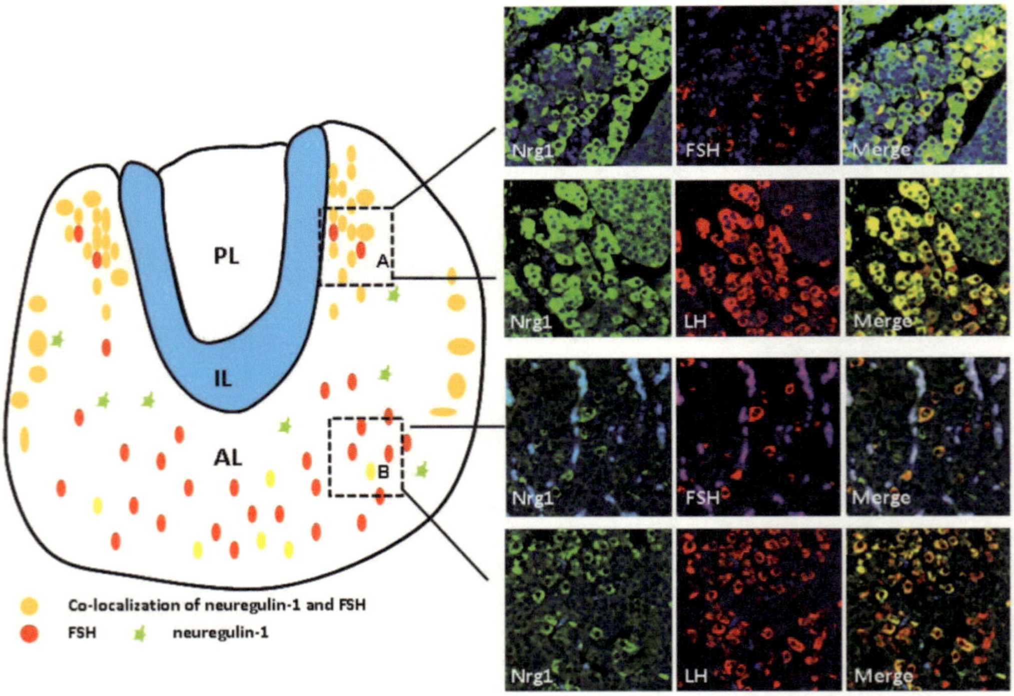

Figure 4. Gonadotrophs are the main source of Nrg1 in the anterior pituitary. PL, posterior lobe; IL, intermediate lobe; AL, anterior lobe. A, pars tuberalis; B, pars distalis. (Zhao et al., 2011a)

In addition, RT-PCR demonstrated varying expression patterns of Nrg 1 isoforms at the mRNA level during the estrous cycle. Type I Nrg1α was expressed at a low level during the proestrous (PE) phase and at a constant level in other phases. In contrast, low levels of type I Nrg1β were observed in the metestrous (ME) and diestrous (DE) phases. Type II Nrg1 was expressed at the highest level during the E1 phase. Both type III Nrg1α and type III Nrg1β were expressed at higher levels during the E1 and E2 phases, when an estrogen surge occurred in response to hypophyseal gonadotrophic hormones. At the protein level, the expression of both 110 kDa and 95 kDa Nrg1s in the anterior pituitary were significantly higher in E1 and E2 phases. No similar expression pattern was observed in the posterior pituitary (Zhao et al., 2011c). In spite of these observations, it is still unclear whether Nrg1 functions in an sex-dependent manner or not in the anterior pituitary, and unfortunately, little is known about the sex-specific expression and function of Nrg1 in the brain (Taylor et al., 2012).

2.1.2. Localization of Nrg1 and ErbB4 receptor in the anterior pituitary of male Rhesus monkeys

In male Rhesus monkeys aged 5-7 years, the existence of Nrg1 and ErbB4 was observed, which showed a partial adjacent pattern, suggesting the existence of Nrg1/ErbB4 juxtacrine signaling in the anterior pituitary in non–human primates (See Figure 5) (Zhao et al., 2011c).

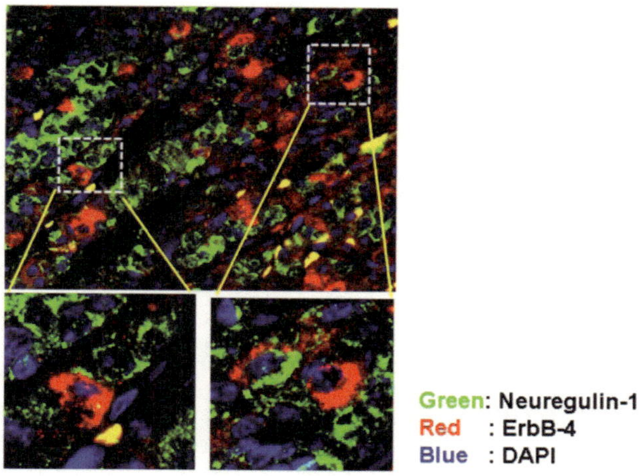

Figure 5. Nrg1 and ErbB4 receptor are expressed in the anteior pituitary of the rhesus monkey. The anterior pituitary of Rhesus monkey was subjected to immunofluorescence staining for both Nrg1 and ErbB4 (Green: Nrg1; Red: ErbB4; Blue: DAPI).

2.2. Expression and Localization of Nrg1 in GH3 cells

Exogenous Nrg1 was first shown to increase PRL mRNA expression and PRL secretion from GH3 cells by activating the ErbB3 receptor and intracellular AKT. In addition, the ErbB3 receptor has been shown to correlate with the malignant transformation of prolactinomas (Vlotides et al., 2008, 2009).

Subsequent investigation demonstrated that administration of siRNA against Nrg1 reduced the expression of multiple isoforms, including the 110-, 60-, 36-, 33-, and 30-kDa proteins, indicating that these bands potentially represented alternatively spliced Nrg1 gene products, post-translationally modified forms, and/or the shed ectodomains from their initial precursors. Immunofluorescence staining also demonstrated the reduced expression of Nrg1α/β in GH3 cells. Nrg1 was detected, with the ErbB2 receptor partially expressed in some human prolactinoma samples. This suggests the existence of Nrg1/ErbB receptor autocrine/paracrine signaling during the development of prolactinoma.

In addition, type III Nrg1 (SMDF) is distinct from the other two types of Nrg1 and contains an extra N terminal transmembrane structure. In type III Nrg1, initial proteolysis frees the EGF-like domain from the membrane, leading to juxtacrine signalling characterised by reciprocal intercellular communication (Bao et al., 2003; Hancock et al., 2008). Further cleavage releases a shorter EGF-like domain-containing peptide, which functions in autocrine / paracrine interactions. Indeed, high levels of ErbB4 receptor and Nrg1 have also been reported to be expressed in K-ras transformed thyroid Kimol and A6 cells, where Nrg1 signals through the ErbB2/ErbB4 heterodimeric complex in an autocrine manner (Mincione et al., 1998). Although Nrg mRNA was present in both tumor and non-tumor tissue, Nrg precursor isoform immunohistochemically showed nuclear immunostaining in most human papillary carcinomas but not in normal thyroid tissue. Cytoplasmic Nrgα, β1 and β3 were also exclusively detected in papillary carcinomas (Fluge et al., 2000). Significant expression of the ErbB2, ErbB3 and ErbB4 receptors, in addition to Nrg1 isoforms, was also detected in the developing murine fetal pancreas, where they potentially contribute to islet development and regrowth (Kritzik et al., 2000). The strong expression of Nrg1 in lactosomatotroph GH3 tumor cells was in sharp contrast with that observed in the anterior pituitary, where Nrg1 was almost undetectable in the prolactotroph (Zhao et al., 2011b). Thus, overexpression of Nrg1 may play a vitally functional role in prolactinoma development.

3. Autocrine/juxtacrine modulation of prolactin (PRL) secretion via Nrg1/ErbB receptor pathway

3.1. Modulating role of Nrg1 on PRL secretion in the anterior pituitary

Previous studies have described the morphological relationship between prolactotrophs and gonadotrophs, which is characterised by conditional gap junctions, and have reported the functional roles of LH on PRL secretion in response to GnRH (Andries et al., 1995; Denef et al., 1983). More recently, Henderson et al. (2008) described GnRH-induced PRL release independent of gonadotrophins.

FSH positive gonadotrophs can form contacts with ErbB3 positive cells and ErbB3 was also shown to be localized on the prolactotroph membrane. These observations, altogether, raised the hypothesis that Nrg1 present in gonadotrophs may function by modulating lactotrophs by interacting with ErbB3 receptor on the membrane. Thus, intrapituitary gonadotrophs and prolactotrophs may partially use gap junctions to form contacts, allowing the binding of gonadotroph-derived membrane-tethered type III Nrg1 to ErbB3 receptors on the prolactotrophic membrane. In addition, both prolactotrophs and gonadotrophs may form contacts through cell adhesion molecules widely distributed in the anterior pituitary, including L1 cell adhesion molecule and neural cell adhesion molecule (Zhao et al., 2010). These molecules may increase the interaction between Nrg1 and ErbB receptors, such as ErbB3 and ErbB4, a process that may activate a series of intracellular signals and also increase enzymatic cleavage of the PRL precursor.

In one study, type I and type III Nrg1α/β as well as membrane-tethered type III Nrg1 were able to be identified using domain-specific primers-based RT-PCR in the mouse gonadotroph αT3-1 cells. Using Western blot assays with an anti-Nrg1 antibody, a cluster of proteins were observed with molecular weights in the range 30–114 kDa. Proteins at 70, 60 and 45 kDa were also detected in serum-free culture medium conditioned by αT3-1 cells. However, commonly recognized soluble Nrg1 with molecular weight ranging from 40–25 kDa were rarely observed, suggesting the precursor is the main form of Nrg1 in this gonadotroph cell line, which may be the base for juxtacrine interaction between Nrg1 and its cognate receptors. Subsequently, PRL and GH secreting GH3 cells were co-cultured with gonadtroph αT3-1 cells pretreated with siRNA against Nrg1. Administration of siRNA against mouse Nrg1 significantly reduced the staining intensities of intracellular Nrg1α/β, as well as their co-localization, as observed with immunofluorescence assays. Nrg1 reduction in αT3-1 cells reduced PRL expression in co-cultured GH3 cells. Co-culturing of GH3 cells with αT3-1 cells treated with siRNA against Nrg1 significantly reduced the secretion of an 18 kDa form of PRL from GH3 cells at 48 h, although it had no significant effect on the secretion of 23-kDa PRL and 22-kDa GH. This result, coupled with the observation that membrane-tethered type III Nrg1 is mainly expressed in the gonadotrophs, suggests the existence of a type III Nrg1-mediated juxtacrine mechanism that affects secretion of a subset of PRL, a process that may also occur in the normal anterior pituitary.

Cleaved full-length PRL has been reported to be a vascular function modulator mainly in the 16-kDa form (Clapp et al., 2006, 2008; Macotela et al., 2006). However, an 18- kDa form was also reported as an intermediate form of the final cleavage product in vitro (Lkhider et al., 2004; Nicoll et al., 1997). We reported that Nrg1 can modulate the release of an 18-kDa cleavage form of PRL, which is typical to GH3 cells. This process may be related to the modulation of Nrg1 on enzymes specific for PRL cleavage, such as cathepsin D and matrix metalloprotease (MMP) family members (Clapp et al., 2006, 2008; Macotela et al., 2006). Indeed, Nrg1 has been shown to promote the expression of MMP-7 and -9 in an ErbB receptor dependent manner in cancer cells (Ueno et al., 2008; Yuan et al., 2006).

3.2. Modulating role of Nrg1 on PRL secretion in rat lactosomatotroph GH3 cells

In one study, siRNA method was used to investigate the autocrine/paracrine effect of Nrg1 on PRL secretion. siRNA of Nrg1 significantly downregulated the release of a soluble form of 36 kDa Nrg1 into the conditioned culture medium. Western blotting analysis showed significantly reduced secretion of both the 23-kDa and the 18-kDa PRLs into the conditioned culture medium in response to the reduced secretion of 36 kDa Nrg1, and a reduction in

ErbB3 receptor activation was also observed. However, downregulation of Nrg1 has no effects on GH secretion. Thus, Nrg1 may modulate PRL secretion from GH3 cells in an autocrine, paracrine/juxtacrine manner (See Fig 6).

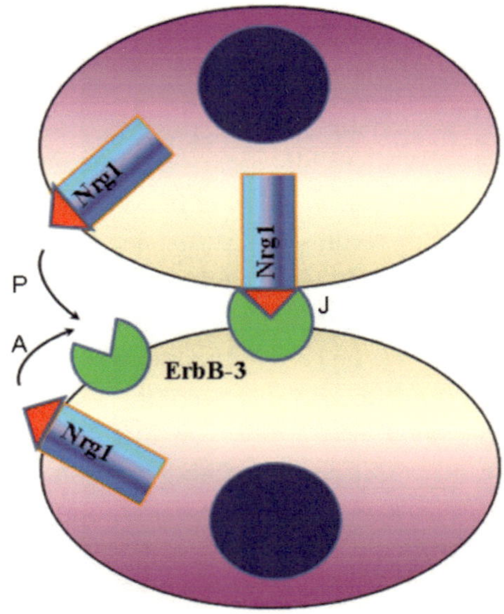

Figure 6. Schematic diagram illustrating the hypothesized model for Neuregulin-1 (Nrg1) on PRL regulation. A, autocrine; P, paracrine; J, juxtacrine.

4. Nrg1/ErbB receptor inhibition as a potential clinical management of prolactinoma

The role of Nrg1-mediated autocrine, paracrine, or juxtacrine signaling in several aspects of cancer biology suggests that it is a potential target for tumor therapy. Success with a combined therapeutic antibody and sheddase inhibitor treatment has been demonstrated in the mammary cancer MCF- 7 cell line, in which the administration of INCB7839 (a second generation sheddase inhibitor) with Lapatinib prevents the growth of ErbB2 positive BT474-SC1 human breast cancer xenografts in vivo (Witters et al., 2008). Gefitinib, a tyrosine kinase inhibitor, has also been reported to suppress Nrg1-mediated ErbB2/ErbB3 signaling to PRL (Vlotides et al., 2008, 2009). A recent investigation has also revealed that Lapatinib, an ErbB2 inhibitor, possesses additional effects in the suppression of PRL expression, and oral Lapatinib treatment triggers the shrinkage of estrogen-induced prolactinomas in rats (Fukuoka et al., 2010). Thus, the co-localization of Nrg1 with ErbB2 in partial prolactinomas suggests that inhibiting Nrg1 expression or abolishing its binding ability might also have similar effects in inhibiting Nrg1-dependent ErbB receptor activation and prolactinoma progression. In one of our studies, five human prolactinoma tissues were stained for both Nrg1 and ErbB2. All samples demonstrated positive staining for Nrg1, and co-expression of both molecules was observed in one sample (Zhao et al., 2011b). Additional prolactinoma samples should be recruited to stress further the role of Nrg1/ErbB receptor singling in future investigations. The findings regarding the endogenous expression of Nrg1 and an Nrg1-mediated autocrine/paracrine mechanism in GH3 cells have expanded previous results and reveal Nrg1 as a potential diagnostic serological marker for prolactinoma. In addition, a therapeutic approach involving the direct functional inhibition of Nrg1 might be a viable clinical treatment for PRL-secreting pituitary tumors.

5. Conclusions and perspectives

Among a series of regulators of PRL, the emerging role of Nrg1 is rather new, but important. Overexpression of Nrg1 and its cognate receptor ErbB2, as well as their co-localization provides the promising therapeutic method to control prolactinoma and hyperprolactinemia. Such a clinical purpose can be achieved by 1) Nrg1 receptor inhibitor, such as Erlotinib, Lapatinib et al.; 2) neutralizing antibody against Nrg1 and 3) their combination. Additionally, Nrg1-mediated autocrine/paracrine mechanism in GH3 cells have expanded previous results and reveal Nrg1 as a potential serological marker not only for prolactinoma diagnosis, but for prognosis evaluation post operation. In addition, a therapeutic approach involving the direct functional inhibition of Nrg1 might be a viable clinical treatment for PRL-secreting pituitary tumors. To avoid the side effects, such as affecting the physiological function of circulating Nrg1 brought by intravenous administration of anti-Nrg1 antibody, the therapeutic hypothesis may be established by intratumoral (i.t.) injection of the therapeutic antibody in patients, whose prolactinomas are highly resistant to chemotherapy or in whom the tumor location can lead to high surgery risk. It has recently been reported that experimental i.t. injections with ErbB2 targeted gold nanoparticles (AuNPs) resulted in high tumor retention with low systemic exposure and represents an attractive delivery strategy (Chattopadhyay et al., 2012).

Author details

Weijiang Zhao
Center for Neuroscience, Shantou University Medical College, Shantou, Guangdong Province, China
Cedars-Sinai Medical Center, Los Angeles, California 90048, USA

Acknowledgement

Publication of this work was supported by National Natural Science Foundation of China (Project 81171138).

6. References

Andries M, Vijver VV, Tilemans D, Bert C, Denef C. Interaction of alpha-T3-1 cells with lactotropes and somatotropes of normal pituitary in-vitro. Neuroendocrinology 1995; 61: 326–336.

Bao J, Wolpowitz D, Role LW, Talmage DA. Talmage. Back signaling by the Nrg-1 intracellular domain. J Cell Biol 2003; 161: 1133–1141.

Bernstein HG, Lendeckel U, Bertram I, Bukowska A, Kanakis D, Dobrowolny H, Stauch R, Krell D, Mawrin C, Budinger E, Keilhoff G, Bogerts B. Localization of Nrg1alpha (Neuregulin-alpha) and one of its receptors, ErbB4 tyrosine kinase, in developing and adult human brain. Brain Res Bull 2006; 69: 546–559.

Borrelli E, Sawchenko PE, Evans RM. Pituitary hyperplasia induced by ectopic expression of nerve growth factor. Proc Natl Acad Sci USA 1992; 89: 2764–2768.

Cai A, Hayes JD, Patel N, Hyde JF. Targeted overexpression of galanin in lactotrophs of transgenic mice induces hyperprolactinemia. Endocrinology 1999; 140: 4955–4964.

Chattopadhyay N, Fonge H, Cai Z, Scollard D, Lechtman E, Done SJ, Pignol JP, Reilly RM. Role of Antibody-Mediated Tumor Targeting and Route of Administration in Nanoparticle Tumor Accumulation in Vivo. Mol Pharm 2012; 9, 2168–2179.

Clapp C, Aranda J, Gonza´lez C, Jeziorski MC, Martı´nez de la Escalera G. Vasoinhibins: endogenous regulators of angiogenesis and vascular function. Trends Endocrinol Metab 2006; 17: 301–307.

Clapp C, Thebault S, Martı´nez de la Escalera G. Role of prolactin and vasoinhibins in the regulation of vascular function in mammary gland. J Mammary Gland Biol Neoplasia 2008; 13: 55–67.

Corfas G, Rosen KM, Aratake H, Krauss R, Fischbach GD. Differential expression of ARIA isoforms in the rat brain. Neuron 1995; 14: 103–115.

Cote GM, Miller TA, Lebrasseur NK, Kuramochi Y, Sawyer DB. Nrg1alpha and beta isoform expression in cardiac microvascular endothelial cells and function in cardiac myocytes in vitro. Exp Cell Res 2005; 311:135–146.

Denef C, Andries M. Evidence for paracrine interaction between gonadotrophs and lactotrophs in pituitary cell aggregates. Endocrinology 1983; 112: 813–822.

Fluge O, Akslen LA, Haugen DR, Varhaug JE, Lillehaug JR. Expression of neuregulins and associations with the ErbB family of tyrosine kinase receptors in papillary thyroid carcinomas. Int J Cancer 2000; 87: 763–770.

Fukuoka H, Cooper O, Mizutani J, Tong Y, Ren S, Bannykh S, Melmed S. HER2/ErbB-2 receptor signaling in rat and human prolactinoma cells: strategy for targeted prolactinoma therapy. Mol Endocrinol 2010; 25:92–103.

Goodearl AD, Davis JB, Mistry K, Minghetti L, Otsu M, Waterfield MD, Stroobant P. Purification of multiple forms of glial growth factor. J Biol Chem 1993; 268: 18095–18102.

Hahn CG, Wang HY, Cho DS, Talbot K, Gur RE, Berrettini WH, Bakshi K, Kamins J, Borgmann-Winter KE, Siegel SJ, Gallop RJ, Arnold SE. Altered neuregulin 1-ErbB4 signaling contributes to NMDA receptor hypofunction in schizophrenia. Nat Med 2006; 12:824–828.

Hancock ML, Canetta SE, Role LW, Talmage DA. Presynaptic type III neuregulin1-ErbB signaling targets a7 nicotinic acetylcholine receptors to axons. J Cell Biol 2008; 181: 511–521.

Harari D, Tzahar E, Romano J, Shelly M, Pierce JH, Andrews GC, Yarden Y. Neuregulin-4: a novel growth factor that acts through the ErbB4 receptor tyrosine kinase. Oncogene 1999; 18: 2681–2689.

Henderson HL, Hodson DJ, Gregory SJ, Townsend J, Tortonese DJ. Gonadotropin-releasing hormone stimulates prolactin release from lactotrophs in photoperiodic species through a gonadotropin-independent mechanism. Biol Reprod 2008; 78: 370–377.

Holmes WE, Sliwkowski MX, Akita RW, Henzel WJ, Lee J, Park JW, Yansura D, Abadi N, Raab H, Lewis GD. Identification of Neuregulin, a specific activator of p185ErbB-2. Science 1992; 256: 1205–1210.

Jacobsen NE, Abadi N, Sliwkowski MX, Reilly D, Skelton NJ, Fairbrother WJ. High-resolution solution structure of the EGF-like domain of Neuregulin- alpha. Biochemistry 1996; 35: 3402–3417.

Jessell TM, Siegel RE, Fischbach GD. Induction of acetylcholine receptors on cultured skeletal muscle by a factor extracted from brain and spinal cord. Proc Natl Acad Sci USA 1979; 76: 5397–5401.

Kritzik MR, Krahl T, Good A, Gu D, Lai C, Fox H, Sarvetnick N. Expression of ErbB receptors during pancreatic islet development and regrowth. J Endocrinol 2000; 165: 67–77.

Lemake GE, Brockes JP. Identification and purification of glial growth. J Neurosci 1984; 4: 75–83.

Liu J, Kern JA. Nrg1 activates the JAK-STAT pathway and regulates lung epithelial cell proliferation. Am J Respir Cell Mol Biol 2002; 27:306–313.

Lkhider M, Castino R, Bouguyon E, Isidoro C, Ollivier-Bousquet M. Cathepsin D released by lactating rat mammary epithelial cells is involved in prolactin cleavage under physiological conditions. J Cell Sci 2004;117:5155–5164.

Macotela Y, Aguilar MB, Guzma´n-Morales J, Rivera JC, Zermen˜o C, Lo´pez-Barrera F, Nava G, Lavalle C, Martı´nez de la Escalera G, Clapp C.Matrix metalloproteases from chondrocytes generate an antiangiogenic16 kDa prolactin. J Cell Sci 2006;119:1790–1800.

Marchionni MA, Goodearl AD, Chen MS, Bermingham-McDonogh O, Kirk C, Hendricks M, Danehy F, Misumi D, Sudhalter J, Kobayashi K. Glial growth factors are alternatively spliced ErbB-2 ligands expressed in the nervous system. Nature 1993; 362: 312–318.

Mincione G, Piccirelli A, Lazzereschi D, Salomon DS, Colletta G. Neuregulindependent autocrine loop regulates growth of K-ras but not erbB-2 transformed rat thyroid epithelial cells. J Cell Physiol 1998; 176: 383–391.

Nicoll CS. Cleavage of prolactin by its target organs and the possible significance of this process. J Mammary Gland Biol Neoplasia 1997; 2:81–89.

Orr-Urtreger A, Trakhtenbrot L, Ben-Levy R, Wen D, Rechavi G, Lonai P, Yarden Y. Neural expression and chromosomal mapping of Neu differentiation factor to 8p12-p21. Proc Natl Acad Sci USA 1993; 90:1867–1871.

Peles E, Ben-Levy R, Tzahar E, Liu N, Wen D, Yarden Y. Celltype specific interaction of Neu differentiation factor (NDF/ neuregulin) with Neu/HER-2 suggests complex ligand-receptor relationships. EMBO J 1993; 12:961–971.

Puricelli L, Proietti CJ, Labriola L, Salatino M, Balañá ME, Aguirre Ghiso J, Lupu R, Pignataro OP, Charreau EH, Bal de Kier Joffé E, Elizalde PV. Neuregulin inhibits proliferation via ERKs and phosphatidyl-inositol 3-kinase activation but regulates urokinase plasminogen activator independently of these pathways in metastatic mammary tumor cells. Int J Cancer 2002; 100:642–653.

Rosnack KJ, Stroh JG, Singleton DH, Guarino BC, Andrews GC. Use of capillary electrophoresis-electrospray ionization mass spectrometry in the analysis of synthetic peptides. J Chromatogr A 1994; 675: 219–225.

Prevot V, Rio C, Cho GJ, Lomniczi A, Heger S, Neville CM, Rosenthal NA, Ojeda SR, Corfas G. Normal female sexual development requires neuregulin-erbB receptor signaling in hypothalamic astrocytes. J Neurosci 2003; 23: 230–239.

Sharif A, Duhem-Tonnelle V, Allet C, Baroncini M, Loyens A, Kerr-Conte J, Collier F, Blond S, Ojeda SR, Junier MP, Prevot V. Differential erbB signaling in astrocytes from the cerebral cortex and the hypothalamus of the human brain. Glia 2009; 57: 362–379.

Spuch C, Diz-Chaves Y. Fibroblast growth factor-1 and epidermal growth factor modualate prolactin responses to TRH and dompamine in prmary cultures. Endocrine 2006; 29: 317–324.

Taylor SB, Taylor AR, Koenig JI. The interaction of disrupted Type II Neuregulin 1 and chronic adolescent stress on adult anxiety and fear related behaviors. Neuroscience 2012; http://dx.doi.org/10.1016/j.neuroscience.2012.09.045

Ueno Y, Sakurai H, Tsunoda S, Choo MK, Matsuo M, Koizumi K, Saiki I. Neuregulin-induced activation of ErbB3 by EGFR tyrosine kinase activity promotes tumor growth and metastasis in melanoma cells. Int J Cancer 2008; 123: 340–347.

Usdin TB, Fischbach GD. Purification and characterization of a polypeptide from chick brain that promotes the accumulation of acetylcholine receptors in chick myotubes. J Cell Biol 1986; 103: 493–507.

Vlotides G, Siegel E, Donangelo I, Gutman S, Ren SG, Melmed S. Rat prolactinoma cell growth regulation by epidermal growth factor receptor ligands. Cancer Res 2008; 68:6377–6386.

Vlotides G, Cooper O, Chen YH, Ren SG, Greenman Y, Melmed S. Neuregulin regulates prolactinoma gene expression. Cancer Res 2009; 69: 4209–4216.

Witters L, Scherle P, Friedman S, Fridman J, Caulder E, Newton R, Lipton A. Synergistic inhibition with a dual epidermal growth factor receptor/HER-2/neu tyrosine kinase inhibitor and a disintegrin and metalloprotease inhibitor. Cancer Res 2008; 68:7083–7089.

Yuan G, Qian L, Song L, Shi M, Li D, Yu M, Hu M, Shen B, Guo N. Neuregulin-beta promotes matrix metalloproteinase-7 expression via HER2-mediated AP-1 activation in MCF-7 cells. Mol Cell Biochem 2008; 318: 73–79.

Zhao W, Zhao X, Peng S, Pan H, Ma Z, Shen Y. Expression and localization of cell adhesion molecules in the pituitary of C57BL/6 mice. J Shantou Univ Med Coll 2010; 23: 65–67.

Zhao W, Ren S. Neuregulin-1 (Nrg1) is mainly expressed in rat pituitary gonadotrope cells and possibly regulates prolactin (PRL) secretion in a juxtacrine manner. Journal of Neuroendocrinology 2011a; 23:1252-1262.

Zhao W, Shen Y, Ren S. Endogenous expression of Neuregulin-1 (Nrg1) as a potential modulator of prolactin (PRL) secretion in GH3 cells. Cell Tissue Res 2011b; 344:313–320.

Zhao W, Ren S. Endogenous Neuregulin-1 expression in the anterior pituitary of female Wistar-Furth rats during the estrous cycle. Journal of Southern Medical University 2011c; 31: 921-927.

Chapter 6

Autocrine and Paracrine Regulation of Prolactin Secretion by Prolactin Variants and by Hypothalamic Hormones

Flavio Mena, Nilda Navarro and Alejandra Castilla

Additional information is available at the end of the chapter

http://dx.doi.org/10.5772/51681

1. Introduction

The synthesis and release of prolactin (PRL) by lactotrophs in the anterior pituitary (AP) are regulated by factors produced in the hypothalamus as well as in the posterior and neurointermediate pituitary lobes, by autocrine and paracrine signals from the anterior pituitary itself (Ben-Jonathan & Hnasko, 2001; Kordon, 1985; Denef, 1988; Denef, 2008; Freeman et al., 2000; Lorenson and Walker, 2001; Schwartz & Cherny, 1992; Schwartz, 2000; Wang & Walker, 1993; Sinha, 1992; Sinha 1995; Moore et al., 2002; Bollengier et al., 1989; Bollengier et al., 1996; Kadowaki et al., 1984; MacLeod et al., 1966; Sgouris & Meites, 1953; Chen et al., 1968; Welsch et al., 1968) and also by gonadal steroids (Maurer & Gorski, 1977; Maurer, 1982). In addition, it has been reported that total PRL and PRL variants (Denef, 2008; Shah & Hymer, 1989) are secreted under different physiological conditions (Denef, 2008; Wang & Walker, 1993; Sinha, 1992; Sinha 1995; Mena et al., 1984; Mena et al., 1992; Boockfor & Frawley, 1987). And, it is known that functional interactions and cytological differences exist among pituitary lactotrophs within the anterior pituitary gland (Denef, 1988; Schwartz & Cherny, 1992; Schwartz, 2000; Boockfor & Frawley, 1987) and that functional variations (Boockfor & Frawley, 1987; Boockfor et al., 1986; Frawley & Boockfor, 1991; Nagy & Frawley 1990), as well as autoregulation (Nagy et al., 1991) and interactions with other pituitary cells (Denef, 2008; Sinha, 1992; Moore et al., 2002; Kadowaki et al., 1984) and with hypothalamic hormones (Ben-Jonathan & Hnasko, 2001; Chen et al., 1968) occur in different circumstances. For instance, lactotrophs from the central AP region of lactating rats, i.e., the region surrounding the neurointermediate pituitary lobe (Boockfor & Frawley, 1987; Frawley & Boockfor, 1991; Papka et al., 1986) are bigger, secrete more PRL than those of the peripheral AP region and after a short period of suckling become more sensitive to the PRL-stimulatory agents, TRH and angiotensin II; moreover, they become unresponsive to dopamine; and interact with lactotrophs in the peripheral region of the gland (Boockfor & Frawley, 1987; Boockfor et al., 1986; Frawley & Boockfor, 1991; Nagy et al., 1991; Nagy & Frawley 1990; Diaz et al., 2002). In these studies, it is possible that the release of PRL variants may have influenced the regulation of PRL release.

In previous reports (Huerta-Ocampo et al., 2007; Mena et al., 2010) we showed that conditioned media (CM) and PRL variants i.e., from 7-14 and 70-97 kDa, from lactating rat APs, characterized by Western blotting and eluted from SDS-PAGE, promoted the *in vitro* vesicular release of the hormone from preformed, mature PRL granules of male rat APs, and that such release was independent of PRL synthesis (Huerta-Ocampo et al., 2007). Autocrine and paracrine types of actions have also been shown to occur within the AP (Denef, 2008; Freeman et al., 2000; Lorenson and Walker, 2001; Schwartz & Cherny, 1992; Schwartz, 2000; Welsch et al., 1968; Diaz, et al., 2002; Huerta-Ocampo et al., 2007; Mena et al., 2010), and were demonstrated when the central and peripheral AP regions of lactating rats were incubated *in vitro* with CM from pituitaries of lactating, pregnant and steroid-treated castrated males or females, but not from untreated castrated rats, intact male rats or by a PRL Standard (Huerta-Ocampo et al., 2007; Mena et al., 2010). Also, more potent effects occurred with CM from APs of early- than from mid- or late- lactating rats and from rats non-suckled for 8 or 16 h than from those non-suckled for 32 h (Mena et al., 2010). These results suggest that, under certain conditions, PRL variants released from lactating and non-lactating rat APs may regulate the release of PRL variants from the lactotrophs.

In the present study, CM proteins, i.e., PRL variants, that were released *in vitro* from the AP regions of lactating rats were separated and electroeluted from SDS-PAGE and tested using *in vitro* incubation techniques. We sought to determine first, whether PRL variants, which are known to occur within the AP (Schwartz & Cherny, 1992; Schwartz, 2000; Wang & Walker, 1993; Sinha, 1992; Bollengier et al., 1989; Huerta-Ocampo et al., 2007; Mena et al., 2010; Mena & Grosvenor, 1972; Asawaroengchai et al., 1978; Nicoll et al., 1969; Mansur & Hymer, 1985), and are released *in vitro* (Mena et al, 1984; Mena et al., 1992; Huerta-Ocampo et al., 2007; Mena et al., 2010; Mena & Grosvenor, 1972; Grosvenor et al., 1967; Grosvenor et al., 1979; Mena et al., 1989; Mena et al., 1993) after the suckling-induced PRL transformation i.e., the transfer of the hormone from a pre-releasable to a releasable state (Mena & Grosvenor, 1972; Grosvenor et al., 1967; Mena et al., 1993) would influence the release of PRL variants from lactating rat lactotrophs; and second, whether the effects of dopamine (DA), thyrotropin-releasing hormone (TRH) and oxytocin (OT) upon PRL release would manifest their effects upon PRL secretion by regulating the release of PRL variants from lactating rat lactotrophs (Mena et al., 2011).

Several reports indicate that PRL has some neuro and gliatrophic properties, and that it mediates the development and maturation of dopaminergic neurons in the hypothalamo-pituitary system (Möderscheim et al., 2007). We showed previously (Morales et al., 2001) that intrathecal injection of PRL in the spinal cord promoted the sympathetic inhibition of milk ejection in lactating rats, and that prolactin variants in CM from the central and peripheral regions of the anterior pituitary from lactating, but not from male rats promoted the *in vitro* release of PRL from pituitary glands of male rats in a dose-dependent manner (Huerta-Ocampo et al., 2007; Mena et al., 2010).

Our results suggest that PRL variants are released into the CM from the central and peripheral AP regions of lactating rats, that they interact and selectively and specifically stimulate or inhibit the *in vitro* release of other PRL variants from lactotrophs of lactating rat APs; that hypothalamic hormones selectively regulate and interact with PRL variants released from AP lactotrophs, and finally, whether in response to CM's from lactating rats, changes in electrical activity (EA) occur in male lactotrophs, as well as in astrocytes from the central nervous system, and in intracellular calcium concentration in sympathetic neurons (Mena et al, 2012b).

2. Materials and methods

2.1 General

Animal studies were performed under a protocol similar to the USPHS Guide for the Care and Use of Laboratory Animals and the Official Mexican Guide from Secretary of Agriculture (SAGARPA NOM-062-Z00-1999) published in 2001. Wistar primiparous lactating rats (8-10 pups per litter) were housed individually in a room with a reversed light-dark cycle (14 h light, 10 h darkness) and constant temperature (23-25°C) and were fed *ad libitum* (Purina Chow, Ralston Purina Co., Chicago IL, USA). On postpartum days 10-12 (7 am, local time) groups of mothers had their pups removed, and 6 h later their pups were or were not returned to the mothers and suckled for 15 min. At the end of the suckling or non-suckling periods, the mothers were killed by decapitation after light ether anesthesia. From all animals employed (see below), the pituitary was removed under a dissecting microscope, the posterior lobe was discarded and, using fine forceps as originally described by Papka et al. 1986, and by Bookfor & Frawley, 1987, the central region around the neurointermediate lobe and the peripheral region i.e., the rest of the AP tissue (Boockfor & Frawley, 1987; Diaz et al., 2002) were dissected independently, and incubated in Earle's medium as described below.

2.2. Preparation of concentrated conditioned media

In individual flasks containing 300 μl of Earle's medium, media were conditioned by incubating tissue fragments corresponding to the central (CR) and peripheral (PR) pituitary regions from lactating rats. The pituitary fragments were incubated immediately after removal to prevent disruption of hormone storage dynamics (Mena et al., 1992; Diaz et al., 2002). Flasks containing the pituitary fragments were gassed with 95% O_2, 5% CO_2, sealed with rubber stoppers and incubated at 37°C in a water bath shaker (American Optical, Buffalo NY, USA) for 1h. CM from pituitary fragments of each group of rats employed was concentrated and desalted in a Centricon micro-concentrator (Centripep, Millipore, Bredford MA, USA) and stored frozen until assayed, along with the corresponding primary cultures of pituitary cells or with cultures of sympathetic neurons.

The dose-response effects of DA (0.5, 1.0, 1.5 μM), TRH (0.1, 1.0, 10 μM) and OT (0.1-10 μM), upon the in vitro release of PRL variants previously exposed to the electroeluted PRL variants from NS and S lactating rat APs were determined by Enzyme-linked immunoabsorbant assay (ELISA).

2.3. SDS-PAGE

The PRL released into the media was determined by non-denaturing SDS-PAGE (12.5% gels) and Western blotting. The gels of SDS-PAGE were divided into 6 fractions which encompassed PRL variants from 6 to 97 kDa. The proteins in each fraction were electrophoretically eluted, dialyzed, lyophilized, and then assayed by ELISA for PRL content, as well as for their effects upon PRL secretion on primary culture of pituitary cells from the lactating rats, different concentrations of hypothalamic hormones, and in central and peripheral cultures of sympathetic neurons and astrocytes from hippocampus.

2.4. Primary cultures of pituitary cells

Pituitary fragments from male APs, or from NS and S lactating rats (n=5) corresponding to the central and peripheral regions of the anterior pituitary were dissected and processed separately. Primary cultures (lactotrophs) were prepared as described by Fiordelisio & Hernandez-Cruz, 2002. The tissue fragments were gently triturated with a Pasteur pipette; the cells were collected by centrifuging for 10 min at 185 x g, and washed twice with Dulbecco's Modified Eagle's Medium (DMEM) containing 10% BSA. The pellet was resuspended in DMEM medium, supplemented with 10% horse serum, 2% Fetal Bovine Serum, 10,000 U penicillin, 10 mg/ml streptomycin, all from Gibco BRL, Grand Island NY, USA. The cultures were maintained for 24 h at 37°C in a humidified atmosphere (95% air and 5% CO_2). The primary cultures were placed in the bottom of 24-multiwell culture plates (Costar, Cambridge, MA, USA) at a density of 2 x10^4 cells per well and three replicates were used in each experiment.

2.5. Cultures of astrocytes from the hippocampal and medial preoptic areas

Astrocyte cultures were obtained as shown previously by Hernández-Morales and García-Colunga, 2009. Two newborn Wistar rats were killed by decapitation and their brains removed. Slices from hippocampal CA1 region, or medial preoptic area were dissected and then the tissue was dissociated (~5000 cells/mL). The suspended cells were placed on a glass coverslip in a 35-mm Petri dish coated with poly-L-ornithine with DMEM supplemented with 10% FBS, 100 U/mL penicillin, 0.1 mg/mL streptomycin and 11 μg/mL piruvate was added. After 24 h, the medium was changed by Neurobasal medium supplemented with G5 (specific for growing astrocytes) and 100 U/mL penicillin, and 0.1 mg/mL streptomycin and 2 mM of L-glutamine. Cultures were kept under controlled air and temperature.

2.6. Cultures of sympathetic neurons

Cultures of sympathetic neurons were obtained as previously reported by Fiordelisio & Hernandez-Cruz, 2002. Briefly, ganglia from 10-day-old rats were removed under aseptic conditions after ether anaesthesia and cervical dislocation. After cleaning and chopping, the neurons were incubated in Ca2+/Mg2+-free Hanks solution with 1 mg/ml trypsin (Worthington Biochem Co.) and 2 mg/ml DNAse I for 30 min at 37ºC. After digestion, trypsin was inactivated by dilution in DMEM containing 10% fetal bovine serum (FBS) and 1 mg/ml trypsin inhibitor (Sigma) and the tissue was incubated in Hanks solution with 2 mg/ml collagenase and 2 mg/ml DNAse I for 30 min at 37ºC. After trituration with a Pasteur pipette, the cell suspension was centrifuged, washed twice in Hanks solution, and resuspended in fresh control culture medium. Cells were seeded on poly L-lysine-treated #1 round glass coverslips (1r105 cells per well), and maintained in control culture medium supplemented with 30 ng/ml of 7S NGF (Sigma) at 37ºC in a humidified atmosphere of 95% air and 5% CO_2. Culture medium was changed three times per week. All experiments were carried out with cultures less than 5 days old.

2.7. Electrophysiology

Astrocyte ion currents were recorded using the whole-cell voltage-clamp technique, as shown previously by Hernández-Morales and García-Colunga, 2009. Primary astrocytes between 4-7 days of culture were placed in a recording chamber and continuously superfused with control solution containing (mM): 136 NaCl, 2.5 KCl, 10 HEPES, 4 $CaCl_2$, 0.5 $MgCl_2$, 10 glucose, pH 7.2. Pipettes were filled with a solution containing (mM): 130 K-gluconate, 10 NaCl, 10 EGTA, 10 HEPES, 2 ATP, 0.2 GTP, pH 7.2, having a resistance of 3-5 MΩ. Astrocytes were held at a potential of -60 mV. The data were analyzed with pClamp 8.2 software and Origin 7. We determined changes in electrical activity (EA) in response to CM's from lactating and from male rats in male lactotrophs, as well as in neurons from the central nervous system.

2.8. Measurements of intracellular Ca^{2+} concentration

Primary astrocytes from hippocampus, medial preoptic area, sympathetic neurons or male rat lactotrophs, between 4-7 days of culture, were incubated for 30 min with the Ca^{2+} indicator Fluo 4-AM. Following this, cells were washed out three times for 10 min with solution containing (mM): 136 NaCl, 2.5 KCl, 10 HEPES, 4 $CaCl_2$, 0.5 $MgCl_2$, 10 glucose, pH 7.2. Cells were recorded on a Confocal Microscope LSM-510. Local application of CM was carried on with U-tube system placed at ~250 μm from the recorded cell. Cells were excited at 488 nm-Ar laser. Fluorescent intensity represents the change in intracellular calcium concentration and is measured in the whole soma. Data are expressed as a change from basal intensity (F0) to maximum intensity reached (%ΔF), %ΔF/F0. Then, we determined fluctuations in intracellular Ca^{2+} concentration, $[Ca^{2+}]_i$, in male lactotrophs in response to CM from lactating and from male rats.

3. Statistical analysis

The PRL concentration was calculated by linear regression and values of PRL concentration obtained by ELISA were averaged for each experimental group. Statistical differences were determined by a one-way analysis of variance (ANOVA), using Dunnett's test, and all treatments were compared versus the control (Earle's medium or Total PRL). Comparisons were analysed with the Graph Pad 5.0 Software, Inc. (San Diego, CA). The significance level was set at $p<0.05$. Each control or test compound was assayed in duplicate, and the assays were performed three times (n=3).

4. Experiments

4.1. Autocrine regulation of prolactin secretion

4.1.1. PRL content of electroeluted (EE) PRL variants released from AP regions of lactating non-suckled (NS) and suckled (S) rats

The PRL variants released from each AP region of NS and S rats were analyzed previously by SDS-PAGE and by Western blotting (32, 33). In the present study these PRL variants were electroeluted i.e., EE PRL from fractions 1-6 after SDS-PAGE; and the PRL content of each fraction was determined by ELISA, as shown in Fig. 1 A-D, and subsequently, to determine whether their increased and/or decreased release of PRL variants, each electroeluted PRL fraction (EE PRL) was incubated with lactotrophs of each AP region of non-suckled and suckled rat APs i.e., Figs. 2-3 (A-D). The fractions contained bands of 7-23 to 97 kDa under NR conditions, and 7-16 to 42 kDa under R conditions, and between 1 and more than 20 ng/μl of PRL variant protein. However, in spite of these variations, similar amounts of total PRL (about 60 ng/μl right panels), were released from each AP regions of NS and S rat, except for the higher amount (80 ng/μl) released from the central AP region of NS rats.

4.1.2. Effects of electroeluted PRL variants (EE PRL), released from AP regions of lactating non-suckled (NS) rats, upon the in vitro release of PRL variants from lactotrophs of NS rats

The EE PRL variants that were released from each AP region of NS rats (Figs. 1 A-B) were tested for their effects upon the amount of PRL release by lactotrophs from AP regions of NS rats, and the results are shown in Fig. 2A-B. CM from the PR region of NS rat APs (Fig. 1 A) contained a low concentration of PRL (< 3 ng/μl) in fraction 2 and high (about 10 ng/μl) in fractions 1 and 3-6; after incubation with the EE PRL variants, lactotrophs of the same region, i.e., the peripheral AP region of NS rats, exhibited increased release i.e., 5-7 ng/μl of PRL variants 1, 2, 4, and 6, and decreased release of PRL variants 3 and 5. When incubated with EE fractions from CM of the central AP region of NS rats, lactotrophs from the same region showed increased release of PRL variants in fractions 1 and 6, and lower release in fractions 2, 3, 4 and 5. Thus, except for the amounts of PRL released from fractions 1 and 6, whose levels were higher or similar to those of the other EE PRL variants, the amounts of other PRL variants released were significantly lower than those of the EE variants. When the central AP

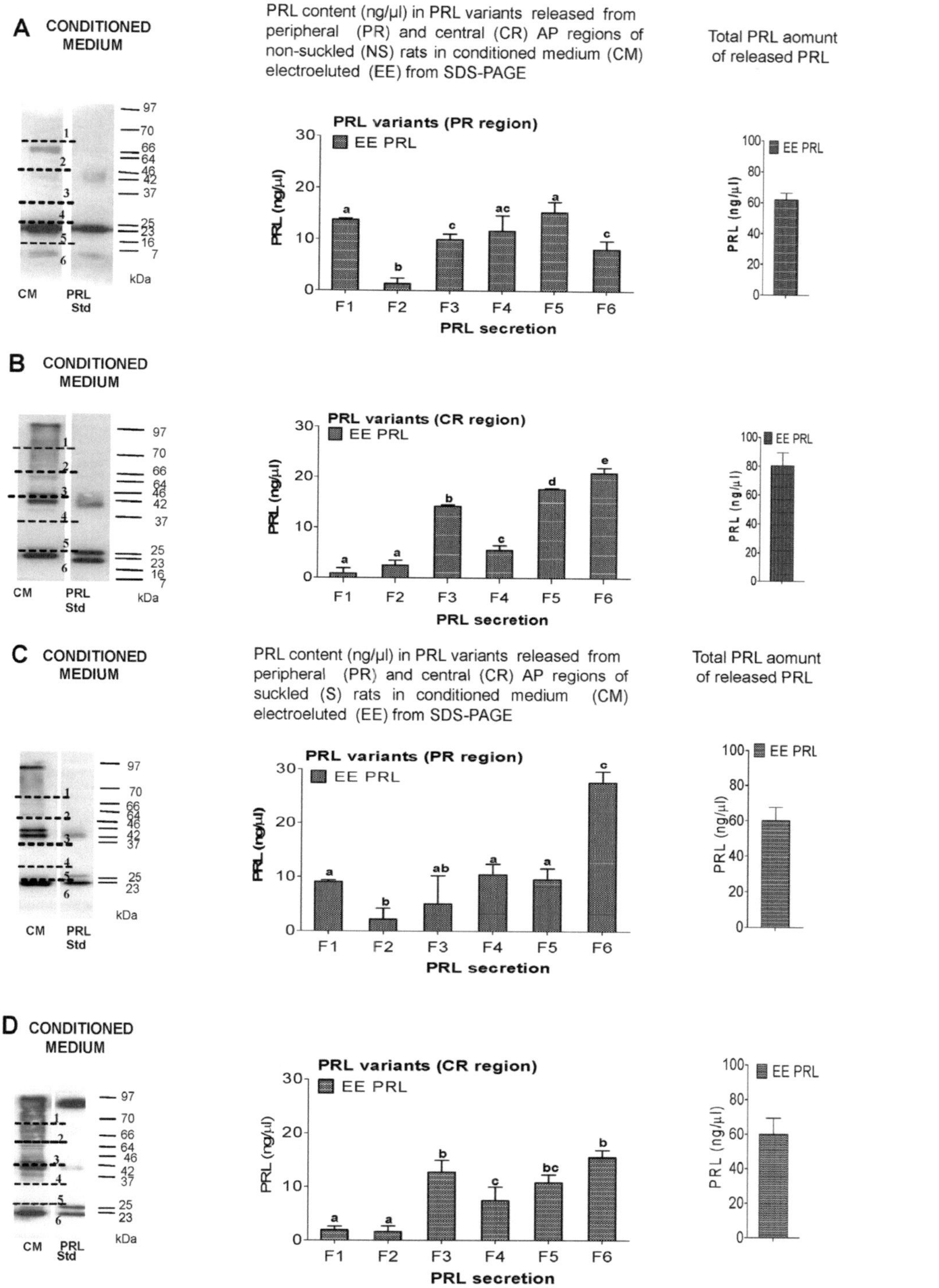

Figure 1. (A-B). SDS-PAGE (left panels) and prolactin (PRL) content (ng/μl) of PRL variants (middle and right panels) released from the peripheral (PR) and central (CR) adenohypophyseal

(AP) regions of non-suckled (NS) rats, and electroeluted (EE PRL) from fractions 1-6 of SDS-PAGE. Data are means ± SEM. Letters (a-d) indicates $P < 0.05$ difference between fractions of EE PRL.
(C-D). SDS-PAGE (left panels) and prolactin (PRL) content (ng/μl) of PRL variants (middle and right panels) released from peripheral (PR) and central (CR) AP regions of suckled (S) rats and electroeluted from fractions 1-6 of SDS-PAGE. Data are means ± SEM. Letters (a-d) indicates $P < 0.05$ for the difference of PRL content between electroeluted fractions.

region of NS rats was incubated with the EE PRL variants from the peripheral AP region of NS rats, medium levels (about 10 ng/μl) of PRL variants 1 and 6, and medium to low levels to PRL variants 2, 3, 4, and 5 were released. As a result of these effects, high levels of total PRL were released from the peripheral but not from the central AP region; indeed, total PRL release from the central AP region was significantly depressed, below the initial level.

In figure 2B, the PRL content of the EE control PRL variants released from the central AP region of NS rats was low in fractions 1, 2 and 4 of CM, and high (>10 ng/μl) in fractions 3, 5 and 6. Also, with respect to the effect of incubating lactotrophs from the central AP region of NS rats with the EE PRL variants from the peripheral AP region, increased release occurred only of PRL variants 1 and 6; and low levels occurred to PRL variants 2-5 from the central AP region; and only the PRL variant 6 was above the zero level, i.e., about 10 ng/μl. Overall, significantly lower levels of PRL than those contained both in the EE PRL variants and in those released from the peripheral region, were released from lactotrophs of both the central and peripheral AP regions.

4.1.3 .Effects of EE PRL variants released from AP regions of lactating non-suckled (NS) rats upon the in vitro release of PRL variants from lactotrophs of suckled (S) rat APs

The effect of incubating lactotrophs from AP regions of S rats with EE PRL variants released from AP regions of NS rats is shown in figures 2 C-D. In figure 2 C the PRL level was low in fraction 2, but medium to high levels, (about 10 ng/ μl) in fractions 1, 3-6; the amount of PRL released from the same AP region of S rats was around zero in fractions 2-5; and low in fractions 1 and 6. Overall, significantly lower amounts of PRL were released from the peripheral AP region of S rats. Also, as shown in figure 2D, the amount of EE PRL released from the central AP region of NS rat APs was low in fractions 1, 2 and 4 and high in fractions 3, 5 and 6; the total amount of released PRL from the peripheral AP region was zero in all fractions, and thus, it was significantly lower than that of the EE PRL. With respect to the amount of PRL released from the central AP region, only fractions 2 and 6 showed high levels and the levels of the other fractions were much lowers (1-3 ng/μl). Thus, as with the effect of CM from the PR of NS rats, the amount of released PRL from the peripheral AP region of S rats, was less than zero, i.e., lower than that of the EE control PRL, and of the still lower amount of PRL released from the central AP region, whose levels also were lower than those of the EE PRL.

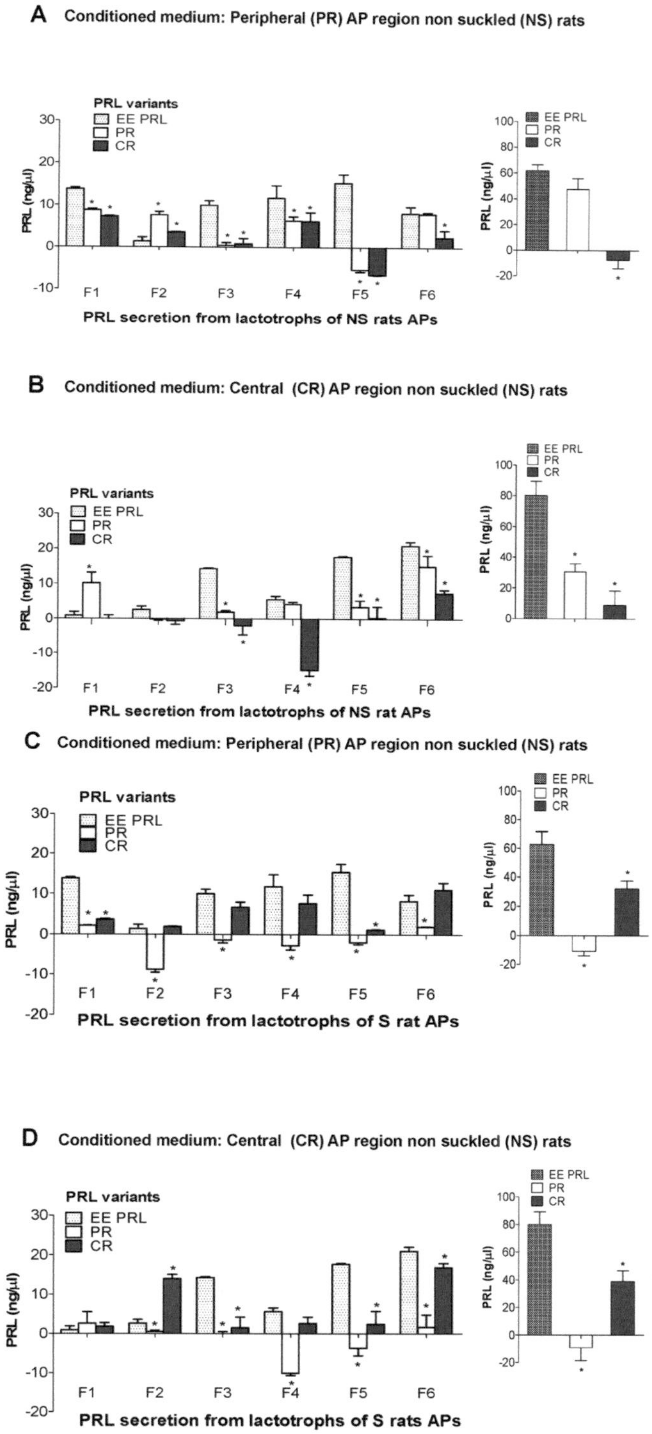

Figure 2. (A-B). Effect of the PRL variants electroeluted (EE PRL) in fractions 1-6 from SDS-PAGE of CM from the peripheral (PR) (panel A), and central (CR) (panel B), AP regions of non-suckled (NS)

lactating rats upon the *in vitro* release of PRL variants by lactotrophs from AP regions of NS lactating rats. Data are means ± SEM. *Differences $P < 0.05$ *versus* control (EE PRL). **(C-D).** Effect of the PRL variants electroeluted (EE PRL) in fractions 1-6 from SDS-PAGE of CM from the peripheral (PR) (panel A), and central (CR) (panel B), AP regions of non-suckled (NS) lactating rats upon the *in vitro* release of PRL variants by lactotrophs from AP regions of suckled (S) lactating rats. Data are means ± SEM. *Differences $P< 0.05$ *versus* control (EE PRL).

4.1.4. Effects of electroeluted PRL variants released from AP regions of lactating suckled (S) rats upon the in vitro release of PRL variants from lactotrophs of suckled (S) rat APs

The effect of incubating lactotrophs from AP regions of S rats, with EE PRL variants released from AP regions of S rats is shown in figures 3 A-B. As shown in figure 3A, the EE PRL content from the peripheral AP region (c.f. Fig. 1C-D) showed medium to high levels (5>20 ng/µl), in all fractions except fraction 2; the amount of PRL released from the peripheral AP region of S rats was medium to high in fractions 1, 3 and 6 and medium to low in fractions 2, 4 and 5; and with respect to the amount of EE PRL released from the central AP region of S rats, (figure 3B), low and medium levels (2 and 8-10 ng/µl), were found in fractions 1, 2 and 3-6, respectively; and with respect to the effect of incubating lactotrophs from the central AP region of S rats with EE PRL variants from the same AP region of S rats, the levels were low in fractions 1 and 2 and higher (around 10 ng/µl) in fractions 3-6; and after incubation with the EE PRL, medium to low levels (1-6 ng/µl) occurred in fractions 1 and 2, reduced levels (-10 ng) in fraction 4 and higher levels (8-10 ng/µl) in fractions 3, 5 and 6 of PRL variants were released from the peripheral AP region of S rats, below zero levels were released from fraction 4 of the same AP region; and there was only a small stimulatory effect on PRL variants 1, 2, 3, 5, and 6. EE control PRL reduced the release of PRL variants from the central AP region to below zero levels in all fractions. As a result of these effects, the total amount of PRL released from the peripheral AP region, and particularly from the central AP region, was significantly lower than that of both the EE PRL variants and of the amount released from the peripheral AP region.

4.1.5. Effects of electroeluted PRL variants, released from AP regions of lactating, suckled (S) rats, upon the in vitro release of PRL variants from lactotrophs of non-suckled (NS) rat APs

The effect of PRL variants released from AP regions of suckled rats upon the release of PRL variants from lactotrophs of the peripheral and the central AP regions of non-suckled rats is shown in figures 3 C-D. In Fig. 3C, the PRL content of the EE fractions from the CM of the peripheral AP regions of S rats was low to medium in fractions 2 and 3, medium to high in fractions 1, 4 and 5, and particularly high in fraction 6; and, as a result of incubation, the amount of PRL released from lactotrophs of the peripheral AP region of NS rats was low in fractions 1, 4-6, and high only in fractions 2 and 3; and from the central AP region of these rats, the amount of PRL released was particularly high in fractions 1 and 6; medium in fractions 2 and 3, and low in fractions 1 and 4-5. As a result of these interactions, the amount of total PRL released from both AP regions was significantly lower than the amount electroeluted from SDS-PAGE, but higher than that shown from NS and S rat AP regions, (c.f. Figs. 2 A-B), due to the effect of CM from NS and S rats.

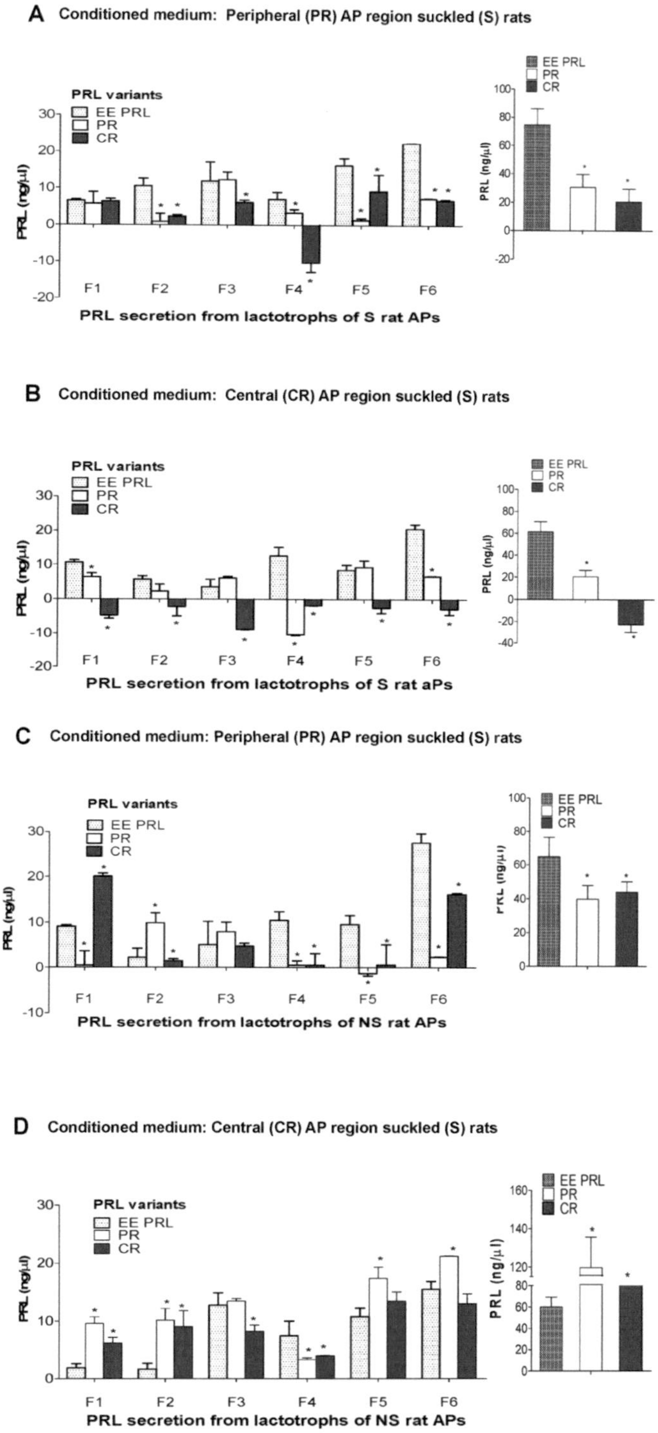

Figure 3. (A-B). Effect of the PRL variants electroeluted (EE PRL) in fractions 1-6 from SDS-PAGE of CM from the peripheral (PR) (panel A), and central (CR) (panel B), AP regions of suckled (S) lactating

rats upon the *in vitro* release of PRL variants by lactotrophs from AP regions of suckled (S) lactating rats. Data are means ± SEM. *Differences $P < 0.05$ *versus* control (EE PRL).
(C-D). Effect of the PRL variants electroeluted (EE PRL) in fractions 1-6 from SDS-PAGE of CM from the peripheral (PR) (panel A), and central (CR) (panel B), AP regions of suckled (S) lactating rats upon the *in vitro* release of PRL variants by lactotrophs from AP regions of non-suckled (NS) lactating rats. Data are means ± SEM. *Differences $P < 0.05$ *versus* control (EE PRL).

The PRL content of the electroeluted fractions from the central AP region of S rats was low in fractions 1 and 2, and high in fractions 3-6 of CM (Figure 3D). However, the amount of PRL released mainly from the peripheral, and in part also by the central AP region, was higher by the peripheral than the EE PRL variants in fractions 1, 2 and 5, 6; this level was about the same in fraction 3, and lower in fraction 4; and with respect to the amount of PRL released from the central AP region it was higher than the electroeluted hormone in fractions 1 and 2, lower in fraction 3 and 4, and about the same high level in fractions 5 and 6. As a result of these effects, an increased release of the hormone occurred from both AP regions, particularly from the peripheral region, whose levels, except from that of fraction 3, were significantly higher than those of the EE PRL as well as of that released from the central AP region, whose levels in fractions 1 and 2 were also higher than those of the EE PRL.

4.2. Effects of hypothalamic hormones upon the release of PRL variants from AP regions of NS and S rats

4.2.1. Dose-response effects of dopamine

The effects of dopamine (DA) upon the release of PRL variants 1-6 from the lactotrophs of the peripheral and central AP regions of non-suckled (NS) and suckled (S) rats are shown in figures 4 A-D. As shown in Fig. 4 A, as compared with the amount of PRL released without DA, the low dose of DA (0.5 μM) inhibited the release of PRL variant 2 and stimulated PRL variants 3 and 5 of the peripheral AP regions of NS rats, and showed no effect upon the release of PRL variants 4 and 6 from the same AP region. Higher doses of DA increased the release of PRL variants in fractions 3 and 5, but 1.5 μM DA inhibited the release of PRL variants 1 and 6. As a result of these effects, the total amount of released PRL from the peripheral AP region of NS rats was decreased only by the highest dose of DA (1.5 μM) but not by the lower and intermediate doses.

The effects of dopamine upon the release of PRL variants from lactotrophs of the central AP regions of non-suckled rats are shown in figure 4 B. The low dose of DA inhibited the release of the PRL variant 1 and showed no effect upon PRL variants 2 and 4, but it promoted a strong release of PRL variants 3, 5 and 6 from the central AP regions of NS rats; 1.0 μM dopamine provoked decreased release of PRL variant 1, and increased release of PRL variants 2, 3, 5 and 6. With 1.5 μM DA, decreased release occurred in fraction 1, and increased release in fractions 3, 5 and 6.

With respect to the effects of DA upon the release of PRL variants from the peripheral AP region of suckled rats APs, as shown in figure 4 C, at the low dose of DA inhibition occurred in fraction 3, stimulation of PRL in fractions 2, 5 and 6, and no effect on PRL variants in fractions

1 and 4. In the presence of 1.0 μM DA there was inhibition of PRL variants in fraction 3, no effect in fraction 4, and stimulation in fractions 2 and 5, 6. The total amount of PRL released from the peripheral AP region of S rats was decreased only by 1.0 and 1.5 μM DA, but not by the lower dose. The effects of DA upon the release of PRL variants from lactotrophs of

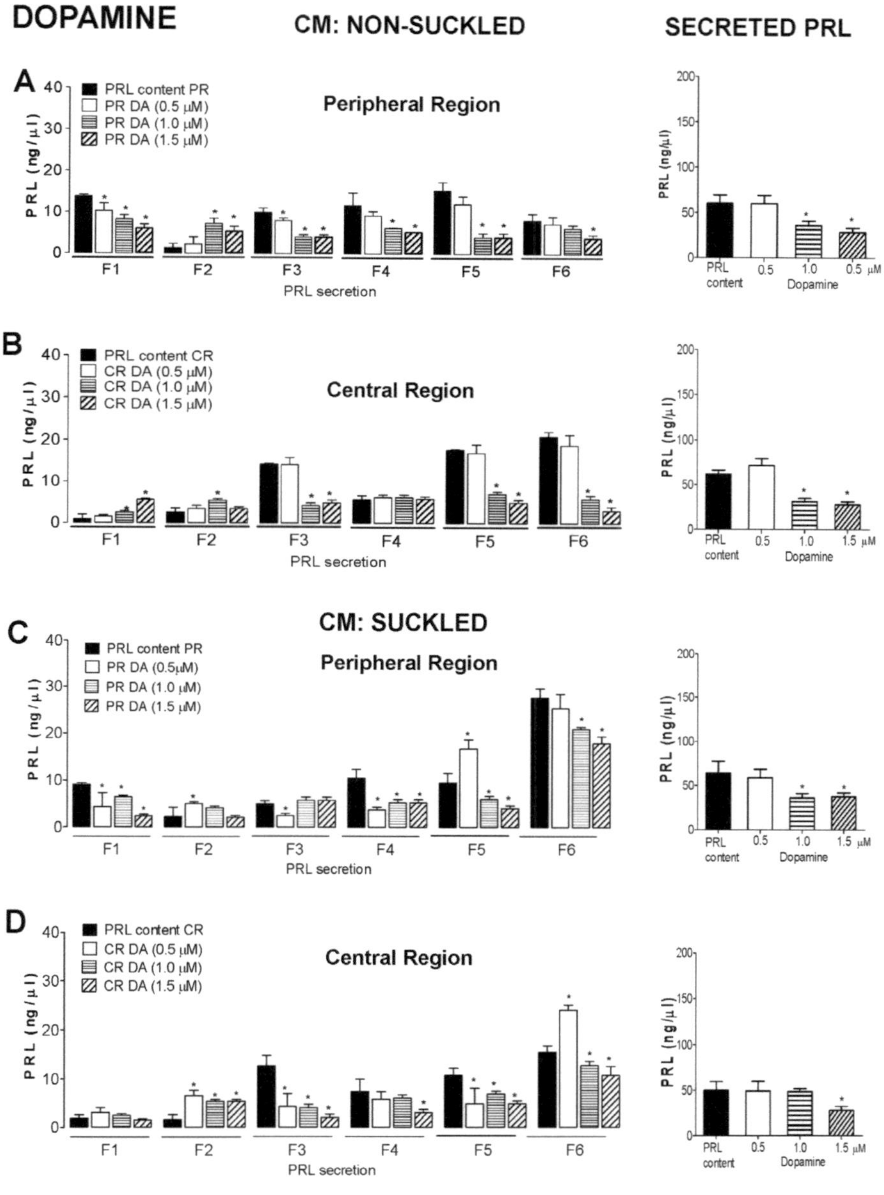

Figure 4. A-D. Effect of dose-response of the PRL variants electroeluted in fractions 1-6 from SDS-PAGE of CM from the peripheral (PR) and the central (CR) regions of adenohypophysis (AP) of suckled (S) and non-suckled (NS) lactating rats incubated with 0.5, 1.0 and 1.5 μM of dopamine (DA), upon the *in vitro* release of PRL variants by lactotrophs from AP regions of NS and S lactating rats. Data are means ± SEM. *Differences $P < 0.05$ *versus* control (PRL content without DA).

the central AP region of suckled rats are shown in figure 4 D. The low dose of DA inhibited the release of PRL in fraction 1, had no effect upon the release of the PRL variant 3, but it promoted the release of PRL variants 2, 4 and 6; the intermediate dose of DA also inhibited the release of PRL from fraction 1, and promoted the release of fractions 2, 4 and 6; 1.5 μM DA inhibited the release of PRL fractions 1 and 2, but it promoted the release of fractions 3-6.

4.2.2. Dose-response effects of TRH

The effects of different doses of TRH, i.e., 0.1, 1.0 and 10 μM, upon the release of PRL variants from AP regions of NS and S rats are shown in Figs. 5 A-D and the values obtained after TRH, are compared with the control values of PRL that were released in the absence of TRH. As compared with control values, without TRH, 0.1 μM TRH provoked increased release, i.e., stimulation of PRL, in fractions 1, 3-6; and inhibition in fraction 2 from the peripheral AP region of NS rats (Fig. 5 A). The effect of 1.0 and 10 μM TRH was to increase the release of all PRL variants 1-6.

The effect of TRH upon the release of PRL variants from the central AP region of NS rats is shown in Fig. 5 B. With 0.1 μM TRH, decreased release of PRL occurred in fraction 1, no change in fractions 2 and 4, and increased release in fractions 3, 5 and 6. Also, with respect to the effect of the higher doses of TRH, increased release occurred to PRL in all fractions 1-6. Fig. 5 C, shows the effect of the low dose of TRH upon the release of PRL variants from the peripheral AP region of S rats. As shown there, release of PRL variants 1, 4, 5 and 6 was stimulated, and there was no effect on PRL variants 2 and 3; and with respect to the effect of the low dose of TRH upon the release of PRL variants from the central AP region of S rats (Fig. 5 D) a decreased release of PRL variant 1; increased release of PRL variants 3, 4 and 6, and no effect upon PRL variants 2 and 5 were observed.

4.2.3. Dose-response effects of oxytocin

The dose-response effects of oxytocin (OT) upon the release of PRL variants from NS rat APs are shown in Figs. 6 A-D. With 0.1 μM oxytocin, increased release of PRL, relative to the control, occurred only for PRL variants 3, 5 and 6 of the PR region of NS rat APs, but the release of PRL in fractions 1, 2 and 4 was inhibited. With respect to the effect of 1.0 μM of oxytocin upon the release of PRL variants from the peripheral AP region of NS rats (Fig. 6 A), there was increased release of PRL variants 3, 5 and 6 and reduce release of PRL variants 1, 2 and 4 from lactotrophs of the peripheral AP region. The high dose of OT, i.e., 10 μM resulted in increased release of PRL variants 2, 3, 5 and 6 from the peripheral AP region and to variants 1-6 from the central AP region of NS rats (Fig. 6 B); and with respect to the effect of the 10 μM OT upon the release of PRL from AP regions of S rats, increased release from the peripheral region occurred for PRL variants 1, 2, 5 and 6; whit no effect on release of PRL variants 3 and 4. Finally, with respect to the effect of the high dose of OT upon AP regions of NS rats, there was increased release of fractions 2, 3, 5 and 6 and no effect on fractions 1 and 3 from the peripheral AP region of NS rats; and with the exception of fraction 5 in which there was no effect, increased release occurred in all the other fractions from the central AP region of the NS rats; and upon the effect of the same dose of oxytocin upon the release of PRL variants from the peripheral AP region of S rats, i.e., Fig. 6 C, also, increased release occurred to PRL variant 5; inhibition to PRL variant 1, and no effect upon PRL variants 2, 3, 4 and 6. And with respect to the effect of the same dose of OT i.e., 1.0 μM upon the release of PRL variants from the central AP region of suckled rats, i.e., Fig. 6 D, lower panel, increased release occurred to PRL variants 1, 2, 5 and 6, and no effect upon PRL variants 3 and 4; and with respect to the effect of the same dose of OT upon the release of PRL variants from the

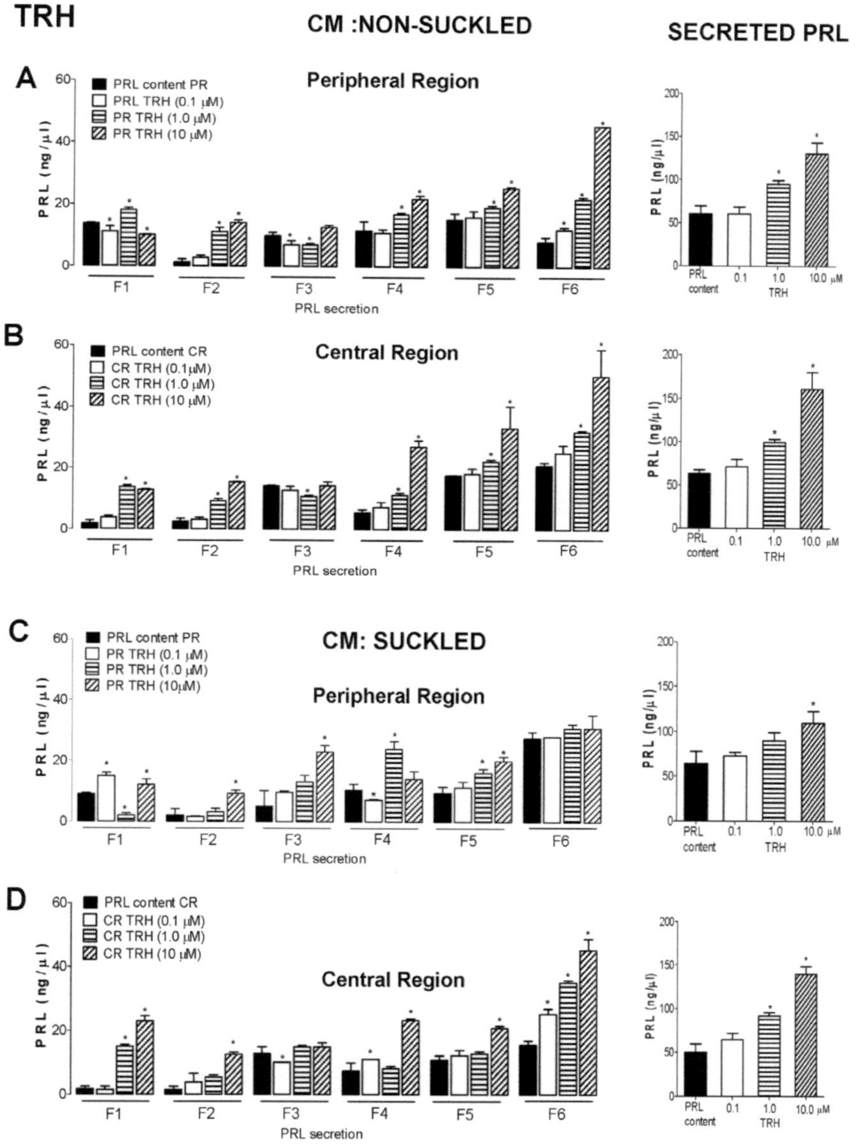

Figure 5. A-D. Effect of dose-response of the PRL variants electroeluted in fractions 1-6 from SDS-PAGE of CM from the peripheral (PR) and the central (CR) regions of adenohypophysis (AP) of suckled (S) and non-suckled (NS) lactating rats incubated with 0.1, 1.0 and 10 μM of TRH, upon the *in vitro* release of PRL variants by lactotrophs from AP regions of NS and S lactating rats. Data are means ± SEM. *Differences $P < 0.05$ *versus* control (PRL content without TRH).

same, i.e., peripheral AP region of S rats, increased release occurred to PRL variants 1, 2 and 5, 6; and no effect upon PRL variants 3 and 4. Finally, with respect to the effect of the high dose of OT upon the release of PRL from lactotrophs of the PR region of S rats, increased release occurred to PRL variants 1, 2, 5 and 6, with no change of PRL variants 3 and 4; the high dose of OT resulted in increased release of all PRL variant from lactotrophs of the central AP region.

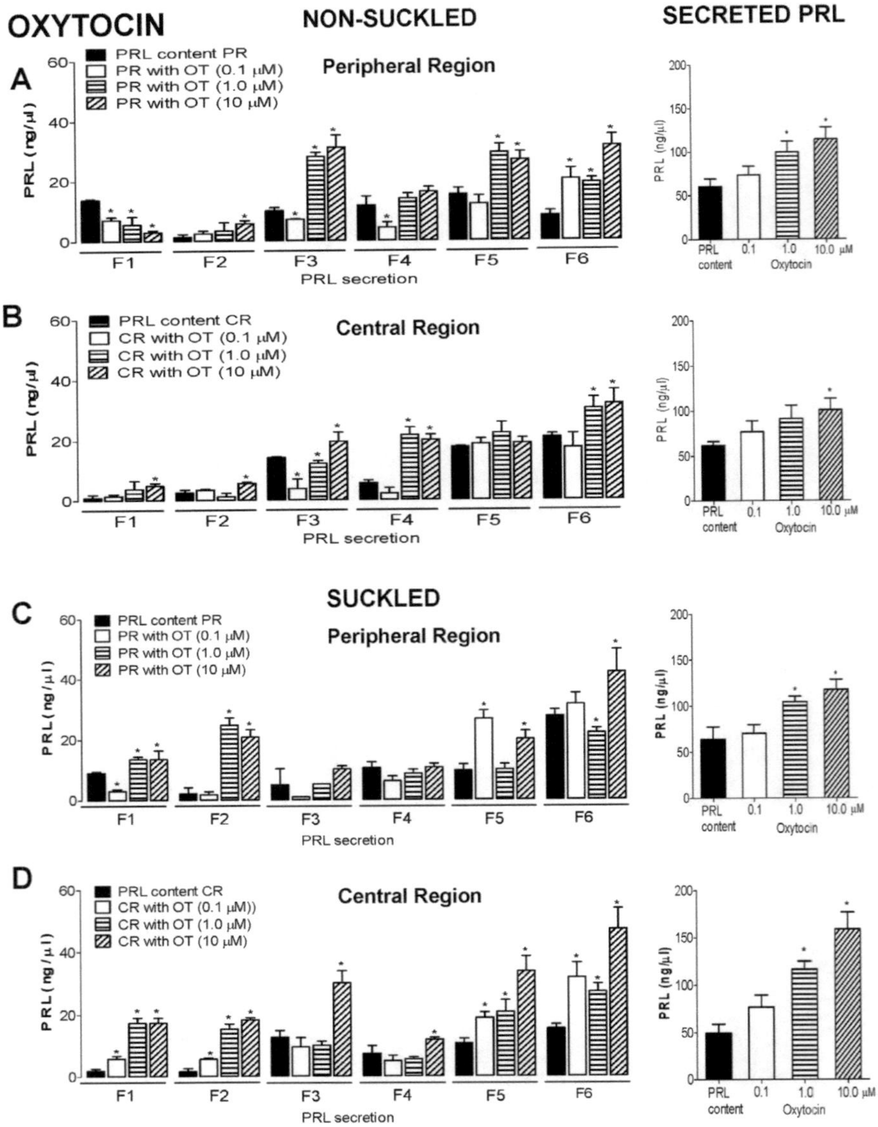

Figure 6. A-D. Effect of dose-response of the PRL variants electroeluted in fractions 1-6 from SDS-PAGE of CM from the peripheral (PR) and the central (CR) regions of adenohypophysis (AP) of suckled (S) and non-suckled (NS) lactating rats incubated with 0.1, 1.0 and 10 μM of oxytocin (OT), upon the *in vitro* release of PRL variants by lactotrophs from AP regions of NS and S lactating rats. Data are means ± SEM. *Differences $P < 0.05$ *versus* control (PRL content without OT).

4.3. Electrical activity upon neurons

4.3.1. Effect of conditioned medium from the lateral and central AP regions of S rats upon cultured sympathetic neurons

Cultured sympathetic neurons, previously incubated with Fluo 4, to record variations of intracellular [Ca^{2+}], showed clear increases of [Ca^{2+}] within 60 sec of adding conditioned medium (CM) from lactating rats, thus indicating that these neurons were activated by the CM (Figure 7). These effects did not occurred when the neurons were incubated with medium from male rat APs (data not shown).

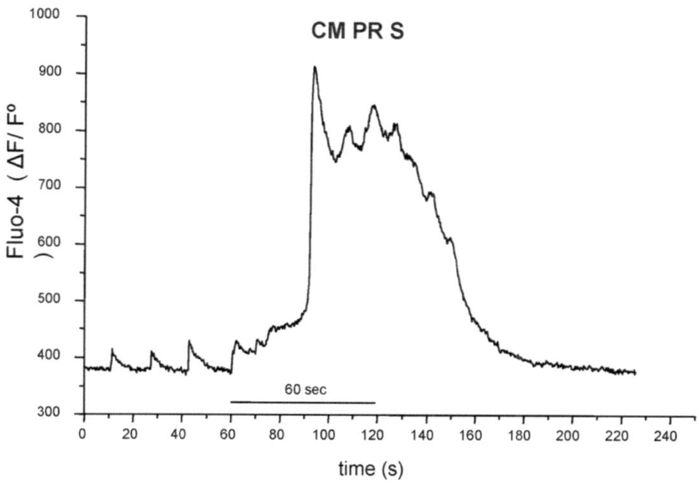

Figure 7. Effect of 60 s exposure of conditioned medium from the peripheral region of suckled rat APs (CM PRS).upon intracellular calcium concentration in cultured sympathetic neurons.

4.3.2. Effect of conditioned medium from the lateral AP region of suckled and of male rat APs upon electrical activity of male rat lactotrophs, and of astrocytes from the hippocampus and medial preoptic area

As shown in Figures 8 A-D, CM of the peripheral region (CMPR) from male rat APs had no effect upon electrical activity of hippocampal astrocytes (Fig. 8A) whereas application of CM from lactating, suckled rats provoked a cationic inward current, shown as a downward deflection in male lactotrophs (Fig. 8C), as well as in astrocytes from the hippocampus and medial preoptic area (Figs. 8B, D). These responses remained for several seconds after washing CMPR out.

4.3.3. Effect of conditioned medium from lactating and male rat APs upon [Ca^{2+}] concentration in astrocytes from the hippocampus

As shown in Figure 9, CM from lactating, suckled rats (Fig. 9A), but not from male rat APs (Fig. 9B) or from non-suckled rats (data not shown) provoked an increased [Ca^{2+}] in hippocampal astrocytes similar to that induced by application of 120 mM K^+ (see Fig. 9C).

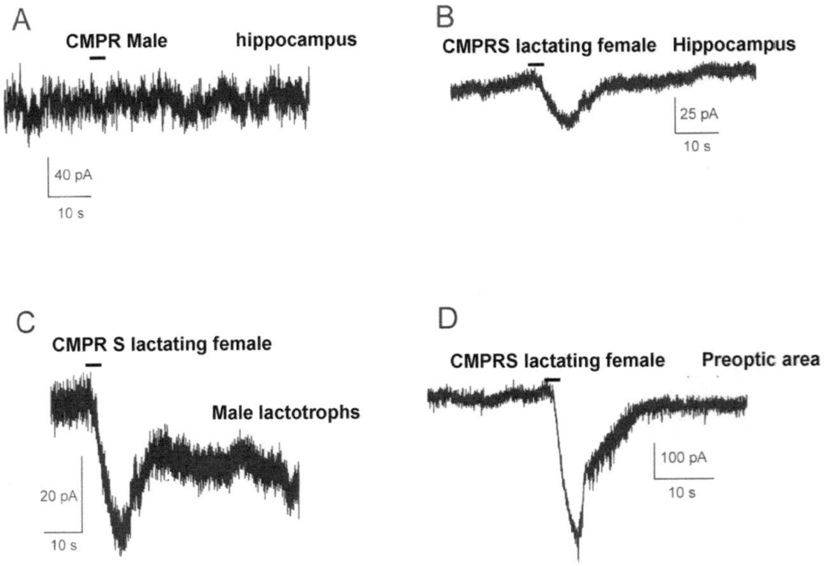

Figure 8. (A-D). Effect of a 1 h incubation with conditioned medium (CM), from the peripheral region (PR) of male rats (A), and from suckled lactating rat APs (B-D) upon hippocampal astrocytes (B), neurons from the preoptic area (D) and upon male rat lactotrophs (C).

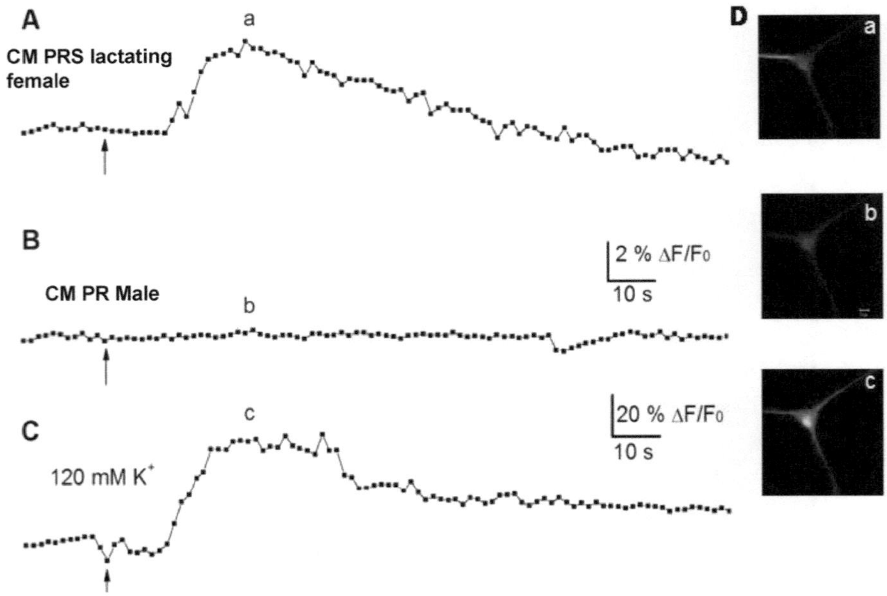

Figure 9. (A-C). Effect of conditioned media from the peripheral AP region of suckled lactating rats (CMPR) and of male rats upon intracellular calcium concentration in hippocampal astrocytes (A-B). Arrow in C indicates the application of 120 mM K^+. Images in D are from astrocytes in A-C.

5. Conclusions

This study confirms that PRL variants ranging from 7 to 97 kDa are released from tissue fragment of each AP region of the anterior pituitary gland of non-suckled and suckled lactating rats. When these variants are electroeluted from SDS-PAGE and then incubated with lactotrophs from each AP region of the same type of rats, they exert different effects (promotion, inhibition or no effect) upon the release of PRL variants from lactotrophs of both AP regions of NS and S lactating rats. In support of this was the fact that the immunoprecipitation of PRL contained in the CM from lactating rats, prevented the effects of PRL variants upon PRL release. Thus, these results indicate that autocrine regulatory effects are exerted by PRL variants upon the release of other variants of the hormone from lactating rat APs, and they are in accord with previous studies showing autoregulation of PRL secretion (Nagy et al., 1991; Nagy & Frawley, 1990; Diaz et al., 2002; Spies & Clegg, 1971; Hebert et al., 1979; Melmed et al., 1980). Similar effects on male lactotrophs by CM from pregnant and lactating females and steroid-treated castrated males or females, but not by CM from intact males or by a PRL standard were reported previously (Huerta-Ocampo et al., 2007; Mena et al., 2010).

Prior to fractionation the total PRL variants from both, the central and peripheral AP regions of NS rats stimulated the release of PRL from the peripheral region, but they inhibited its release from the central AP region. However, when CM from lactating rats was fractionated by SDS-PAGE, eluates of fractions 5 and 6 containing 23-25 kDa PRL had the greatest effect on PRL release, although weaker immunoreactive bands with lower, or even inhibitory activity, were also detected in the upper gel fractions. In addition, separation by SDS-PAGE and electroelution of PRL variants indicated that CM from the lactating rat pituitary contains 37 to 46 kDa PRL variants as well as 23 to 25 kDa PRL variants, that exert different effects upon the release of other PRL variants from the lactating rat pituitary and from APs of rats in different conditions Huerta-Ocampo et al., 2007; Mena et al., 2010). Therefore, the present study shows that the lactating rat pituitary produces PRL variants that are absent or deficient in the male pituitary gland and in the PRL Standard, even though the AP of male and of other types of rats, do respond to stimulatory factors released from the anterior pituitary of lactating rats (Mena et al., 2010). The results presented here, together with those in our previous study, also indicate that several PRL variants are produced and released by the lactating rat pituitary (Denef, 1988; Sinha 1992; Asawaroengchai et al., 1978); this hormonal heterogeneity may be physiologically very relevant in the context of autoregulatory mechanisms determining the wide range of PRL effects under different physiological conditions (Schwartz & Cherny, 1992; Schwartz, 2000; Sinha, 1992) and upon different structures (Ben-Jonathan et al., 2001; Lorenson & Walker, 2001; Ho et al., 1993; Celotti et al., 1997).

In addition to the regulatory effects of PRL variants from lactating rats upon the release of the hormone, further evidence of these effects was obtained when CM's from lactating rats were treated with phosphatase or with endoglycosidase which increased their ability, i.e., that of the PRL variants present in them to stimulate PRL release from lactating rat APs, similar to the effect shown previously upon male rat lactotrophs (Mena et al., 2010). These effects of dephosphorylation and deglycosylation of CM provide additional evidence that PRL variants in CM are responsible for the effects upon lactating rat lactotrophs. PRL released from the AP of lactating and non-lactating rats is phosphorylated and glycosylated and thus, it is less bioactive than the dephosphorylated and deglycosylated variants (Ho et al., 1993a; Sinha, 1995, Ho et al., 1993b).

In the present study we also analyzed whether the ability of the hypothalamic hormones dopamine, TRH and oxytocin, as established by many previous *in vivo* and *in vitro* studies (Mena et al., 1989), to regulate the release of AP PRL, would be manifest by their direct action upon the lactotrophs and interaction with the autocrine actions of PRL variants; and whether these effects would finally promote or inhibit the release of PRL variants, thereby regulating the release of the hormone. The results obtained showed that the effects of the hypothalamic hormones were exerted upon the lactotrophs both by interacting with the autocrine actions of the PRL variants, and also by regulating the release of PRL variants from these cells. Thus, when a high dose (1.5 μM) of DA was applied directly upon the lactotrophs of NS and S rats, the secretion of most PRL variants from both AP regions of non-suckled and suckled rats was inhibited, as previously reported by others (Nagy et al., 1991), whereas the lower dose (0.5 μM) slightly stimulated the release of PRL variants, mainly from the central AP region of suckled rats. TRH provoked an increased release of some PRL variants from both the central and peripheral AP regions of NS and S rats, and OT at 1 and 10 μM, showed an intense stimulatory effect, particularly of 23-34 kDa PRL, from both AP regions of non-suckled and suckled lactating rat APs. Thus, these effects of hypothalamic hormones upon the release of PRL variants may also regulate, and thus interact with, the autocrine effects exerted by the PRL variants and lead to an integrative regulation of PRL secretion (Mena et al., 1989; Mena et al., 2011).

This study shows that when pituitaries from male rats are incubated for a short period of time in conditioned media from each pituitary region of lactating rats, either suckled or non-suckled, there is a significant dose-dependent increase of PRL release from male rat lactotrophs. Also, as shown previously (Mena et al., 2010) our results obtained by Western blotting confirm that CM from lactating rat pituitary contains several prolactin variants, i.e., 37-46 kDa as well as 16-25 kDa, capable of stimulating PRL release from male rat pituitary. In addition, CM obtained from male rat pituitary regions as well as PRL standard have no significant stimulatory effect on PRL secretion of pituitary regions from either lactating or male rats (Huerta-Ocampo, 2007; Mena et al., 2010), this suggests that the male pituitary gland is deficient in the same PRL variants, and of other possible factors, that are released by the lactating rat AP, even though it does contain receptors for stimulating factors released from the anterior pituitary of lactating rats (Mena et al., 2011; Mena et al., 2012a).

Based upon these results, it was of interest to determine whether production and release of pituitary prolactin variants contained in CM from lactating rats under different conditions, and their effects upon PRL release from incubated male AP regions, vary depending on the animal's physiological condition, and whether CM's from lactating or male rats exert effect upon brain structures, i.e., astrocytes in the hippocampus and medial preoptic area, and of sympathetic neurons (Fiordelisio & Hernandez-Cruz, 2002). The results obtained from Electrical recording of these astrocytes showed that astrocytic activation occurred upon exposure to CM from the lateral and central regions of lactating suckled rat APs (Hernández-Morales M & García-Colunga, 2009).

In conclusion, the results of the present and previous studies suggest that, in addition to regulation by hypothalamic and other influences, the release of PRL variants from the lactating rat AP is also regulated by autocrine influences exerted upon the gland by the previously released PRL variants; furthermore in parallel and interacting with such autocrine regulation, the effect of the hypothalamic hormones on PRL release is also regulated through the same mechanism i.e., the stimulation or inhibition of the release of PRL variants from the pituitary gland. Moreover, the present results confirm previous findings (Huerta-Ocampo, 2007; Mena et al., 2010; Mena et al., 2011; Möderscheim et al., 2007, Mena et al., 2012a), that CM from lactating rats, contain prolactin variants capable of inducing rapid release of PRL from the untreated male rat pituitary, and that they can also activate of astrocytes and neurons in different areas of the central and peripheral nervous system (Mena et al, 2012b).

Abbreviations

AP	Anterior pituitary
$[Ca^{2+}]$	Intracellular calcium concentration
CM	Conditioned media
CR	Central region
DA	Dopamina
EE	Electroeluted
EA	Electrical activity
ELISA	Enzyme-linked immunoabsorbant assay
KDa	Kilodalton
NR	Non-reducing
NS	Non-suckled
OT	Oxytocin
PR	Peripheral region
PRL	Prolactin
S	Suckled
TRH	Thyrotropin releasing hormone

Author details

Flavio Mena, Nilda Navarro and Alejandra Castilla
Departamento de Neurobiología Celular y Molecular, Instituto de Neurobiología, Universidad Nacional Autónoma de México, Campus Juriquilla, Querétaro, México

Funding

This work was supported by Grants from PAPIIT-DGAPA-UNAM (IN201808 and IN206711), and by from CONACyT (No. 128037).

Acknowledgement

We gratefully acknowledge Dr. A.F. Parlow and the National Hormone and Pituitary Program of the National Institute of Diabetes and Digestive and Kidney Diseases for the generous gift of rat PRL, and the corresponding antiserum. Finally, we gratefully acknowledge the help of Martin Garcia Servín Head of the Animal Facilities at INB (Universidad Nacional Autónoma de México), and in particular to Dr. Dorothy Pless for reading and correcting the manuscript.

6. References

Asawaroengchai, H., Russell, S.M., & Nicoll, C.S. (1978). Electrophoretically separable forms of rat prolactin with different bioassay and radioimmunoassay activities. *Endocrinology*. 102(2):407-414.

Ben-Jonathan, N., & Hnasko, R. (2001). Hypotalamic control of prolactin synthesis and secretion. *In*: Horseman ND. Amsterdam (ed.), *Prolactin*, Kluwer Academic, pp. 1-24.

Bollengier, F., Mahler, A., Matton, A., & Vanhaelst, L. (1996). Molecular heterogeneity and glycosylation modulation of rat pituitary isoforms synthesized and secreted In vitro in postnatal ontogeny, gestation, lactation and weaning. *Neuroendocrinology*. 8(9):721-730.

Bollengier, F., Velkeniers, B., Hooghe-Peters, E., Mahler, A., & Vanhaelst, L. (1989). Multiple forms of prolactin and growth hormone in pituitary cell subpopulations separated using a Percoll gradient system: disulphide-bridge dimers and glycosylated variants. *J Endocrinol*. 120(2):201-206.

Boockfor, F.R., & Frawley, L.S. (1987). Functional variations among prolactin cell from different pituitary regions. *Endocrinology*. 120(3):874-879.

Boockfor, F.R., Hoeffler, J.P., & Frawley, L.S. (1986). Estradiol induces a shift in cultured cells that release prolactin or growth hormone. *Am J Physiol*. 250(1Pt1):103-105.

Celotti, F., Negro-Cesi, P., & Poletti, A. (1997). Steroid metabolism in the mammalian brain: 5alpha-reduction and aromatization. *Brain Res Bull*. 44(4):365-375.

Chen C.L, Voogt, J.L. & Meites, J. (1968). Effect of median eminence implants of FSH, LH or prolactin on luteal function in the rat. *Endocrinology*. 83(3):1273-1277.

Denef, C. (1988). Autocrine/Paracrine intermediates in hormonal action and modulation of cellular responses to hormones. In: Cellular Endocrinology. Section 7: *The Endocrine System*, New York, Oxford University Press, Vol 1. pp. 461-514.

Denef, C. (2008). Paracrinicity: The Story of 30 Years of Cellular Pituitary Crosstalk. *J Neuroendocrinol*. 20(1):1-70

Diaz, N., Huerta-Ocampo, I., Marina, N., Navarro, N., & Mena, F. (2002). Regional mechanisms within anterior pituitary of lactating rats may regulate prolactin secretion. *Endocrine*. 18(1):41-46.

Fiordelisio, T., & Hernandez-Cruz, A. (2002). Oestrogen regulates neurofilament expression in a subset of anterior pituitary cells of the adult female rat. *J Neuroendocrinol*. 14(5):411-424.

Frawley, L.S., & Boockfor, F.R. (1991). Mammosomatotropes: presence and functions in normal and neoplastic pituitary tissue. *Endocr Rev*. 12(4):337-355.

Freeman, M.E.,. Kanyicska, B., Lerant, A., & Nagy G. (2000). Prolactin: structure, function and regulation of secretion. *Physiol Rev*. 80(4):1523-1631.

Grosvenor, C.E., Mena, F. & Schaefgen, D.A. (1967). Effect of non-suckling interval and duration of suckling upon the suckling-induced fall in pituitary prolactin concentration in the rat. *Endocrinology*. 81(3):449-453.

Hebert, D.C., Ishikawa, H., & Rennels, E.G. (1979). Evidence for the autoregulation of hormone secretion by prolactin. *Endocrinology*. 104(1):97-105.

Hernández-Morales, M., & García-Colunga, J. (2009): Effects of nicotine on K+ currents and nicotinic receptors in astrocytes of the hippocampal CA1 region. *Neuropharmacology.* 56(6-7):975-983.

Ho, T.W., Leong, F.S., Olaso, C.H., & Walker, A.M. (1993). Secretion of specific nonphosphorylated and phosphorylated rat prolactin isoforms at different stages of the estrous cycle. *Neuroendocrinology.* 58(2): 160-165.

Huerta-Ocampo, I., Fiordelisio, T., Díaz, N. Navarro, N., Castilla, A., Cárabez, A., Aguilar, A.M., Morales, T., Hernández-Cruz, A., & Mena, F. (2007). Vesicular release of prolactin from preformed prolactin granules is stimulated by soluble factor(s) from pituitaries of lactating rats. *Neuroendocrinology.* 85(1):1-15.

Kadowaki, J., Ku, N., Oetting, W.S., & Walker, A.M. (1984). Mammotroph autoregulation: Uptake of secreted prolactin and inhibition of secretion. *Endocrinology.* 114(6):2060-2067.

Kordon, C. (1985). Neural mechanisms involved in pituitary control. *Neurochem Int.* 7(6):917-925.

Lorenson, M.Y., & Walker, AM. (2001). Structure–function relationships in prolactin. In: Horseman ND. Amsterdam (ed.), *Prolactin.* Kluwer Academic, pp.189-217.

MacLeod, R.M., Smith, M.C., & Dewitt, G.W. (1966). Hormonal properties of transplanted pituitary tumors and their relation to the pituitary gland. *Endocrinology.* 79(6):1149-1156.

Mansur, G., & Hymer, W.C. (1985). Characterization of immunoreactive and bioactive forms of prolactin in the rat pituitary. In: McCleod RM, Thorner M, Scapagnini U. Padova (eds.), *Prolactin,* Basic and Clinical Correlates, Liviana Press, pp. 501-507.

Maurer, R.A. (1982). Estradiol regulates the transcription of the prolactin gene. *J Biol Chem.* 257(5):2133-2136.

Maurer, R.A., & Gorski, J. (1977). Effects of estradiol-17beta and pimozide on prolactin synthesis in male and female rats. *Endocrinology.* 101(1):76-84.

Melmed, S., Carlson, H.E., Briggs, J., & Hershman J.M. (1980). Autofeedback of prolactin in cultured prolactin-secreting pituitary cells. *Horm Res.* 12(6):340-344.

Mena, F., & Grosvenor, C.E. (1972). Effect of suckling and of exteroceptive stimulation upon PRL release in the rat during late lactation. *J Endocrinol.* 52(1):11-22.

Mena, F. Martinez-Escalera, G., Clapp, C., & Grosvenor, C. (1984).In-vivo and in-vitro secretion of prolactin by lactating rat adenohypophyses as a function of intracellular age. *J Endocrinol.* 101(1):27-32.

Mena, F., Clapp, C., Aguayo, D., Morales, M.T., Grosvenor, C.E., Martinez de la Escalera, G. (1989). Regulation of prolactin secretion by dopamine and thyrotropin-releasing hormone in lactating rat adenohypophyses: influence of intracellular age of the hormone. *Endocrinology.* 125(4):1814-1820.

Mena, F., Hummelt, G., Aguayo, D., Clapp, C., Martinez de la Escalera, G., Morales, T. (1992). Changes in molecular variants during in vitro transformation and release of prolactin by the pituitary gland of the lactating rat. *Endocrinology.* 130(6):3365-3377.

Mena, F., Montiel, J.L., Aguayo, D., Morales, M.T., & Aramburo, C. (1993). Recent findings on prolactin transformation by the lactating rat pituitary. *Endocr Regul.* 27(3):105-113.

Mena, F., Navarro, N., & Castilla, A. (2011). Regulatory effects of dopamine, oxytocin and thyrotropin-releasing hormone on the release of prolactin variants from the adenohypophysis of lactating rats. *International Journal of Endocrinology & Metabolism.* 9(3):382-390.

Mena, F., Navarro, N., & Castilla, A. (2012a). Autocrine regulation of prolactin secretion by prolactin variants released from lactating rat adenohypophysis. *Acta Endocrinologica,* In press.

Mena, F., Navarro, N., Castilla, A., Fiordelisio, T., Morales, T., Hernández-Morales, M., & García-Colunga, J. (2012b). Release of prolactin (PRL) from pituitary lactotrophs of male rats and functional activity of astrocytes from hippocampal and medial preoptic area, and of sympathetic neurons, are stimulated by PRL variants released from the anterior pituitary (AP) of lactating rats. *Neuroendocrinology*. Envoy.

Mena, F., Navarro, N., Castilla, A., Morales, T. Fiordelisio, T. Cárabez, A., Aguilar, M.B., Huerta-Ocampo, I. (2010). Prolactin released In vitro from the pituitary of lactating, pregnant, and steroid-treated female or male rats stimulates prolactin secretion from pituitary lactotrophs of male rats. *Neuroendocrinology*. 91(1):77-93.

Möderscheim, T.A.E., Gorba, T., Pathipati, P., Kokay, I.C., Grattan, D.R., Williams, C.E., & Scheepens, A. (2007). Prolactin is involved in glial responses following a focal injury to the juvenile rat brain. *Neuroscience*. 145(3):963-973.

Moore, H.P., Andresen, JM., Eaton, BA., Grabe, M., Haugwitz, M., Wu, MM., & Machen, TE. (2002). Biosynthesis and secretion of pituitary hormones: dynamics and regulation. *Arch Physiol Biochem*. 110(1-2), 16-25.

Morales, T., Shapiro, E., & Mena, F. (2001). Beta-adrenergic mechanisms modulate central nervous system effects of prolactin on milk ejection. *Physiol Behav*. 74(1-2):119-126.

Nagy, G.M., & Frawley, L.S. (1990). Suckling increases the proportions of mammotropes responsive to various prolactin-releasing stimuli. *Endocrinology*. 127(5):2079-2084.

Nagy, G.M., Bookfor, F.M., & Frawley, L.S. (1991). The suckling stimulus increase the responsiveness of mammotropes located exclusively within the central region of the adenohypophysis. *Endocrinology*. 128(2):761-764.

Nicoll, C.S., Parsons, J.A., Fiorindo, R.P., & Nichols, C.W. (1969). Estimation of prolactin and growth hormone levels by polyacrylamide disc electrophoresis. *J Endocrinol*. 45(2):183-197.

Papka, R.E., Yu, S.M., & Nikitovitch-Winer, M.B. (1986). Use of immunoperoxidase and immunogold methods in studying prolactin secretion and application of immunogold labelling for pituitary hormones and neuropeptides. *Am J Anat*. 175(2-3):289-306.

Schwartz, J, & Cherny, R. (1992). Intercellular communication within the anterior pituitary influencing the secretion of hypophyseal hormones. *Endocr Rev*. 13(3):453-475.

Schwartz, J. Intercellular communication in the anterior pituitary. *Endocr Rev*. 21(5):488-513.

Sgouris, J.T., & Meites, J. (1953). Differential inactivation of prolactin by mammary tissue from pregnant and parturient rats. *Am J Physiol*. 175(2):319-321.

Shah, G.N., & Hymer, W.C. (1989). Prolactin variants in the rat adenohypophysis. *Mol Cell Endocrinol*. 61(1):97-107.

Sinha, Y.N. (1992). Prolactin variants. *Trends Endocrinol Metab*. 3(3):100-106.

Sinha, Y.N.(1995). Structural variants of prolactin: occurrence and physiological significance. *Endocr Rev*. 16(3):354-369.

Spies, H.G., & Clegg, M.T. (1971). Pituitary as a possible site of prolactin feedback in autoregulation. *Neuroendocrinology*. 8(3):205-212.

Wang, Y.F., & Walker, A.M. (1993). Dephosphorylation of standard prolactin produces a more biologically active molecule: evidence for antagonism between nonphosphorylated and phosphorylated prolactin in the stimulation of Nb2 cell proliferation. *Endocrinology*. 133(5):2156-2160.

Welsch, C.W., Sar, M., Clemens, J.A., & Meites, J. (1968). Effects of estrogen on pituitary prolactin levels of female rats bearing median eminence implants of prolactin. *Proc Soc Exp Biol Med*. 129(3):817-820.

Chapter 7

The Effect of Physiological and Environmental Factors on the Prolactin Profile in Seasonally Breeding Animals

Edyta Molik, Tomasz Misztal and Dorota A. Zieba

Additional information is available at the end of the chapter

http://dx.doi.org/10.5772/51465

1. Introduction

Light, being an environmental factor, has a significant effect on reproductive functions of animals exhibiting sensitivity to changes of the day length [1]. Among mammals there are many species displaying seasonality of reproduction, and given that, two models of seasonal sensitivity were distinguished. The first one refers to long-day animals (horses), in which reproductive processes are induced by lengthening days, i.e. in the spring. The other model concerns short-day animals, which include sheep, goats and deer; in these animals the reproduction system is stimulated and estrus takes place in the autumn and winter period [2]. In sheep the phenomenon of seasonality relates not only to reproduction but also to lactation. Following the process of mammogenesis in mammals, a mammary gland is developed, which is a complex cutaneous acinotubular gland [3]. The endocrine mechanism of entering and maintenance of lactation in sheep involves a number of hormones, which proves that the process relies basically on the activity of hypothalamus and pituitary gland [4,5,6]. One of the principal hormones conditioning both triggering and maintenance of lactation, synthesis of milk proteins, fat and immunoglobulins is prolactin (PRL), which is secreted chiefly by lactotroph cells of the anterior pituitary gland [7]. Prolactin is also produced locally by the mammary gland of mammals and does not differ immunologically from prolactin produced by the pituitary gland [8]. An important role in the process of mammogenesis and lactogenesis is assigned also to glycocorticoids, insulin and growth hormone and estrogens [9].

The fundamental feature of all living organisms is the ability to receive and process information about changes in the environment. Succession of physiological changes is synchronized with changes of environmental conditions and conditioned by the activity of the biological clock [10,11]. It is confirmed via seasonal changes of the activity of the hypothalamic-pituitary axis in animals kept under permanent light conditions. Thanks to constant and cyclical factors physiological processes can be synchronized with a relevant season of the year. The synthesis of melatonin is a biochemical signal informing the organism about changing light conditions [12,13,14]. Numerous studies go to show the existence of a molecular mechanism involved in deciphering of the melatonin signal which is found in the SCN (Suprachiasmatic Nucleus) and in the PT (Pars Tuberalis). Both in the SCN and PT there are several dozens of genes of the biological clock such as *Per1, Per2* or *Cry 1, Cry2,* which are associated with each other [15,16]. The melatonin profile changing in a 24-hour cycle affects the rhythmical changes in the expression of the clock genes, which is reflected via their different amounts of mRNA in the PT and SCN. The maximum expression of the *Cry1* gene occurs during the dusk period parallel to the growth of the melatonin concentration, whereas the expression of the *Per1* gene is induced at dawn [17,18].

2. The effect of diverse photoperiod and exogenous melatonin on the secretion of prolactin under *in vivo* conditions

According to Misztal et al. (1999) [19] the modulating effect of melatonin on the secretion of prolactin can be exerted via two various mechanisms. The first one refers to the circadian rhythm and applies probably only to the prolactin stored in lactotrph cells of the pituitary gland. Tuberalin - a factor produced in the infundibular part of the gland probably triggers the expression of the PRL gene in lactotroph cells [20]. The daily secretion of prolactin is also controlled by the dopaminergic system because even the short-lasting growth of prolactin under the influence of melatonin is observed only in a situation when the activity of the dopaminergic system is weakened [21]. It must be stressed that the daily rhythm of prolactin displays a high seasonal variability; in the spring a higher concentration of the hormone is observed in morning and evening hours, and in the summer the daily secretion peak falls at night. In the autumn the rhythm has a two-phase character, like in the spring, whereas the concentration rises in morning and evening hours. In the winter, though, no specific release of prolactin is observed at all.

The other mechanism for regulation of the prolactin secretion is related to its circannual secretion rhythm, when melatonin, owing to its lipophilic, exerts a direct effect on lactotroph cells of the pituitary gland and, accordingly, on the secretion of prolactin [19,22,23]. Under natural conditions the maximum PRL concentration in the sheep's bloodstream is recorded in the long-day period; whereas at this time the melatonin level drops. The lowest level of prolactin is observed during short days, when the melatonin level is the highest [24,25] Shortening of the day length or prolonged administration of melatonin in the period of physiologically increased concentration of prolactin leads to a reduced secretion of this hormone [1,13]. Seasonal changes in the prolactin secretion in the lactation period in sheep undoubtedly affect milk yields. Rhythmical changes of the level of prolactin and melatonin throughout the year were observed mainly in barren sheep and rams; however, studies carried out in the group of sheep used for dairy production confirmed the presence of the seasonal rhythm of these two hormones. The experiments demonstrated a definite influence of the day length on the parameters of ewes' milk yields. Mothers entering lactation in the period of shortening days yielded 50% less milk as compared to ewes milked in the long-day period. The drop in milk yields in the shortening photoperiod resulted from the change in the prolactin secretion. The highest PRL concentration in sheep milked in the long-day period was identified in May 312.6 ± 45.2 ng/ml, at this time the concentration of melatonin amounted to 33.5± 11.2 ng/ml. As lactation progressed and days became shorter, the concentration of prolactin declined, and that of melatonin increased (table 1).

Months	May		June		July		August		September	
	$\bar{x}$	SE	$\bar{x}$	SE	$\bar{x}$	SE	$\bar{x}$	SE	$\bar{x}$	SE
Melatonin pg/ml	133.5	11.3	77.8	18.9	73.3	15.1	124.7	21.6	91.3	22.2
Prolactin ng/ml	312.6	45.2	185.7	34.7	247.0	48.9	151.6	33.9	43.9	10.1

Table 1. Changes in the concentration of melatonin and prolactin in sheep milked in the long-day period

As regards sheep lambed and milked in the short-day period and kept under the natural photoperiod conditions the highest level of prolactin was observed in August, i.e. 124.0 ± 48.8 ng/ml. In the first month of milking the concentration of prolactin in sheep corresponded to its seasonal rhythm and declined in subsequent months (table 2).

Months	August		September		October		November	
	$\bar{x}$	SE	$\bar{x}$	SE	$\bar{x}$	SE	$\bar{x}$	SE
Melatonin pg/ml	87.8	15.5	82.3	15.0	77.5	16.1	93.2	17.4
Prolactin ng/ml	124.6	48.8	60.5	11.1	30.8	9.7	16.8	4.1

Table 2. Changes in the concentration of melatonin and prolactin in sheep milked in the short-day period

As the light day shortened, the secretion of PRL declined as the level of the hormone in September was lower by 15% as compared to the concentration observed in August. A distinct drop in the prolactin level was observed in the period of the last two months of lactation, i.e. in October and November, and amounted respectively to 30.8 ± 9.7 ng/ml and 16.8 ± 4.1 ng/ml. The low concentration of prolactin already in the first month of milking and systematic growth of the melatonin secretion in the period of shortening days exerted an impact on the parameters of sheep milk yields, causing a drop of ewes' milk yields. In the group of sheep kept under artificially simulated long-day conditions, 16 hours of light and 8 hours of darkness (16L:8D), in the period from August to November, the concentration of PRL already in the second month of milking, i.e. from September to November, decreased. In October and November a sharp drop in the concentration of prolactin was observed. The parameters of milk yields of sheep kept under conditions of artificially extended light day decreased proportionately to the drop in the concentration of prolactin (table 3).

Months	August		September		October		November	
	$\bar{x}$	SE	$\bar{x}$	SE	$\bar{x}$	SE	$\bar{x}$	SE
Melatonin pg/ml	60.4	19.8	17.6	7.6	4.4	1.1	17.0	5.5
Prolactin ng/ml	132.7	37.4	147.9	22.4	84.3	12.5	38.3	15.2

Table 3. Changes in the concentration of melatonin and prolactin in sheep kept under simulated long-day conditions -16L:8D

In the short-day period even in lactating sheep it is highly difficult to maintain an appropriately high concentration of prolactin. Studies carried out by Molik et al. (2007) [26] demonstrated that in sheep under artificially extended long-day conditions (16L:8D) it is impossible to maintain a high concentration of prolactin as well as to maintain lactation during shortening days.

Subsequent studies conducted on sheep milked in the long-day period showed that introduction of exogenous melatonin and initiation of artificial short-day conditions (16D:8L - 16 hours of darkness 8 hours of light) in the long-day period gave rise to reduction of the prolactin concentration (table 4).

Months	Concentracion of prolactin ng/ml									
	May		June		July		August		September	
	$\bar{x}$	SE	$\bar{x}$	SE	$\bar{x}$	SE	$\bar{x}$	SE	$\bar{x}$	SE
Control group milked in the long day period	220.5 2	8.1	199.1	5.6	137.8	9.4	125.7	9.2	84.3	4.4
Sheep with melatonin implants	160.8	5.6	155.3	5.4	117.1	9.3	84.6	11.3	60.3	4.7
Sheep group under artificial short-day conditions 16D:8L	192.8	9.3	82.8	4.2	163	6.2	78.6	8.6	52.8	2.7

Table 4. Changes in the concentration of prolactin in sheep exposed to the effects of exogenous melatonin and simulated short-day conditions 16D:8L

In the first month of milking, in May, the highest concentration of prolactin was identified in sheep kept under natural day length conditions, with its level amounting to 220.52 ± 8.1 ng/ml. As lactation progressed and days shortened, the secretion of prolactin dropped and in the last two months it amounted respectively to 125.7 ± 9.21 ng/ml and 84.3 ± 4.4 ng/ml. Use of subcutaneous melatonin implants in ewes caused a drop in the concentration of prolactin. Already in the first month of milking, in May, the concentration of prolactin amounted to 160.8 ± 5.6 ng/ml. In subsequent 60 days of lactation (June) a further bigger decrease of the concentration of prolactin was recorded, reaching the level of 82.8 ± 4.2 ng/ml. As lactation progressed and melatonin implants started to exert their effects, a further drop in the secretion of prolatin was observed. In the group of sheep exposed to the effects of artificially simulated short-day conditions (16D:8L), the highest concentration of prolactin was identified in May, equaling 192.8 ± 9.3ng/ml. In subsequent months of lactation keeping sheep under 16D:8L conditions caused a drop in the secretion of prolactin. In the fourth and fifth month of milking the secretion of prolactin decreased again, reaching in August the level of 78.97± 8.63 ng/ml, and in September 52.83 ± 2.73 ng/ml. The studies revealed that simulation of the long signal of melatonin in the spring and summer period contributes to disturbance of the endogenous rhythm of prolactin.

In studies carried out to date no differences have been identified as to the amount of milk obtained in the period of lambs rearing. In the early lactation period sucking is an important factor stimulating the PRL secretion in the mother's organism [27]. The sucking impulse induces release of serotonin [28] and oxytocin in the central nervous system (CNS) which give rise to the release of prolactin from the pituitary gland into the peripheral blood [29]. Experiments conducted on lactating rat females demonstrated that intravenous administration of specific oxytocin antagonist (desGly-NH2-d(CH2)5[D-Tyr2,Thr4]OVT) completely inhibits the release of prolactin triggered by the sucking impulse [30]. Another important compound stimulating the release of prolactin induced by sucking is represented by salsolinol produced by the dopaminergic system in the lactation period. Infusion of exogenous salsolinol into the CNS in the group of lactating sheep gave rise to the release of prolactin into blood [31].

With that in mind, further experiments were carried out, which aimed at determining changes in the secretion of prolactin in sheep feeding lambs in the period of lengthening and shortening days, and verifying the hypothesis that melatonin can modify the secretion of prolactin despite strong stimulation of the mammary gland by sucking in the early lactation period [32]. Results of these studies demonstrated that administration of exogenous melatonin to ewes feeding lambs in the long-day period caused a significant drop in the concentration of prolactin. The identified changes in the PRL concentration in sheep entering lactation in the long-day period are comparable with the studies by Rhind et al. (1991) [33] which proved that in mothers rearing lambs in the period of lengthening days the concentration of prolatin rises. The studies conducted showed that despite intensive sucking the secretion of prolactin in sheep with melatonin implants dropped significantly. It must be stressed that the melatonin signal, acting as a marker of the biochemical biological clock, is evolutionarily so strong that the secretion of prolactin is reduced despite the stimulating sucking impulse.

Introduction of melatonin implants for sheep rearing lambs in the short-day period did not cause significant changes in the profile of the prolactin secretion. By analyzing the profile of the PRL secretion in both sheep groups, a conclusion can be drawn that in sheep lambed in November the concentration of prolactin in the first control sample drawn was lower by 50% as compared to the control sample drawn in March. In the long-day period the concentration of prolactin in the control group increased, and the secretion of melatonin decreased. In the autumn and winter period, though, as natural conditions set in, the concentration of melatonin increased and the level of prolactin dropped. The extending signal of melatonin observed in the autumn and winter period causes under natural conditions a decrease of the concentration of prolactin in sheep [34,35].

3. The effect of the day length and exogenous melatonin on the secretion of prolactin under *in vitro* conditions

Studies carried out on a group of lactating sheep under in vivo conditions showed modulating effects of melatonin with respect to the secretion of prolactin. The above mentioned relations demonstrate that melatonin can modulate the seasonal rhythm of the prolactin secretion affecting directly the pituitary gland. The highest concentration of melatonin receptors in the sheep's pituitary gland was identified in the pars tuberalis [36]. This structure is located precisely between the eminentia medialis of the hypothalamus and the distal part of the gland, which enables its mediation in the communication of the brain with the pituitary gland. In the sheep's PT only a MT1 melatonin receptor is found, and surgical separation of the pituitary gland from the hypothalamus does not have any influence on the concentration and location of this receptor and its sensitivity to binding melatonin [37]. Despite the fact that it was demonstrated that the activity of PT secretory cells is seasonal and melatonin-dependent, it was not to confirmed that it is involved in the control of seasonal changes in the sexual activity.

The presence of melatonin receptor limited to the PT of the pituitary gland, and lack of direct effects of melatonin both on the prolactin gene expression and release of prolactin in cultures of lactotroph cells under in vitro conditions [38] suggests that melatonin regulates the seasonal secretion of prolactin by way of a specific compound synthesized in the PT. The presence of such a compound in the PT, with a peptide structure and stimulating secretion of prolactin from lactotroph cells of the pituitary gland, was confirmed in experiments, and the peptide itself was called tuberalin [36,39]. Own studies carried out under in vitro conditions demonstrated that both the day length and administration of exogenous melatonin affect the profile of the prolactin secretion. In vitro incubations of pituitary explants taken from sheep on 30th day of lactation were held in three periods: in the period of lengthening days (March), in the period of shortening days (August) and in the short-day period (November). The pituitaries taken were divided along the sulcus into two halves so that each one contained the adenohypophysis and the neurohypophysis. In vitro incubation was held during 3 hours in the Parker medium at a temperature of 37^0C. The control group (G1) was incubated in a medium without any hormonal additives, whereas the experimental group (G2) was incubated in a medium with exogenous melatonin. The experiments performed demonstrated that administration of exogenous melatonin in the long-day period caused a decrease of the secretion of prolactin in the pars tuberalis (table 5)

Group	Secretion of prolactin µg/ml					
	March		August		November	
	$\bar{x}$	SE	$\bar{x}$	SE	$\bar{x}$	SE
Parst tuberalis – control group (G1)	145.4	21.2	65.4	15.7	13.1	2.8
Parst tuberalis – with melatonin (G2)	105.0	11.4	45.4	9.2	13.7	2.2

Table 5. Effects of the day length and exogenous melatonin on the secretion of prolactin under in vitro conditions.

The concentration of prolactin in the period of lengthening days (March) in the control group was at the level of 145.45 ± 21.2 µg/ml, whereas in the group incubated with melatonin it was lower and amounted to 105.06 ± 11.4 µg/ml. In the period of shortening days (August), the concentration of prolactin in the medium with exogenous melatonin was lower, equaling 45.4 ± 9.2 µg/ml, as compared to the control group, being at the level of 65.4 ± 15.7 µg/ml. The lowest concentration of prolactin both in the control group and experimental one was recorded in the short-day period. The experiments conducted confirmed the seasonal rhythm of prolactin, because the highest concentration of this hormone was observed in the period of lengthening days (145.45 ± 21.2 µg/ml). At the same time the lowest one was recorded in the short-day period (13.1 ± 2.8 µg/ml). The experiments conducted under in vitro conditions showed that in the long-day period melatonin exerted a strong inhibitory effect on the secretion of prolactin. The studies confirmed also a direct influence of melatonin on cells of the sheep's pars tuberalis. It was demonstrated that the secretory activity of lactotroph cells of the pituitary gland under in vitro conditions is closely linked to the day length, and at the same time to the secretion of melatonin. It must be stressed at this point that the obtained seasonal distribution of prolactin concentrations in lactating sheep resembles a seasonal rhythm of the prolactin secretion in barren sheep [19]. However, it should be noted that in the group of lactating sheep the secretion of prolactin is much more intensive. Melatonin administered on the 30th day of lactation contributed to the reduction of the prolactin secretion [40].

4. The role of orexins and leptin in the regulation of the secretion of prolactin in sheep

The process of entering and maintenance of lactation in sheep involves a great number of hormones, with prolactin playing a key role. In recent years, though, a focus has been placed on orexins and their role in the secretion of prolactin in sheep. In 1998 a new group of neuropeptides was identified. It was demonstrated that they exert a significant influence on food intake, and in this manner they were dubbed orexins (Greek *orexis* – appetite) [41].

Orexins derive from the same precursor – prepro-orexin, but they are a product of different posttranslational modifications. It is a protein built of 130 amino acid residues (mouse, rat) or 131 amino acid residues (human). In terms of the amino acid sequence a rat's prepro-orexin displays 83% homology with a human protein and 95% with a mouse's protein [41]. Two forms of the newly discovered compounds are distinguished: orexin A (OxA) and orexin B (OxB), which are molecules whose amino acid composition is similar to the gut hormone - secretin [42]. Orexin A and orexin B bind specifically and activate two GPCR receptors (G-protein coupled receptors), which – before discovery of the ligands - were called orphan receptors, and now they are known as orexin receptors – 1 and – 2 (Ox1R and Ox2R). Studies carried out in 2000 by Date et al. [43] confirmed that matrix RNA of Ox1R and Ox2R exhibits strong expression in the middle, anterior (adenohypophysis) and posterior (neurohypophysis) lobe of the rats' pituitary. At the same time it was noticed that in the anterior part of the pituitary gland Ox1R is subject to stronger expression than Ox2R. The observations go to show that the rat's pituitary is a gland capable of receiving the orexin signal.

Studies related to the synthesis of orexins and distribution of their receptors reveal that they are found in numerous brain sections and confirm the theory, according to which these compounds are regulatory proteins active in the central nervous system [41,44].

Experiments conducted on rats demonstrated that administration of exogenous orexin causes increased intake of food by animals [41]. OxA stimulates appetite in a dose-dependent manner and this effect prevails even for up to 4 hours after injection. The effect of OxB injection does not prevail as long as that of OxA; after two hours stimulation of food intake is low. The longer effects of OxA probably are attributable to the molecular structure, thanks to which it is more resistant than OxB to an attack of inactivating peptidases [41].The experiments also displayed functions of orexins – other than the metabolic one. It was confirmed that orexins play a modulating role in the regulation of the hypothalamic-pituitary-thyroid axis [45], - adrenal axis [46] and – gonadal axis [47].

Results of *in vivo* studies conducted in 2000 by Russell et al. [48] showed for the first time that injection of orexin A reduced the level of prolactin in rats' blood. Moreover, it was concluded that the mechanism is not connected with the activity of TIDA neutrons synthesizing dopamine (PRL inhibitor). In *in vitro* experiments it was proven that OxA exerts a direct influence on the secretory activity of explants of the hypothalamus and pituitary gland. Orexin A is also described as an inhibitor of the PRL secretion by lactotroph cells of the pituitary anterior lobe by Dusza and Ciereszko (2007) [49]. However, results of studies carried out on immature female rats under primary culture conditions are completely different as they reveal a statistically significant growth of the prolactin secretion depending on a dose and time of incubation of pituitary glands [50].

The orexin gene expression in ruminants was defined for the first time only in 2002 and it was shown that the location of the mRNA of prepro-orexin in the hypothalamus in sheep corresponds with the published pattern for rodents. Results of the studies confirmed also that the orexin gene expression is sensitive to changes in the day length (higher during shorter days). However, no starving-induced changes were identified, which questions the key role of orexins in the regulation of appetite in sheep [51,52].

In the light of the presented results of the studies orexins can be perceived as a link integrating the processes of maintaining energy, hormonal and reproductive balance. Orexin A can be of special importance to animals exhibiting sensitivity to changes in the day length, which include sheep. The process of entering and maintenance of lactation in the animals involves a number of factors, whereas the key role is attributed to prolactin and growth hormone. Unfortunately, mechanisms regulating secretion of these compounds in sheep in the lactation period still remain unclear. It is certain, though, that defining functions of orexins - above all - in the regulation of the prolactin secretion will make it possible to understand the process of maintaining lactation in sheep, in particular in the short-day period. Thus, the purpose of the initiated studies was to determine the role of orexin A in the regulation of the prolactin secretion in sheep under different day-length conditions in in vitro experiments.

The experiments were performed on 15 sheep. Pituitary glands were taken from sheep on the 30th day of lactation in the long-day period (May n=5), in the period of shortening days (August n=5) and in the short-day period (December n=5). The pituitaries taken were divided along the sulcus into two halves so that each one contained the adenohypophysis and the neurohypophysis. *In vitro* incubation was held during 3 hours in the Parker medium at a temperature of 37^{0}C. The control group (G1) was incubated in a pure medium, whereas the experimental group (G2) was incubated in a medium with exogenous orexin A. Injection of exogenous orexin caused an increase of prolactin secretion already in the first hour of incubation (451.6±9.4 μg/ml) (table 6).

Group	Secretion of prolactin μg/ml					
	Hours of incubation					
	First hour		Second hour		Third hour	
	$\bar{x}$	SE	$\bar{x}$	SE	$\bar{x}$	SE
Parst tuberalis – control group (G1)	401.8	6.0	344.6	8.2	155.8	3.6
Parst tuberalis – with orexin A (G2)	451.6	9.4	346.5	7.0	196.3	4.7

Table 6. Effects of orexin on the secretion of prolactin in the long-day period

In the control group in the second hour of incubation the concentration of prolactin was lower (344.6±8.2 μg/ml) than in the group with orexin (346.5±7.0 μg/ml). But in the third hour of incubation the concentration of prolactin in the experimental group was higher by 40.5 μg/ml than in the control group. In general, the PRL concentration in the long-day period during three-hour incubation in the group with orexin A equaled (331±15.2ng/ml) and was higher as compared to the control group (300.0±16.6 ng/ml). The experiments demonstrated that irrespective of how the secretory capabilities of cells deteriorated in the course of incubation, exogenous orexin A stimulates the PRL secretion in the long-day period in lactating ewes (53).

Studies conducted in the period of shortening days (August) showed that administration of orexin A can modulate prolactin secretion (table 7).

Group	Secretion of prolactin µg/ml					
	Hours of incubation					
	First hour		Second hour		Third hour	
	$\bar{x}$	SE	$\bar{x}$	SE	$\bar{x}$	SE
Parst tuberalis – control group	38.05	12.1	32.1	9.6	19.2	7.3
Parst tuberalis – with orexin A	40.6	13.5	38.7	10.1	28.6	9.7

Table 7. Effects of orexin on the secretion of prolactin in the period of shortening days (August)

While analyzing changes in the prolactin secretion in sheep during 3-hour incubation, the highest secretory activity of cells was observed in the first two hours of the experiment. In the first hour of incubation the concentration of prolactin in the group incubated with orexin A equaled (40.6±13.5 µg/ml) and was higher as opposed to the control group (38.05±12.1 µg/ml). The concentration of prolactin in the second hour of the experiment was still higher than that in the control group and equaled respectively (38.7±10.1, 32.1±9.6 µg/ml). In the third hour of the experiment it was demonstrated that in the experimental group the concentration of prolactin was higher (28.6±9.7 µg/ml) as compared to the control group (19.2±7.3 µg/ml).

In the period of shortening days, when the concentration of prolactin under natural conditions is reduced, administration of orexin A caused a growth of the prolactin secretion; similarly, injection of exogenous orexin A in the short-day period caused an increase of the prolactin secretion (table 8)

Group	Secretion of prolactin µg/ml					
	Hours of incubation					
	First hour		Second hour		Third hour	
	$\bar{x}$	SE	$\bar{x}$	SE	$\bar{x}$	SE
Parst tuberalis – control group	135.1	8.4	107.8	7.5	65.7	5.9
Parst tuberalis – with orexin A	158.9	9.2	164.8	7.5	79.9	7

Table 8. Effects of orexin on the secretion of prolactin in the short-day period (December)

In the first hour of incubation of the pituitaries in the short-day period it was observed that the prolactin secretion in the experimental group increased (158.9±9.2 pg/ml) as contrasted with the control group (135.1±8.4 pg/ml). In the second hour of incubation it was recorded that the concentration of prolactin in the experimental group grew (164.8±7.5 pg/ml), whereas in the control group the concentration of prolactin amounted to (107.8±4.0 pg/ml).

Results obtained in the third hour of incubation revealed that the concentration of prolactin in the control group equaled (65.7±5.9 pg/ml), whereas in the group treated with exogenous orexin it amounted to (79.9±7.0 pg/ml). Despite the fact that secretory capabilities of cells deteriorated in the course of incubation, the PRL concentration in the examined samples grew.

The experiments conducted under in vitro conditions confirmed that the annual rhythm of the PRL secretion in sheep is characterized by a higher concentration in the long-day period (summer) and lower concentration in the short-day period (winter).

Orexin exerts its effects on the PRL secretion in sheep, like in case of rodents, thanks to the presence of specific receptors Ox1R and Ox2R in the cytoplasmatic membrane of cells. Their existence in the sheep's adenohypophysis was described in 2002 by Xu et al.[54], who identified a high homology of the structure of a gene encoding sheep's Ox1R and a gene of the receptor in a rat (87%) and human being (89%). The presence of both of these forms of orexin receptors in the sheep's pituitary gland was also confirmed by Zhang et al. in 2004 [55].

Studies carried out to date with a view to explaining the relations between orexin and prolactin have been conducted mainly on rats. Thus, results of experiments on sheep in the period of lactation offer new information about the role of orexins in seasonally breeding animals. The conducted experiments proved that orexin A exerts a greater stimulating effect on the level of the PRL secretion in the summer season than in the winter season. The weaker response of sheep's pituitaries to orexin during short days as compared to the response during long days is a phenomeon of resistance of lactotroph cells to the orexin signal. Such a reaction of endocrine cells can be explained by the seasonal rhythm of biosynthesis and secretion of orexin in sheep, regulated by the photoperiod. It was proven that under conditions of shortening light days the expression of the orexin precursor gene in these ruminants is on a higher level than during long days [51]. As a result, an increased concentration of the mRNA of prepro-orexin in the winter season is observed, followed by an increased concentration of orexin in the organism. It is probable that at this time the saturation degree of orexin receptors of lactotroph cells with endogenous ligand is so high that adding exogenous orexin A does not cause such a distinct response as that occurring during long days. While attempting to identify interactions between the secretion of prolactin and growth hormone and the level of melatonin in lactating sheep an analogous phenomenon was noticed. Despite the fact that ewes lambed in June were kept under artificial long-day conditions, as the day became shorter, a drop in the PRL level was observed. In consequence, it was concluded that the secretion of the hormones retained its endogenous seasonal rhythm. The effect of the loss of the pituitary cells' sensitivity to the summer signal of the hormone of darkness repeating for too long does not allow for extension of sheep's lactation to the autumn and winter period [57].

In experiments conducted in 2006 it was proven for the first time that leptin exerts an effect on the melatonin secretion both under *in vitro* [57] and *in vivo* [58] conditions. It was observed that the day length (photoperiod) is one of the factors which modulate the effects of leptin directly in the sheep's pineal gland, with an inhibitory effect of leptin on melatonin secreted by explants of the pineal gland in the period of lengthening days. However, during shortening days leptin stimulated the melatonin secretion by the gland explants [57]. Results of the *in vitro* experiments were confirmed in *in vivo* experiments, in which leptin was injected into the 3rd brain chamber. They demonstrated that exogenous leptin has an inhibitory effect on the concentration of melatonin during long days and a stimulating dose-dependent effect – during short days [58].

Seasonal insensitivity to leptin is observed in sheep in the spring and summer period, making it possible for the ruminants to make energy reserves, and despite increasing fatness intake of food in sheep is not reduced. Increased intake of food and a growth of the body weight during long days – LD (*Long Days*) spring - summer – is characterized by a high concentration of leptin in blood plasma, which "loses" then its anorectic features. In the short-day period – SD (*Short Days*) autumn - winter, when the availability of food dwindles, the sensitivity of centres regulating food intake in the hypothalamus to the concentration of leptin returns to normal. This paradox is explained by leptin resistance occurring during LD, whereas the neuroendocrinological basis of leptin resistance has not been fully understood yet. One of the phenomena underlying leptin resistance is auto-supression of the transfer of signal from the receptor to the cell centre resulting from the leptin-induced expression of SOCS-3 factors, being inhibitors of cytokine sygnalisation [58]. The phenomenon is observed in particular in the area of ventromedial hyopothalamus [58], where long-form receptors of leptin Ob-Rb are found in the highest concentration.

Orexigenic and anorexigenic systems are linked in terms of morphology and functionality. It confirms the hypothesis about the existence of a nervous network regulating hunger, located in nervous centres of the hypothalamus. The area of receptors and nerve endings for orexigenic factors overlaps with the area of receptors for anorexigenic factors, which also reveals mutual interactions of the two systems. In animals with strong seasonal breeding characteristics the network of the above described relations overlaps additionally with effects of the photoperiod, which by way of a biological signal in the form of melatonin interferes with the developed relations. The suprachiasmatic nucleus (SCN), which is a part of the biological clock, generates signals adjusting food intake to the circadian rhythm. This element is considerably weakened in the primates, and in particular in humans, but it is very efficient in ruminants. The objective of the conducted experiments was to investigate interactions between the day length and leptin and orexin B in sheep under *in vivo* conditions.

The experiments were carried out on 24 sheep of the Polish sheep breed. The first stage of experiments (n=12) was conducted in the period of lengthening days (spring – summer). The second stage (n=12) was held under conditions of shortening days (autumn – winter). Three weeks prior to the initiation of the planned experiments metal stainless cannulas were inserted surgically into the third brain chamber of ewes (using the stereotactic method by Traczyk and Przekop [1963] [59]). The tests were started at the sunset, and were continued during subsequent 6 hours. The experiments were performed so that each ewe received in a

2-week interval intraventricular infusion of Ringer-Locke's fluid – control, recombinant sheep leptin (roleptin) – in a dose of 0.5 µg/kg body weight (Leptin 1), and roleptin in a dose of 1.0 ug/kg body weight (Leptin 2). On the day of the experiment animals were put in individual cattle crushes, the Ringer-Locke's fluid (control) and roleptin were injected intraventricularly for the first time directly after drawing time-zero blood samples and in the 60th and 120th minute of the 6-hour experiment. During the experiment blood samples were drawn every 15 minutes. Blood was poured into test tubes containing 100 µl of heparin solution (1000 IU/ml).

During lengthening days the total PRL concentration in the plasma of control sheep was significantly higher ($P < 0.001$) than during shortening days (132.28 ± 19.87 vs. 44.41 ± 8.27 ng/ml). Intraventricular infusions of two doses of exogenous leptin reduced the concentration of prolactin during SD ($P < 0.001$) as compared to the values observed in control ewes. It was concluded that the day length is one of the factors which modulate the effects of leptin on the prolactin secretion in sheep. It was observed that central infusions of leptin into the 3rd brain chamber significantly decreased the concentration of prolactin in sheep during short days in a dose-dependent manner; whereas the effect was opposite during a long photoperiod.

In subsequent experiments a test of the hypothesis about season-dependent effects of leptin and orexin B on the endocrine activity of sheep was performed. Six weeks prior to the start of the experiments ewes were subjected to an ovariectomy procedure, and subcutaneous estradiol implants were inserted into each of them. Three weeks prior to the initiation of the planned experiments metal stainless cannulas were inserted surgically into the third brain chamber of ewes (using the stereotactic method by Traczyk and Przekop [1963] (59). Like in the previous experiment, the tests were started at the sunset, and were continued during subsequent 6 hours. The experiments were performed so that each ewe received in one-week interval intraventricular infusion: 1. Control group (CG) - Ringer-Locke's fluid (pH=7.4); 2. Experimental group 1 (Gr 1) – recombinant sheep leptin (PLR Laboratory, Israel) in a dose of 0.5 µg/kg, the dose was selected based on experiments [58]; 3. Experimental group 3 (Gr 3) – orexins B (PolyPeptides Laboratories, Strasbourg, France) in a dose of 0,3 µg/kg., 4. Experimental group 5 (Gr 5) - superantagonists of leptin (D23L/L39A/D40A/F41A; PLR Laboratory Israel) in a dose of 50 µg/kg, and then orexin B in a dose used previously. In the control group and experimental group 1, 2, and 3 infusions of selected factors were performed three times, every 60 minutes from the start of the experiment, in group 5 the leptin antagonist was infused twice, in the zero and 1st hour of the experiment, and ghrelin/orexin B was infused 15 and 60 minutes after administration of leptin antagonist. During the 6-hour experiment blood samples were drawn every 15 minutes. The average concentration of melatonin in the plasma of ewes from the control group was higher ($P < 0.001$) during LD as compared to the values recorded in animals during short days (87.28 ± 1.2 vs. 59.70 ± 3.1 pg/ml). In the seasons of lengthening days exogenous recombinant sheep leptin significantly reduced the concentration of melatonin ($P < 0.001$) in relation to the values observed in ewes from the control group, whereas during a short day it significantly increased ($P < 0.01$) the concentration of melatonin. Orexin B did not have any impact on the concentration of melatonin during a short day, but it caused a significant growth ($P < 0.05$) of the concentration of melatonin on a long day.

During a lengthening day the total PRL concentration in the plasma of sheep from the control group was markedly higher ($P < 0.001$) as contrasted with shortening days (132.28 ± 19.87 vs. 44.41 ± 8.27 ng/ml). Intraventricular infusions of exogenous leptin reduced the concentration of prolactin during SD ($P < 0.001$) as compared to the values observed in ewes from the control group. The average concentration of endogenous orexin was higher ($P < 0.01$) during short days (0.59 ± 0.05 ng/ml) as opposed to LD (0.39 ± 0.01 ng/ml) in the control group of sheep. Exogenous orexin caused a growth ($P < 0.05$) of the plasma concentration of endogenous orexin respectively on a long and short day (0.62 ± 0.01 ng/ml and 0.71 ± 0.03 ng/ml), whereas the effects of leptin reduced ($P < 0.05$) the concentration of orexin during LD and SD. Based on the conducted experiments it was concluded that orexin B and anorectic hormone – leptin directly interact closely with each other, regulating not only the processes of metabolism but influencing jointly release of melatonin and prolactin, and the interactions additionally depend on the prevalent photoperiod.

5. Summary

So far it has been believed that milk yields in mammals are determined by genetic and environmental factors. In recent years, though, a special focus has been placed on light, being the modulator of the prolactin level. In farm animals changes of the light day play a very important role as they determine their yields. The length of the light day, and in particular the melatonin profile, is of special importance in sheep as they determine reproductive processes, in which lactation is the last stage of reproductive physiology. Experiments carried out on sheep demonstrated that both the melatonin profile and prolactin profile retain features of a seasonal rhythm depending on the day length. The synthesis of melatonin by the pineal gland is a biochemical signal informing the organism about the break of the day or night. This hormone regulates activities of numerous organs. Until now the activity of melatonin has been associated with the impact on the reproductive system. Experiments carried out in recent years have shown that melatonin can modulate the level of prolactin. Under natural conditions the maximum concentration of prolactin in sheep blood is observed in the long-day period, and at this time the level of melatonin drops. The lowest concentration of prolactin is recorded during short days, when the level of melatonin is the highest. Shortening of the day length or long-term injection of melatonin in the period of physiologically increased concentration of prolactin leads to a reduced secretion of this hormone. Lactation in sheep involves a number of hormones, and for that reason in recent years a special focus has been placed on the role of orexins in the regulation of the prolactin secretion. Experiments conducted demonstrated that orexin A exerts a greater stimulating effect on the level of the PRL secretion in the summer season than in the winter season. The weaker reaction of sheep's pituitaries to orexin during short days as compared to the response during long days is a phenomenon of resistance of lactotroph cells to the orexin signal. Such a reaction of endocrine cells can be explained by the seasonal rhythm of biosynthesis and secretion of orexin in sheep, regulated by the photoperiod.

Author details

Edyta Molik and Dorota A. Zieba
Agricultural University in Krakow, Poland

Tomasz Misztal
The Kielanowski Institute of Animal Physiology and Nutrition, Polish Academy of Sciences, Poland

Acknowledgement

This research was supported by projects MNiSZW NN311245033 and DS/KHiOK/3242/2010.

6. References

[1] Misztal T. Melatonina – hormon sezonowości rozrodu u owiec. Postępy Nauk Rolniczych 1996; 6: 43- 58.
[2] Thiery JC, Chemineau P, Hernandez X, Migaud M, Malpaux B. Neuroendocrine interactions and seasonality. Domestic Animal Endocrinology 2002; 23: 87-100.
[3] Smith White SS, Ojeda SR. Maternal modulation of infantile ovarian development and available ovarian luteinizing hormone realizing hormone (LHRH) receptors via milk LHRH. Endorinology 1984; 115: 1973-1983.
[4] Peaker M, Neville MC. Hormones in milk: chemical signals to the offspring's'. Journal of Endocrinology 1991; 131: 1-6.
[5] Freeman ME, Kanyicska B, Lerant A, Nagy G. Prolactin structure, function and regulation of secretion. Reviews of Physiology 2000; 80: 1523-1631.
[6] Grattan DR. The actions of prolactin in the brain during pregnancy and lactation Programme Brain Ressearch 2001; 133: 153-171.
[7] Schams D, Rüsse J, Schallenberger E, Prokopp S, Chan JSD. The role of steroid hormones, prolactin and placental lactogen on mammary gland development in ewes and heifers. Journal of Endocrinology 1984; 102: 121-130.
[8] Flavoner IR, Vacek AT. Degradation of J^{125} labelled prolactin in the rabbit: effect of nephrectomy and prolactin infusion. Journal of Endocrinology 1983; 99: 360-377.
[9] Campbell PG, Frey DM, Baumrucker CR. Changes in bovine mammary insulin binding during pregnancy and lactation. Comparative Biochemistry and Physiology 1987; 87B: 649-653.
[10] Hastings M, Maywood ES. Circadian clocks in the mammalian brain. Bioessays 2000; 22: 23–31.
[11] Lewczuk B. Siatkówka, jądro skrzyżowania oraz szyszynka jako elementy zegara biologicznego ssaków. Medycyna Weterynaryjna 2007; 63 (5) 506-511.
[12] Wilkinson M, Arednt J, Bradtke D, Deziegler. Determination of a dark-induced increase in pineal N-acetyltransferase activity and simultaneous radioimmunoassay of melatonin in pineal, serum and pituitary tissue of the male rat. Journal of Endocrionology 1977; 72: 243-244.
[13] Arendt J. Role of the pineal gland and melatonin seasonal reproductive function in mammals. Reviews of Reproductive Biology 1986; 8: 266-320.

[14] Lincoln GA. Photoperiod- pineal- hypothalamic realy in sheep. Animal of Reproductive Science 1992; 28: 203-217.

[15] Lincoln G. Messager S, Andersson H, Hazlerigg D. Temporal expression of seven clock gens in the suprachiasmatic nucleus and the pars tuberalis of the sheep: evidence for an internal coincidence timer. Proceedings of the National Academy of Sciences of the United States of America 2002; 99(21) 13890 - 13895

[16] Hazlerigg DG, Andersson H, Johnston JD, Lincoln G. Molecular characterization of the long - day response in the soay sheep, a seasonal mammal. Current of Biology 2004; 14: 334 - 339

[17] Hazlerigg DG. What is the role of melatonin within the anterior pituitary?. Journal of Endocrinology 2001; 170: 493 - 501

[18] Lincoln GA. Decoding the nightly melatonin signal through circadian clockwork. Molecular and Cellular Endocrinology 2006; 252: 69 - 73

[19] Misztal T. Romanowicz K, Barcikowski B. Rola melatoniny w sekrecji prolaktyny u owiec. Postępy Biologii Komórki 1999; 26: 117- 123.

[20] Johnston JD. Photoperiodic regulation of prolactin secretion: changes in intra-pituitary signaling and lactotroph heterogeneity. Journal of Endocrinology., 2004; 180: 351-356.

[21] Thiery JC. Monoamine content of the stalk-median eminence and hypothalamus in the adult fenale sheep as affected by day length. Journal of Neuroendocrinology 1991; 3: 407-411.

[22] Lincoln GA, Short RV. Seasonal breeding: Nature's contraceptive', Recent Progress in Hormone Research 1980; 36: 1-52.

[23] Morgan PJ, Barret P, Davidson G, Lawson W. Melatonin regulates the synthesis and secretion of several proteins by pars tuberalis cells of the ovine pituitary. Journal of Neuroendocrinology 1992; 4: 557-563.

[24] Reiter RJ. Neuroendocrinology of melatonin. In: Melatonin Clinical Perspectives. editors: Miles A, Philbrick DRS, Thomson C, Oxford: Oxford University Press 1988; 1-42

[25] Robinson JJ. S, Wigzell RP, Aitken JM, Wallace S, Ireland and IS, Robertson. Daily oral administration of melatonin from March on wards advances by 4 months the breeding season of ewes maintained under the ambient photoperiod at 57^0 N'. Animal of Reproductive Science 1992; 27: 141-160

[26] Molik E, Misztal, T, Romanowicz K, Wierzchoś E. Dependence of the lactation duration and efficiency on the season of lambing in relation to the prolactin and melatonin secretion in ewes. Livestock Science 2007; 107: 220-226.

[27] Grattan DR. Behavioral significance of prolactin signaling in the central nervous system during pregnancy and lactation. Reproduction 2002; 123(4) 497-506.

[28] Wachs EA, Gorewit RC, Currie WB. Half-life clearance production rate foe oxytocin in cattle during lactation and mammary involution. Domestic Animal Endocrinology 1984; 1: 121-140.

[29] Sanchez-Andrade G, Kendrick KM. The main olfactory system and social learning in mammals. Behavior of Brain Resarche 2009; 200(2) 323-335.

[30] Egli M, Bertram R, Sellix MT, Freema, ME. Rythmic secretion of prolactin in rats: action of oxytocin coordinated by vasoactive intenstinal polypeptyde of suprachiasmatic nucleus origin. Endocrinology 2004; 145(7) 3386-3394.

[31] Misztal T, Górski K, Tomaszewska-Zaremba D, Molik E, Romanowicz K. Ientification of salsolinol in the mediobasal hypothalamus of lactating ewes and its relation to suckling-induced prolactin and GH release. Journal of Endocrinology 2008; 198: 83-89.
[32] Molik E, Misztal T, Romanowicz K, Zięba DA. The effects of melatonin on prolactin and growth hormone secretion in ewes under different photoperiods, during the early post partum period. Small Ruminant Research 2010; 94: 137-141
[33] Rhind S, Bass J, Doney M, Hunter E. Effect of litter size on the milk production, blood metabolite profiles and endocrine status of ewes lambing in January and April. Animal Production 1991; 53: 71-80
[34] Lincoln GA, Clarke IJ. Evidence that melatonin acts in the pituitary gland through a dopamine- independent mechanism to mediate effects of daylength on the secretion of prolactin in the ram. Neuroendocrinology 1995; 7: 637-643.
[35] Leong DA, Frawley LS, Neill JD. Neuroendocrine control of prolactin secretion. Annual Review of Physiology1983; 45; 109-127.
[36] Morgan PJ, Williams LM. The pars tuberalis of the pituitary: a gateway for neuroendocrine output. Reviews of Reproduction 1996; 1: 153-161.
[37] Williams L, Lincoln GA, Mercer JG, Barrett P, Morgan PJ, Clarke IJ. Melatonin receptors in the brain and pituitary gland of hypothalamo-pituitary disconnected Soay rams. Journal of Neuroendocrinology 1997; 9: 639-643.
[38] Stirland JA, Johnston JD, Cagampang FRA, Morgan PJ, Castro MG, White MRH, Davis JRE, Loudon ASI. Photoperiodic regulation of prolactin gene expression in the Syrian hamster by a pars tuberalis-derived factor. Journal of Neuroendocrinology 2001; 13: 147-157.
[39] Hazlerigg DG, Hastings MH, Morgan PJ. Production of prolactin realizing factor by the ovine pars tuberalis. Journal of Neuroendocrinology 1996; 8: 489-492.
[40] Molik E, Misztal T, Romanowicz K, Ciuryk S, Kisielewska A. Wpływ melatoniny na sekrecję prolaktyny u laktujących owiec – badania in vitro. Roczniki Naukowe Zootechniki 2005; 22: 253-256.
[41] Sakurai T, Amemiya A, Ishii M, Matsuzaki I, Chemelli RM, Tanaka H, Williams SC, Richardson JA, Kozlowski GP, Wilson S, Arch JRS, Buckingham RE, Haynes AC, Carr SA, Annan RS, McNulty DE, Liu WS, Terrett JA, Elshourbagy NA, Bergsma DJ, Yanagisawa M. Orexins and orexin receptors: a family of hypothalamic neuropeptides and G protein-coupled receptors that regulate feeding behavior. Cell 1998; 92: 573-585.
[42] De Lecea L, Kilduff TS, Peyron C, Gao XB, Foye PE, Danielson PE, Fukuhara C, Battenberg ELF, Gautvik VT, Bartlett FS, Frankel WN, Van den Pol AN, Bloom FE, Gautvik KM, Sutcliffe JG. The hypocretins: hypothalamus-specific peptides with neuroexcitatory activity Proceedings of the National Academy of Sciences of the United States of America 1998; 95: 322-327.
[43] Date Y, Mondal MS, Matsukura S, Ueta Y, Yamashita H, Kaiya H, Kangawa K, Nakazato M. Distribution of orexin/hypocretin in the rat median eminence and pituitary. Molecular Brain Research. 2000; 76 (1) 1-6.
[44] Taheri S, Mahmoodi M, Opacka-Juffry J, Ghatei MA, Bloom SR. Distribution and quantification of immunoreactive orexin A in rat tissues. FEBS letters 1999; 457: 157-161.
[45] Mitsuma T, Hirooka Y, Mori Y, Kayama M, Adachi K, Rhue N, Ping J, Nogimori T. Effects of orexin A on thyrotropin-releasing hormone and thyrotropin secretion in rats. Hormone and Metabolic Research 1999; 31 (11) 606-9.

[46] Spinazzi R, Andreis PG, Rossi GP, Nussdorfer GG. Orexins in the regulation of the hypothalamic-pituitary-adrenal axis. Pharmacological Review 2006; 58: 46–57.
[47] Russell SH, Small CJ, Kennedy AR, Stanley SA, Seth A, Murphy KG, Teheri S, Ghatei MA, Bloom SR. Orexin A Interactions in the hypothalamo-pituitary gonadal axis. Endocrinology 2001; 142 (12) 5294–5302.
[48] Russell SH, Kim MS, Small CJ, Abbott CR, Morgan DG, Taheri S, Murphy KG, Todd JF, Ghatei MA, Bloom SR. Central administration of orexin A suppresses basal and domperidone stimulated plasma prolactin. Journal of Neuroendocrinology 2000; 12 (12) 1213-8.
[49] Dusza L, Ciereszko R. Regulacja sekrecji gonadotropin i prolaktyny oraz ich oddziaływanie na tkanki docelowe. Wydawnictwo Uniwersytetu Warmińsko-Mazurskiego 2007; 95-138.
[50] Martyńska L, Polkowska J, Wolińska Witort E, Chmielowska M, Wasilewska-Dziubińska E, Bik W, Baranowska B. Orexin A and its role in the regulation of the hypothalamo-pituitary axes in the rat. Reproductive Biology 2006; 6 (2) 29-35.
[51] Archer ZA, Findlay PA, Rhind SM, Mercer JG, Adam CL. Orexin gene expression and regulation by photoperiod in the sheep hypothalamus. Regulatory Peptides 2002; 104 (1-3) 41-45.
[52] Iqbal J, Henry BA, Pompolo S, Rao A, Clarke IJ. Long-term alteration in bodyweight and food restriction does not affect the gene expression of either preproorexin or prodynorphin in the sheep. Neuroscience 2003; 118 (1) 217-26.
[53] Molik E, Zięba DA, Misztal T, Romanowicz K, Wszoła M, Wierzchoś E, Nowakowski M. The role of orexin A in the control of prolactin and growth hormone secretions in sheep – in vitro study. Journal of Physiology and. Pharmacology 2008; 59 (9) 91-100.
[54] Xu R, Wang Q, Yan M, Hernandez M, Gong C, Boon WC, Murata Y, Ueta Y, Chen C. Orexin-A augments voltage-gated Ca2+ currents and synergistically increases growth hormone (GH) secretion with GH-releasing hormone in primary cultured ovine somatotropes. Endocrinology 2002; 143 (12) 4609–4619.
[55] Zhang S, Blache D, Vercoe P E, Adam CL, Blackberry MA, Findlay PA, Eidne KA, Martin GB. Expression of orexin receptors in the brain and peripheral tissues of the male sheep', Regulatory Peptides 2004; 124 (1-3) 81-86.
[56] Molik E, Misztal T, Romanowicz K, Wierzchoś E. The Influence of length day on melatonin secretion during lactation in seasonal sheep. Archiv fur Tierzucht 2006; 49: 359-364.
[57] Zieba DA, Klocek B, Williams GL, Romanowicz K, Boliglowa L, Wozniak M. In vitro evidence that leptin suppresses melatonin secretion during long days and stimulates its secretion during short days in seasonal breeding ewes. Domestic Animal Endocrinology 2007; 33(3) 358-365.
[58] Zieba DA, Szczesna M, Klocek-Gorka B, Molik E, Misztal T, Williams GL, Romanowicz K, Stepien E, Keisler DH, Murawski M. Seasonal effects of central leptin infusion on melatonin and prolactin secretion and on SOCS-3 gene expression in ewes. Journal of Endocrinology 2008; 198: 147-155.
[59] Traczyk W, Przekop F. Methods of investigation of the function of the hypothalamus and hypophysis in chronic experiment in sheep. Acta Physiolica Polonica 1963; 14: 217-226.

Chapter 8

The Role of Prolactin in the Regulation of Male Copulatory Behavior

Toru R. Saito, Márk Oláh, Misao Terada and György M. Nagy

Additional information is available at the end of the chapter

http://dx.doi.org/10.5772/55515

1. Introduction

In developed countries, the elderly population increases at an accelerated rate due to a decrease in the birth rate and the prolongation of life through medical development. Moreover, increases in the elderly population allow the prediction of an increase in hyperprolactinemia caused by aging. It is well known that hyperprolactinemia decreases libido and causes oligozoospermia [1]. On the other hand, hyperprolactinemia is caused by or associated with, a variety of pathogenic stages: pituitary adenoma, hypothalamic disorders, hypogonadism and hypothyroidism, and is detected in patients with infertility [2, 3], impotence and hypogonadism [4]. PRL is a polypeptide hormone that is synthesized and secreted from mammotropes in the anterior lobe of the pituitary gland [5]. Many studies have documented a critical role of PRL in the maintenance of lactation in women and female animals [6, 7] as well as in immunregulation in both, males and females [8], however, its role in sexual behavior is not entirely clear [9-16].

It has been also shown that DAerg agonists facilitate several aspects of copulatory behavior and *ex copula* genital responses [10]. DAerg neurons, locating in the medial preoptic area (MPOA), and the zona incerta (incertohypothalamic DAerg system) are the key centers in the stimulatory control of sexual functions [17-18]. (R)-salsolinol (SAL), a DA related and derived tetrahydroisoquinoline, has been recently identified as a strong candidate for being the endogenous PRL releasing factor (PRF) synthesized in both the hypothalamus and the neurointermediate lobe (NIL) of the pituitary gland. Analysis of SAL concentrations revealed parallel increase and decrease with the elevation and reduction of plasma PRL, respectively. SAL is sufficiently potent and selective *in vivo* to account for the massive discharge of PRL that occurs after physiological changes. At the same time, parallel with its DA depleting effect in sympathetically innervated peripheral organs, SAL can reduce testosterone secretion both *in vivo* and *in vitro* from Leydig cells [19-20]. Based upon all of these data, the aim of our present studies was to confirm the suppressive effects of hyperprolactemia induced by grafting pituitary glands under the kidney capsule and to investigate the effect of a single injection of SAL on the elevation of plasma PRL and on sexual behavior in male rats.

Sexually experienced male rats of the Wistar-Imamichi strain (Imamichi Institute for Animal Reproduction, Tsuchiura, Japan), approximately 10 weeks old at the start of the experiments, were used. The animals were kept in a room with a temperature of 22-26 Celsius and subjected to a light-schedule of 14 hrs light and 10 hrs darkness (lights off at 19:00). They were provided with pellet diet CRF-1 (Charles River Laboratories Japan, Atsugi, Japan) and water ad libitum. Stimulus females of the same strain were rendered sexually receptive by treatment with estradiol benzoate (10μg/0.1 ml sesame oil, Sigma Chemical Co. Ltd., St. Louis, USA) 48 hrs prior to, and progesterone (500μg/0.1 ml sesame oil, Sigma Chemical Co. Ltd., St. Louis, USA) 4 hrs prior to exposure to males.

One group of experimental animals were anesthetized with Nembutal (40 mg/kg, i.p.) and implanted one and two whole pituitaries from male donors with the same age in the same strain under the left kidney capsule [21]. Rats having 1 or 2 pituitary grafts were sacrificed by decapitation between 19:30 and 20:30 in a week after the test. It was carried out in 30 seconds after taking animals out from their cages [22-23].

In a separate group of animals, intravenous (i.v.) cannula have been inserted into the jugular vein of male Sprague-Dawley rats for injection of SAL, and being able to take blood samples. Saline or SAL (4 mg/kg body weight i.v.) have been injected to the animals prior to expose them to females being in estrus.

Copulatory behavior test have been conducted four weeks after the surgery. After a male rat was placed in the semi-circular observation cage (radius 40, height 50 cm) faced with Plexiglass under low-level red-light illumination for a few minutes, a sexually receptive female was introduced to its cage. Tests lasted 60 min from the introduction of the female. Behavioral testing was conducted between 19:30 and 20:30. The behavior categories scored included the following [24]. *Mounting frequency* (MF): number of mounts without intromission preceding ejaculation. *Intromission frequency* (IF): number of mounts with intromission preceding ejaculation. *Ejaculation frequency* (EF): number of ejaculations during 60 min. *Mount latency* (ML): time from the presentation of the female to the male's first mount. *Intromission latency* (IL): time from the presentation of the male's first intromission. *Ejaculation latency* (EL): latency from the first intromission until ejaculation. *Post-ejaculatory interval* (PEI): latency from ejaculation to the next intromission.

Blood collected and centrifuged at 3,000 g for 15 minutes for the analysis of serum hormone. The serum was stored at -80 Celsius until analyzed by RIA for determination of serum PRL, LH and FSH. Serum concentrations of PRL, LH and FSH were measured by RIA using the method of Furudate et al. [25] with reagents provided from NIADDK. The standard references used were, rPRL-RP-3 for PRL, rLH-RP-2 for LH and rFSH-RP-2 for FSH. The intra- and inter-assay coefficients of variation were 9.6 and 15.9 for PRL, 3.5 and 5.3 for LH, and 5.3 and 9.8 for FSH, respectively. Testosterone levels were also measured by direct RIA.

All data are presented as mean ± SEs. The results from the copulatory behavior testing were analyzed using Fisher's exact probability test and the Mann-Whitney U test and the data for hormone levels and organs weights were analyzed by Duncan's multiple t-test.

2. Effect of pituitary transplants induced hyperprolactinaemia on copulatory behavior

The results of serum hormone levels in two pituitaries grafted and sham animals are shown in Table 1. Prolactin (PRL) concentration in rats having two pituitary grafts was significantly higher than sham operated animals ($p < 0.05$). There were no significant differences in the serum levels of luteinizing hormone (LH), folliculostimulating hormone (FSH) and testosterone between the same groups of animals.

Group	LH (ng/ml)	FSH (μg/ml)	Prolactin (ng/ml)	Testosterone (ng/ml)
Graft	1.3 ± 0.16	65.3 ± 13.60	31.1 ± 3.40[a]	2.1 ± 0.29
Sham	1.3 ±0.20	97.4 ± 9.84	7.2 ± 1.51[b]	2.6 ± 0.24
All data represent mean ± S.E. *p<0.05 a vs. b				

Table 1. Serum hormone levels in grafted male rats

As it is shown on Fig. 1, the mean number of mount in rats having one-, two grafted pituitaries and non was 76.5 ± 5.35, 66.8 ± 6.37 and 40.2 ± 3.43, respectively. The mount frequency (MF) showed a tendency to be higher in grafted, compared with sham-operated animals. The mean frequency of intromission (IF) was lower for one (18.0 ± 1.27) and two pituitaries grafted males (10.0 ± 2.00), compared to sham-operated controls (29.0 ± 2.00). There were significant differences in IF between two pituitaries grafted and sham-operated males ($p < 0.05$). Ejaculation could be detected in all one-pituitary grafted and sham-operated males, while did not in 4 out of 6 two-pituitaries grafted males. The mean ejaculation frequency (EF) of one, two pituitaries grafted and sham males was 3.5 ± 0.33, 0.8 ± 0.20 and 5.2 ± 0.20, respectively. The EF of two pituitaries grafted males is significantly lower than sham males ($P < 0.01$).

As shown on Fig. 2, having two pituitary grafts resulted in a significant prolongation in the mean latency of intromission, compared with sham-operated animals (1,014.4 ± 206.12 versus 67.8 ± 7.72 sec, $p < 0.05$). The mean latency to the first ejaculation showed a tendency to extend in animals having one (652.1 ± 56.06 sec), two (1,367.5 sec) pituitary grafts, compared with sham-operated males (369.7 ± 25.28 sec). The post-ejaculatory interval (PEI) tended to extend in animals having one (425.7 ± 27.40 sec) or two (487.5 sec) pituitary grafts, compared with sham-operated animals (341.7 ± 3.27 sec).

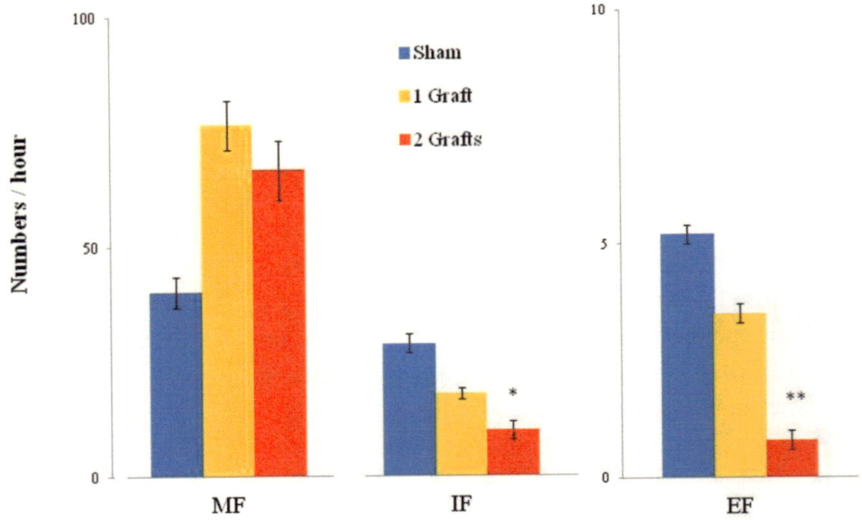

MF: Mount frequency. IF: Intromission frequency. EF: Ejaculation frequency. *p<0.05:2 Grafts vs. Sham; **p<0.01:2 Grafts vs Sham

Figure 1. Copulatory behavior in pituitary-grafted male rats.

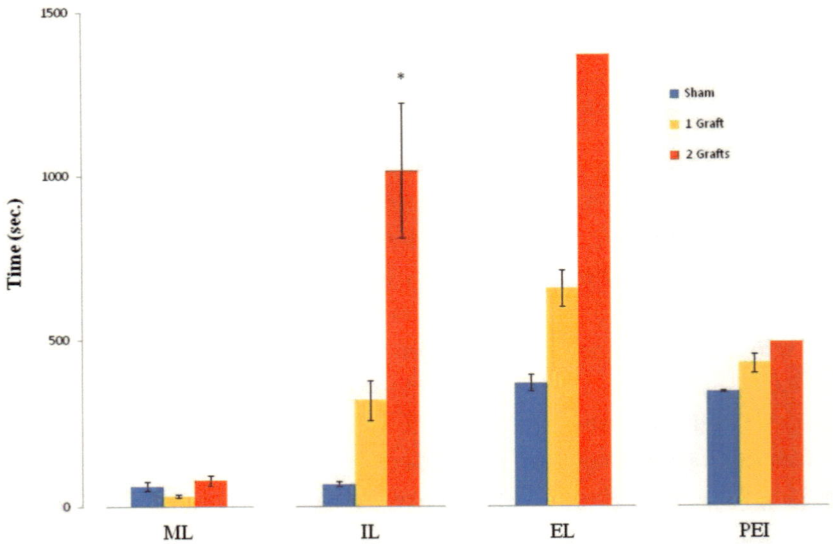

MF: Mount frequency. IF: Intromission frequency. EF: Ejaculation frequency.PEI: Post-ejaculatory interval *p<0.052 Grafts vs. Sham;

Figure 2. Copylatory behavior in pituitary-grafted male rats

3. Effect of SAL on copulatory behavior

Plasma PRL concentrations of control and SAL groups at 15 min before exposure to females were 7.3 ± 2.0 and 8.0 ± 1.5 ng/ml, respectively. Moreover, plasma PRL concentrations in males immediately after exposure to the females were 7.4 ± 1.2 and 68.0 ± 5.9 ng/ml, respectively. All (8 out of 8) of the control animals ejaculated in the presence of the female, whereas only 33% (2 out of 6) of the SAL group ejaculated. An increasing tendency for mount latency and intromission latency as well as a decreasing tendency for intromission frequency has been observed in the SAL injected group compared to the controls.

Group	Basal (ng/ml)	After Exposure (ng/ml)	Ejaculation Frequency
Control	7.3 ± 2.0	7.4 ± 1.2[a]	100%
SAL	8.0 ± 1.5	68 ± 5.9[b]	33%
All data represent mean ± S.E. *$p<0.05$ a vs. b			

Table 2. Effect of SAL on Plasma PRL levels and copulatory behaviour

4. Discussion

In male subjects, parallel with the age related testosterone depletion, there is a gradual increase of plasma PRL, generally referred as hyperprolactinemia, which is strictly related with a decrease of libido, erectile dysfunctions and oligozoospermia. It is an important issue in humans, because the proportion of elderly generation increases in developed countries, therefore, they also face to the same problems. Our data confirm previous results that only a mild but sustained elevation of PRL secretion is enough for inhibiting copulatory behavior. However, the exact neuronal and/or endocrine background of these age-related changes is not completely known. Our results underline the relationships between DA and its metabolite, SAL, in the regulation of sexual behavior and put a new player into the focus of this field. SAL cannot pass the blood-brain barrier, therefore, it likely affects copulatory behavior out of this barrier. In theory, anterior lobe of the pituitary gland may be one of the sites. In spite of the well documented PRL releasing activity of SAL *in vivo*, it has been also shown that SAL does not have a significant PRL releasing activity *in vitro*. Therefore, it can be hypothesized that SAL induces an elevation of plasma PRL as well as inhibition of the copulatory behavior through indirect pathways, which can communicate with each other. Short time elevation of plasma PRL that can be detected after SAL treatment just before copulation may be enough to inhibit copulatory behavior, but it needs further investigations.

Interestingly enough, SAL is also supposed to be formed after taking alcohol, and negative effect of alcohol on sexual behavior is also well known. Based on all of these, if we can learn more about the role of SAL in the regulation of sexual behavior, it shall be advantageous not only for basic research but it may give a chance to find the way to use agonists or antagonists of this molecule for using them in the medical or clinical fields. Although some progress has been made in identifying neurotransmitter-receptor effects on behavioral components of the copulatory behavior, but it is rather complex, and no drug has been found yet to affect only a single component.

Author details

Toru R. Saito and Misao Terada
Behavioral Neuroscience Section, Nippon Veterinary and Life Science University, Tokyo, Japan

Márk Oláh and György M. Nagy*
Cellular and Molecular Neuroendocrine Research Laboratory, Department of Human Morphology, Semmelweis University, Budapest, Hungary

Acknowledgement

This work was supported by OTKA-81522 for GMN. Thanks are due to Mariann Akocsi for her excellent technical help preparing this manuscript.

5. References

[1] Weizman A, Weizman R, Hart J Maoz B, Wijsenbeek H, Ben David M (1983) The correlation of Increased Serum Prolactin levels with Decreased Sexual Desire and Activity in Elderly Men. J am geriatr soc 31: 485-488.

[2] Segal S, polishhuk WZ, Ben-David M. (1976) Hyperprolactinemic Male Infaertility. Fertil steril 27: 1425-1427.

[3] Segal S, Yaffe H, Laufer N, Ben-David M (1979) Male Hyperprolactinemia: effects on Fertility. Fertil steril 32: 556-561.

[4] Thoener MO, Besser GM (1978) Bromocriptine Treatment of Hyperprolactinaemic Hypognadism. Acta endocrinol 88: 131-146.

[5] Maki A (1988) Prolactin and Male Sexual Dysfunction. Nippon hinyokika gakkai zasshi. 79: 1002-1010.

[6] Bridges RS, DiBiase R, Loundes D (1985) Prolactin Stimulation of Maternal Behavior in Female Rats. Science 227: 782-784.

[7] Molz H, Lubin M, Leon M Numan M (1970) Hormonal Induction of Maternal Behavior in the Ovariectomized Nulliparous Rat. Physiol behave 5: 1373-1377.

[8] Bole-Feysot C, Goffin V, Edery M, Binart N, Kelly PA (1998) Prolactin (PRL) and its receptor: actions, signal transduction pathways and phenotypes observed in PRL receptor knockout mice. Endocr Rev. 19(3):225-68.

[9] Bartke A, Morgan WW, Clayton RN, Banerji TK, Brodie AM, Parkening TA, Collins TJ (1987) Neuroendocrine Studies in Hyperprolactinaemic Male Mice. J Endocrinol. 112:215-20.

---

* Corresponding Author

[10] Bitran D, Hull EM (1987) Pharmacological Analysis of Male Rat Sexual Behavior. Neurosci Biobehav Rev. 11:365-89.

[11] Doherty PC, Baum MJ, Todd RB (1986) Effects of Chronic Hyperprolactinemia on Sexual Arousal and Erectile Function in Male Rats. Neuroendocrinology 42:368-75.

[12] Doherty PC, Bartke A, Smith MS, Davis SL (1985) Increased Serum Prolactin Levels Mediate the Suppressive Effects of Ectopic Pituitary Grafts on Copulatory Behavior in Male Rats. Horm Behav. 19:111-21.

[13] Kalra PS, Simpkins JW, Luttge WG, Kalra SP (1983) Effects on Male Sex Behavior and Preoptic Dopamine Neurons of Hyperprolactinemia Induced by MtTW15 Pituitary Tumors. Endocrinology 113:2065-71.

[14] Weber RF, Ooms MP, Vreeburg JT (1982) Effects of Prolactin-Secreting Tumour on Copulatory Behaviour in Male Rats. J Endocrinol 93:223-9.

[15] Bailey DJ, Herbert J (1982) Impaired Copulatory Behaviour of Male Rats with Hyperprolactinaemia Induced by Domperidone or Pituitary Grafts. Neuroendocrinology 35:186-93.

[16] Svare B, Bartke A, Doherty P, Mason I, Michael SD, Smith MS (1979) Hyperprolactinemia Suppresses Copulatory Behavior in Male Rats and Mice. Biol Reprod. 21:529-35.

[17] Giuliano, F; Allard (2011) Dopamine and sexual function. International Journal of Impotence Research 13 (S3): S18-S28

[18] Juan M. Dominguez, Elaine M. Hull (2005) Dopamine, the medial preoptic area, and male sexual behavior Physiology & Behavior 86: 356 – 368.

[19] Stammel W, Thomas H, Staib W, Kühn-Velten WN (1991) Tetrahydroisoquinoline alkaloids mimic direct but not receptor-mediated inhibitory effects of estrogens and phytoestrogens on testicular endocrine function. Possible significance for Leydig cell insufficiency in alcohol addiction. Life Sciences 49 (18):1319–1329

[20] Oláh M, Bodnár I, Daniel G, Tóth EB, Vecsernyés M, Nagy GM (2011) Role of salsolinol in the regulation of pituitary prolactin and peripheral dopamine release. Reproductive Medicine and Biology 10 (3): 143-151

[21] Aoki S, Saito TR, Otaka S, Amao H, Tagawa M, Umeda M, Sugiyama M, Takahashi KW (1992) Improvement of Pituitary Homograft under the Kidney Capsule in Mice. Exp. anim. 41: 87-91.

[22] Dunn JD, Arimura A, Scheving LE (1972) Effect of Stress of Circadian Periodicity in Serum LH and Prolactin Concentration. Endocrinology 90: 29-33.

[23] Raud HR, Kiddy CA, Odell, WD (1971) The Effect of Stress upon the Determination of Serum Prolactin by Radioimmunoassy. Proc. soc. exp. biol. med. 136: 689-693.

[24] Heimer L, Larsson K (1967) Mating Behavior of Male Rats after Olfactory Bulb Lesions. Physiol. behav. 2: 207-209.

[25] Furudate S, Nakano T (1989) Prolactin Secretion and its Response to Stress during the Estrous Cycle of the Rats. Exp. anim. 38: 313-318.

Chapter 9

Prolactin and Infertility

Gokalp Oner

Additional information is available at the end of the chapter

http://dx.doi.org/10.5772/55557

1. Introduction

Prolactin (PRL) is one of several hormones that are produced by the pituitary gland. PRL has many different roles throughout the body, and most of those are clearly shown as clinical symptom. Perhaps the most important classical role of prolactin is to stimulate milk production in women after the delivery of a baby. Prolactin levels increase during pregnancy causing the mammary glands to enlarge in preparation for breastfeeding and ready to secrete colostrums closely after delivery. Later on the elevated prolactin levels help with the sustained production of milk during nursing. The somatomammotrop cells of the anterior pituitary gland synthesize and secrete prolactin, which is under the control of hypothalamic factors, mainly the tonic inhibition of Dopamine (DA). There are several other sources of PRL-like substances in the periphery such as placental lactogens, (similar to pituitary PRL), mammary gland (produced within the mammary epithelial cells), or PRL variants of immune cell origin (that modulates the immune system). (Gellersen,1989; Andersen 1990; Lkhider, 1996; Kurtz,1993; Gala, 1994, Montgomery,1990; Ben-Jonathan 1996; Yu-Lee LY 1997)

It is important to underline that serum PRL in normal individuals is considered as almost entirely pituitary PRL sources, the above mentioned extra pituitary-PRL may contribute significant amounts but either carries as specific function and target mainly to the local environment acting via paracrine/autocrine manner. (Yu-lee 1997; Bachelot 2007)

During the first several months of breastfeeding, the higher basal prolactin levels also serve to suppress ovarian cyclicity , through the inhibition of pituitary hormones, mainly via LH suppression (Taya 1982) This is the reason why women who are breastfeeding do not get their periods and therefore do not often become pregnant. In actively breastfeeding mothers the related hyperprolactinaemia persisting even over a year. It was observed that extended lactational amenorrhea is associated with low LH levels, and interestingly suckling induced PRL elevation as a response has a positive effect on prolongation. (Diaz 1991; Diaz 1995).

Menstruation and ovulation may only occasionally occur before the drop of elevated basal PRL levels. As time goes on with less frequent breastfeeding, e.g. during weaning however, the PRL levels do not stay as high and the woman may start to ovulate. In cases of nonlactating/ nonbreastfeeding mothers, that may happen between 2-3 month after delivery. (Baird 1979)

Similarly, elevated PRL levels are shown during gestation, but mechanisms to inhibit ovulation is related to elevated estardiol and progesterone levels and a consequent depression of pituitary FSH secretion (Marrs 1981).

Generally, the lactogenic hormones play role also in regulation of reproductive function. On one hand, PRL is essential to maintain regular oestrus cycles. PRL knock out mice are completely infertile (Horsemann 1997). One of the other actions of PRL is to stimulate ovarian production of progesterone. That is required in the process of preparation for embryo implantation and it is dependent on a continued estrogen and progesterone secretion by the corpus luteum, which is supported by a functional pituitary during the first half of pregnancy in rodents. (Binart 2000)

On the other hand, high prolactin levels are associated with anovulation or may cause directly or indirectly infertility. In young women, hyperprolactinemia is probably one of the most common endocrine disorders related to pituitary function. Women who are not pregnant and are not breastfeeding should have lower levels of basal PRL (typically 10–28 μg/L in women and 5–10 μg/L in men are defined as "normal levels") If a non-pregnant woman has abnormally high levels of PRL, it may cause her difficulty in becoming pregnant. It is considered as the most frequent cause of anovulatory sterility, although spontaneous pregnancy may occur occasionally. The prevalence of hyperprolactinemia varies in different patient populations, stays below 1% (0.4% in an unselected normal population) but can be as high as 17% of women with reproductive disorders shown at the clinics (Crosignani 1999)

The suppression of pituitary hormones by PRL, similar that described during lactation has an indirect anovulatory effect. PRL however, acts also directly on the ovary to inhibit the hCG-induced follicle rupture, resulting in the inhibition of ovulation. (Yoshimura 1989).

Clinically significant elevation of PRL levels may cause infertility in several different ways. First, prolactin may stop a woman from ovulating. If this occurs, a woman's menstrual cycles will stop. In less severe cases, high prolactin levels may only disrupt ovulation once in a while. This would result in intermittent ovulation or ovulation that takes a long time to occur. Women in this category may experience infrequent or irregular periods. Women with the mildest cases involving high prolactin levels may ovulate regularly but not produce enough of the hormone progesterone after ovulation. This is known as a luteal phase defect. Deficiency in the amount of progesterone produced after ovulation may result in a uterine lining that is less able to have an embryo implant. Some women with this problem may see their period come a short time after ovulation (Shibli-Rahhal,2011)

Hyperprolactinemia is commonly found in both female and male patients with abnormal sexual and/or reproductive function or with galactorrhea. If serum prolactin levels are above 200 μg/L, a prolactin-secreting pituitary adenoma (prolactinoma) is the underlying cause, but if levels are lower, differential diagnoses include the intake of various drugs, compression of the pituitary stalk by other pathology, hypothyroidism, renal failure, cirrhosis, chest wall lesions, or idiopathic hyperprolactinemia. When a pituitary tumour is present, patients often have pressure symptoms in addition to endocrine dysfunction, such as headaches, visual field defects, or cranial nerve deficits (Wang, 2012). The objectives of therapy are to improve the symptoms associated with high PRL levels and to reduce the size of a pituitary tumour.

Pharmacotherapy is available to reduce the tumour size and consequently decrease PRL levels. The large majority of patients with prolactinomas, both micro- and macroprolactinomas, can be successfully treated with dopamine D2 receptor agonists as first-line treatment, with normalization of prolactin secretion and gonadal function, and with significant tumour shrinkage in a high percentage of cases, to prevent the need for surgery. In cases when the only cause of infertility is chronic anovulation due to hyperprolactinemia, a 60-80% pregnancy rate can be achieved. Surgical resection of the prolactinoma is the option for patients who may refuse or do not respond to long-term pharmacological therapy. Radiotherapy and/or estrogens are also reasonable choices if surgery fails. In patients with asymptomatic microprolactinoma no treatment needs to be given and a regular follow-up with serial prolactin measurements and pituitary imaging should be organized (Asa 2002; Crosignani 1999, Molitch 2003).

The most commonly used dopamine agonists are bromocriptine, pergolide, quinagolide and cabergoline. When comparing the plasma half-life, efficacy and tolerability of these drugs are different, there is also important to evaluate the risk/ benefits profile of each product. As the current clinical practice, pharmacological treatment with dopamine agonist plays an important role. The recommendations on the most effective dosages and the advantages of a long term efficacy of products have been evaluated summarizing the results of case histories of the last decades.

2. Clinical diagnosis of hyperprolactinemia

A variety of etiological factors including disorders of the hypothalamo-pituitary axis, interruption of dopamine synthesis, stress, pituitary tumours, polycystic ovary syndrome, primary hypothyroidism, and various medications may lead to hyperprolactinemia (5). Hyperprolactinemia in girls causes delayed puberty, hypogonadotropic hypogonadism, primary or secondary amenorrhea, and galactorrhea (Fideleff, 2000). Hyperprolactinemia in men may result in as a first signs of decreased libido or impotence, however also cause inefficient sperm production and infertility (Colao, 2004).

As one of the fist signs in women with high prolactin levels may have irregular periods or no periods at all. Another common symptom is "galactorrhea", which is the occurrence of a milky discharge from the breast in a woman who has not recently been pregnant. The discharge is the result of persistant high PRL levels stimulating the mammary gland for milk production. Some women may see galactorrhea occur spontaneously. Others may see it only if they squeeze their nipples.

As diagnostic practice, after signs and labtests have been evaluated the magnetic resonance imaging (MRI) of the pituitary gland should be performed in all patients. A pituitary adenoma with a diameter of less than 1 cm is defined as "microadenoma" and one above 1 cm in diameter as "macroadenoma".

3. Measurement of prolactin

Prolactin can be measured with a simple blood test drawn at the fertility doctor's office. In order to get accurate results, prolactin should be drawn first thing in the morning. Since PRL may serve as a hormone to affect reproductive functions, sexual contact, stimulation of nipples in human may cause a not just immediate but also next-day-long alterations of the PRL secretory pattern. (Kruger 2012) These fluctuations are measured on the next day to produce a PRL elevation around noon, additional of the regular circadian rhythm of PRL levels, as the peak on the morning. Accordingly it is important to note that the woman should have the instructions to eat nothing from the night before and to avoid any stimulation of the breast and nipples, included sexual intercourse as well, from the day before also.

Since stimulation of the breast /nipples (stress such as physical exam) may cause immediate release of PRL one common mistake that doctors make is to draw a prolactin blood test immediately after a patient has had a breast exam in the office. These women will have high prolactin levels because of the exam and therefore they may show false (i.e. transient) increase of PRL levels. Prolactin should also be drawn early in the menstrual cycle - before ovulation. This is because prolactin levels are naturally higher after ovulation.

A prolactin level of 5-20 ng/mL is considered normal in both sexes, according to some laboratories and test references the male and female (a bit higher) normal range may differ. A level above 20 ng/mL in two successive measurements is defined as hyperprolactinemia (7). According to WHO standards: 1 μg/L = 21.2 mIU/L. PRL levels > 250 ng/mL usually indication for prolactinoma, when PRL > 500 ng/mL it is considered as diagnosis for macroprolactinoma. (Melmed, 2011)

There are cases when false positive and elevated PRL levels are measured: two high molecular mass forms of prolactin (PRL) in serum have been identified: macroprolactin (big-big PRL, > 100 kDa) and big PRL (40-60 kDa). Big PRL is a consistent "normal" component of total serum PRL but rarely cause of hyperprolactinemia. Macroprolactin is usually a complex of PRL and IgG in composition, it is formed in the circulation from monomeric PRL with a molecular mass of 150-170 kDa, but may have some additional variability in composition. In labor tests the PRL in the complex remains reactive to a variable extent in immunoassays. Individuals may show a different pattern of % of these variants, or even can be a predominant immunoreactive component of circulating PRL and the cause of apparent hyperprolactinemia, but it has minimal bioactivity in vivo and is not of pathological significance. As necessary the reference technique of gel filtration chromatography at the laboratory should be available for confirmation and request on investigation of samples to avoid confusion of diagnostics. (Fahie-Wilson 2005)

4. Causes of high prolactin levels

4.1. Pituitary tumours

Pituitary adenomas are the most common tumour type in the pituitary gland. There is approximately 10% incidence was shown obtained by post-mortem autopsy, with similar ratio of male and female patients. The most frequently detected tumours (over 39%) are sparsely granulated PRL cell adenomas. The others types are GH cell or mixed PRL/GH adenoma, ACTH cell adenoma/Crooke's cell adenoma (~14%) ; Gonadotroph cell adenoma (6.6%); Null cell adenoma/oncocytoma (~32%) and other or unclassified types (Buurman, 2006).

Invasive tumours with multiple recurrences are only classified as aggressive tumours or "atypical adenomas". Tumours with systemic metastasis must be considered as carcinomas, and "only" make up 0.1% to 0.2% of all pituitary tumours, but with very poor prognostics of 66% mortality (Oh, 2012). However it was suggested that a full picture inlcuded clinical signs (gender, DA-resistant hyperprolactinemia, etc) , radiological status (invasive macro or giant tumour) and histological signs of angiogenesis, mitoses level, vascular invasion and molcular biology parameters (Ki-67 > 3 %, p53 positive, up-regulation of genes related to invasion and proliferation, and allelic loss of chromosome 11) should be taken into account considering the potential malignancy, prognosis of prolactin secreting tumours and identify the optimal therapy as early as possible. The key question is to identify factors associated with tumour aggressiveness. The approach combined genomic and transcriptomic analysis focus to the subtype of pituitary tumour able to identify molecular events associated with the aggressive and malignant phenotypes. Allelic loss in certain loci of chromosome 11 has been detected in tumours with signs of malignancy, potentially responsible for triggering the aggressive and malignant phenotypes. Within the recent years there are an increasing number of genes or molecular signs that has been associated with pituitary tumorigenesis to develop predictive and potential prognostic markers. (Zemmoura, 2012; Dworakowska, 2012; Wierinckx 2011)

About one-third of all pituitary tumours are not associated with hypersecretory syndromes but, rather, present with symptoms of an intracranial mass, such as headaches, nausea, vomiting or visual field disturbances. Only rare cases of pituitary tumours are considered as malignant prolactinoma. Tumours that produce growth hormone (GH) may also secrete prolactin in nearly 25% of cases. This is a common source of misdiagnosis, as the features of prolactin excess may capture attention while the more subtle features of GH excess go unnoticed.

4.1.1. Characteristics of pituitary adenomas

In some people, a small group of cells may form a cyst in the pituitary gland which produces elevated levels of prolactin. These cysts are called prolactinomas or pituitary adenomas. It is unclear exactly how these cysts get started. Recent investigations on pituitary tumours reported that approximately 12% of pituitary glands (obtained by autopsy of 3048 patients) are shown histologically diagnosed but clinically inapparent adenoma. Among the mean tumour size is approx 1.9mm. According to published data two-thirds of adenomas has a tumour size <3 mm, half of them were smaller than 1 mm in diameter and ~23% was between 3-10mm. In this study only few (3/76) tumours were identified as macroadenomas corresponding to a tumour size >10 mm. (Buurman, *2006)*

The prevalence of clinically apparent prolactinomas ranges from 6–50/ 100,000 in reported populations (Daly, 2006; Fernandez 2010). The prevalence of "ever-treated" hyperprolactinemia is approximately 20 /100,000 in male patients and approximately 90 /100,000 in female patients. (Kars, 2009)

The adenomas can be seen and measured using MRI and classified based on their size.

Small adenomas are known as microadenomas. They measure less than one centimetre in diameter. This is the most common type of adenoma found. Microadenomas can even be present in healthy people who do not have high prolactin levels. Microadenomas can be treated with medication. They do not grow large and do not need to be treated if hormone levels are normal. Microprolactinomas usually follow a benign course and rarely progress to macroprolactinomas. However, in rare cases microadenoma may transform to other tumours.

- A case history it was reported that a microadenoma transformed to macroprolactinoma within 10 month, probably due to estrogen therapy applied. The case report emphasizes the role of dopaminergic agonist in treatment of hyperprolactinemia. (Garcia, 1995)
- A case history of a 22 -year-old woman with the signs of galactorrhea and slight hyperprolactinemia , showed 7-mm intrapituitary lesion which responded to treatment with cabergoline. This PRL-secreting microadenoma has a sudden change within 4 years of diagnose. The case represents a rapid evolution from a microprolactinoma initially responding to dopamine agonists to a fatal pituitary carcinoma. (Guastamacchia, 2007)

Adenomas larger than 1 centimetre are called macroadenomas. If untreated, macroadenomas can grow further and start to compress the nearby tissues and structures causing life-threatening events or even fatal outcome. The closest structures are the optic nerves, internal carotid arteries. If a macroadenoma causes compression of the optic nerves, partial blindness can result. For this reason, it is important to treat macroadenomas whether or not a woman is interested in getting pregnant. Medication can be used to treat them but if that fails, surgery may be necessary.

- According to a recent clinical study in Japan, treatment with Cabergoline achieved a high pregnancy rate with uneventful outcomes in infertile women with prolactinoma, independent of tumour size and bromocriptine resistance or intolerance. Over 90% of patients in the study conceived pregnancies, and one-third of the macroprolactinomas disappeared. Cabergoline monotherapy could serve as an alternative of the conventional combination bromocriptine therapy with surgery or irradiation in macroprolactinomas. (Ono, 2010)

4.2. Hypothyroidism

The hyperprolactinemia of hypothyroidism is related to several mechanisms. In response to the hypothyroid state, a compensatory increase in the discharge of central hypothalamic thyrotropin releasing hormone (TRH) results in increased stimulation of prolactin secretion.

Although TRH was originally named for its ability to trigger the release of thyroid-stimulating hormone (TSH) in mammals, it became apparent that TRH exerts multiple hypophysiotropic activities also in human. Stimulation with TRH will provide a diagnostic test to demonstrate a TSH release curve typical of the subclinic hypothyroidism. PRL is under tonic inhibition by the hypothalamus by way of the PRL inhibitory factor, DA. PRL-releasing factors include TRH., Increased release of TRH may also cause a sustained stimulation of prolactin release from the pituitary gland. There are several clinical reports presented the correlation between subclinic hypothyroidism-hyperprolactinemia and sterility. Treatment with thyroid hormone supplements will result in correction of both the thyroid feedback and the high prolactin levels.

4.3. Macroprolactinemia

Asymptomatic patients with intact gonadal and reproductive function and moderately elevated prolactin levels may have macroprolactinemia (Vallette-Kasic, 2002). Hypersecretion of PRL by lactotroph cells of the anterior pituitary cause hyperprolactinemia. Patients with hyperprolactinemia may have radiologically undetected microprolactinomas, but some of them may present other causes of hyperprolactinemia characterised as a symptom of macroprolactinemia, with a predominance of higher molecular mass prolactin forms (big-big prolactin, MW > 150 kDa). This term should not be confused with macroprolactinoma, which refers to a large pituitary tumour greater than 10 mm in diameter.

The prevalence of macroprolactinemia varies between 15-46% in hyperprolactinemic populations, and it may because confusing tests results that could not be differentiated from true hyperprolactinemic patients, on the basis of clinical features alone. The pathophysiology of macroprolactinemia is based on a mechanisms of the increased antigenicity of these molecules, leading to the appearance of autoantibodies against PRL, which can consequently reduce the bioactivity of PRL and provide extended half-life. Therefore macroprolactinemia is manifested with less frequent clinical symptoms in macroprolactinemic patients and the tests results mainly due to the delayed clearance of

PRL. According to recent publications of Isik et al, evaluating over 300 hyperprolactinemic patients, over 26% of them resulted in elevated macroprolactin levels, with the less frequent signs of galactorrhea or abnormal MRI results compared those to patients with predominant monomer hyperprolactinemia. The other symptoms and frequency of amenorrhea, infertility, irregular menses, gynecomastia, and erectile dysfunction were similar in both groups. (Isik, 2012)

Macroprolactinemic patients have no clinical symptoms of hyperprolactinemia and may have no pituitary adenomas. It is still controversial whether macroprolactinemia is a benign condition that does not need further investigation and treatment. Patients can be screened for macroprolactinemia by PEG (polyethylene glycol) precipitation as a standard laboratory test with a results of recovery of ≤40% to normal monomeric PRL level is used as an indication of macroprolactinemia (Tamer, 2012). The clinical importance of this test is based on the lower prevalence of pituitary adenomas in this group, compared to "true hyperprolactinemic" patients.

4.4. PCOS (polycystic ovary syndrome)

PCOS is a common problem that can cause infertility by inhibiting ovulation, affecting 3.5-10% of the reproductive age of women. For unknown reasons, some women with PCOS may have slightly high PRL levels. PCOS similar to hypoprolactinemic are both common causes of secondary amenorrhoea in women. The relationship between PCOS and hyperprolactinemia so far has been reported still with controversial results: it seems that PCOS is very prevalent with hyperprolactinemia, nevertheless there are different reasons of altered regulation of gondotropin secretion, and suggests that these conditions have independent origins. Recent investigators using serial serum sampling have excluded transient elevations of PRL and have shown a less frequent association of these two disorders. According to clinical guidelines PCOS patients with increased PRL levels must be investigated for other causes of hyperprolactinemia, because hyperprolactinemia may be due to a reason of concomitant disease, but not proved the cause-relationship to PCOS. Treatment of infertility associated with PCOS has changed in the last decade due to the introduction of new medications such as insulin-sensitizing drugs, aromatase inhibitors, gonadotropin treatment etc. (Bracero 2001, Urman, 2006, Escobar-Morreale, 2004)

- In a study conducted in Brazil, among the 82 PCOS women, 13 (16%) presented high PRL levels (over 100 microg/l). There were several reasons of hyperprolactinemia: pituitary adenoma; drug-induced hyperprolactinemia, or macroprolactinemia. The non-hyperprolactinemic PCOS patients (over 80%) represented normal PRL levels. The authors concluded that hyperprolactinemia is not a clinical manifestation of PCOS. (Filho, 2007)

4.5. Medications

Some medications can cause higher levels of prolactin to be produced. The most common medications that do this are known as anti-psychotic medications. The antipsychotics mostly act as dopaminergic neurotransmitters/ receptor blockers can also cause endocrine side effects, as hyperprolactinaemia and it is most common side effect of first-generation antipsychotics. The second- and thirdgeneration antipsychotics have a weaker affinity for D2 dopamine receptors, thus hyperprolactinemia is less common when such medication is used. (Uzun et al. 2005). The risk of side effects caused by antipsychotics is individual and it does not depend solely on the therapeutic dose and may have influence on some predisposing conditions. (Ružić 2011)

Other medications which may increase prolactin levels:

- Some types of anti-depressants, serotonin reuptake inhibitors, SRIs (fluvoxamine; fluoxetine; paroxetine, duloxetine etc)
- Some types of sedatives
- Catecholamine depletor
- Dopamine synthesis inhibitor
- Neuropeptides
- Anticonvulsants
- Opiates and opiate antagonists
- Estrogen Oral contraceptives (birth control pills)
- Some types of blood pressure medications (methyldopa, verapamil)
- A medication for nausea (Reglan, metoclopramide)
- Antacids (cimetidine)

4.6. Stress

A high prolactin level can sometimes be related to physical stress. Even drawing blood can by itself cause someone to produce and immediate prolactin-release. PRL eleveation can also detected in response to strong or sudden external stimuli in general, such as stressful environmental conditions, or can be related to physchological reasons. This latter can be evaluated by stress profile or measured by experimental conditions, such as "Screamer Index", which is shown resulting in values to be parallel to levels of hyperprolactinemia in women. (Harrison, 1988; Cepisky, 1992). On the other hand, anxiety and irritability maybe a result of hyperprolactinemia. In rat models PRL increased the stimulatory effect of ACTH-induced corticosterone secretion (Jaroenporn, 2007).

- Endocrine abnormalities are frequently associated with a wide range of psychological symptoms. These symptoms may reach the level of psychiatric illness (mainly mood and anxiety disorders) or just being identified by the subclinical forms of assessment provided by the Diagnostic Criteria for Psychosomatic Research (DCPR). In a population study reported by Sonino et al, (2007), the majority of patients suffered from at least one of the three DCPR syndromes considered: irritable mood (over 45%), demoralization, persistent somatization. Long-standing endocrine disorders may imply a degree of irreversibility of the pathological process. Endocrine treatment may cause even the worsening of psychological symptoms. The methodology and assessment score provided by DCPR tests have been demonstrated to be a valuable tool for psychological assessment in endocrine disease from diagnostic to follow-up periods. (Sonino 2007)

- In clinical environment the variability of PRL concentration in random estimations underline the need for special testing to rule out stress-related hyperprolactinemia and diagnostic pitfalls. It was recommended by the results, that two or three serial PRL determinations in resting conditions provide more reliable results (Muneyyirci-Delale, 1989).
- In experimental conditions, hyperprolactinemia and stress interact differentially according to the length of the stimuli and that is connected to the immune response modulated by PRL. Surgical or restraint stress induce marked (2x- 4x) increase of plasma PRL of control rats, but interestingly did not change the PRL levels of hyperprolactinemic rats. In both cases the plasma glucose levels reported elevated (Reis, 1996).
- It is suggested as a result of a retrospective observational study, that life events such as changes in subject's social or personal environment indicated that these stressful conditions may provoke hyperprolactinemia. Even an exposure during childhood to a stressful environment maybe associated with hyperprolactinemia and/or galactorrhea later in life as a response to specific environmental changes (Sobrinho, 1984). Patients with hyperprolactinemia reported significantly more life events, these events rated as being of „moderate", marked or severe „negative" impact compared with control subjects (Sonino, 2004).
- There is evidence that several external stress-factors may contribute to the occurrence of hyperprolactinemia. In theory, stress might have been involved in facilitation of a clonal proliferation of a single mutated cell and cause prolactinomas. Patients in functional hyperprolactinemic status, stress might trigger neuroendocrine changes involving DA and/or serotonin, which both can consequently affect PRL release. (Verhelst, 2003; Freeman, 2000; Fava, 1981.)

5. Hyperprolactinemia and infertility

Prolactin is a pituitary-derived hormone that plays an important role in a variety of reproductive functions. It is an essential factor for normal production of breast milk following childbirth. Additionally, prolactin negatively modulates the secretion of pituitary hormones responsible for gonadal function, including luteinizing hormone and follicle-stimulating hormone. Clnincally significant hyperprolactinemia may result in hypogonadism, infertility, and galactorrhea, or in some cases it may remain asymptomatic for a long period. (Klibanski 2010) The most commonly cited indications for treatment of microprolactinomas is infertility and hypogonadism. Hypogonadism and infertility associated closely with the treatment: DA agonists can restore normal PRL levels and consequently the normal gonadal function . According to the date of a meta-analyis, patients treated with bromocriptine had normalization of prolactin levels and it was successful in 53% of patients with infertility. Studies with cabergoline showed similar results: cabergoline was shown more effective than bromocriptine reducing PRL levels, or in symptoms of amenorrhea/oligomenorrhea, or in some of the patient-important outcomes. (Gillam 2006; Wang 2012)

Prolactin is under dual regulation by hypothalamic hormones delivered through the hypothalamic–pituitary portal circulation. The differential diagnosis and causes of pathological hyperprolactinemia are summarized in Figure 1.

The predominant signal is inhibitory, preventing prolactin release, and is mediated by the neurotransmitter dopamine. The stimulatory signal is mediated by the hypothalamic TRH. The balance between the two opposite signals determines the amount of prolactin released from the anterior pituitary gland (Verhelst; 2003).

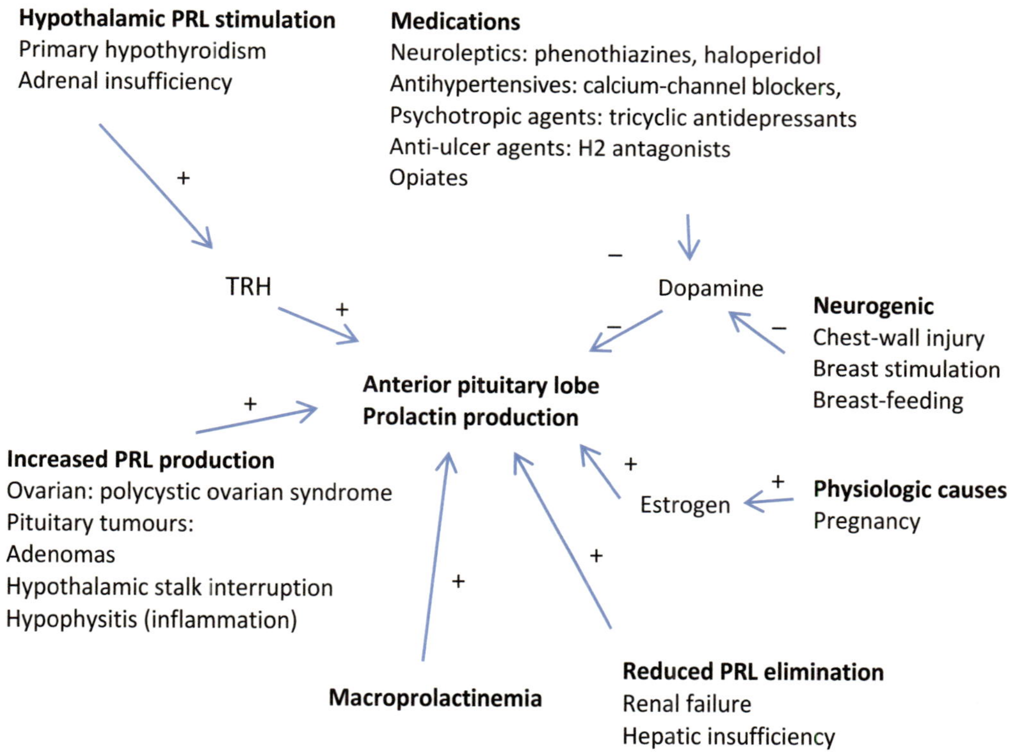

Figure 1. Prolactin is under dual control from the hypothalamus.

6. Hyperprolactinemia management

- The first steps in cases of signs of hyperprolactinemia should be a critical diagnosis, as discussed above, may involve dynamic testings, assessment for macroprolactinemia and further laboratory tests to eliminate false positive or negative results.

- Consider other underlying causes, such as suspected drug-induced hyperprolactinemia, hypothyroidism, elimination/renal failure, other persistent pituitary and parasellar tumours, etc.
- Identify the size of pituitary tumour and other anatomical circumstances.
- Apply pharmacotherapy treatment specified to patient

The major steps of diagnosis of hyperprolactinemia is summarized in Figure 2.

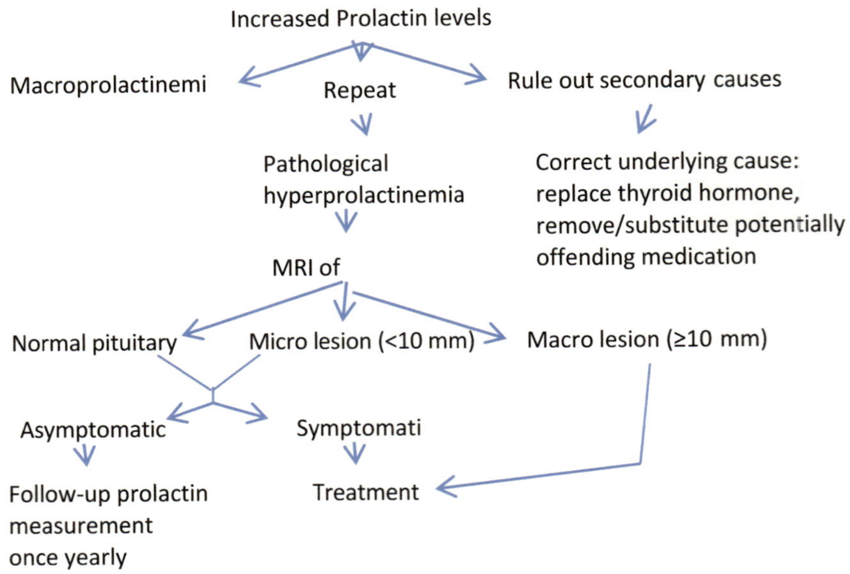

Figure 2. Approach to diagnosis of hyperprolactinemia.

7. Recommendations for the diagnosis of hyperprolactinemia

Specific recommendations for diagnosis of hyperprolactinemia include the following (Melmed 2011):

- A single measurement of serum prolactin level can confirm the diagnosis if the level is above the upper limit of normal and the serum sample was obtained without excessive venipuncture stress. Dynamic testing of prolactin secretion is not recommended to diagnose hyperprolactinemia.
- Macroprolactin evaluation is recommended in patients with asymptomatic hyperprolactinemia.
- When there is a discrepancy between a very large pituitary tumour and a mildly elevated prolactin level, serial dilution of serum samples is recommended to eliminate the "hook effect," or an artifact that can occur with some immunoradiometric assays leading to a falsely low prolactin value.

8. Recommendations for drug-induced hyperprolactinemia

Specific recommendations for management of drug-induced hyperprolactinemia are as follows (Melmed 2011):

- In a symptomatic patient with suspected medication-induced hyperprolactinemia, the drug should be discontinued for 3 days or an alternative drug substituted, and the serum prolactin measurement should then be repeated. However, the patient's physician should be consulted before an antipsychotic agent is discontinued or substituted. If the drug cannot be discontinued and the onset of the hyperprolactinemia does not coincide with starting therapy, magnetic resonance imaging (MRI) of the pituitary gland may distinguish medication-induced hyperprolactinemia from symptomatic hyperprolactinemia caused by a pituitary or hypothalamic mass.
- Patients with asymptomatic medication-induced hyperprolactinemia should not be treated. Estrogen or testosterone can be used in patients with long-term hypogonadism (hypogonadal symptoms or low bone mass) caused by medication-induced hyperprolactinemia.
- If it is not possible to stop the drug causing medication-induced hyperprolactinemia, cautious administration of a dopamine agonist should be considered, in consultation with the patient's physician.

9. Treatment of hyperprolactinemia

As noted above, prolactin levels can often be corrected by stopping suspected medication or switching to a different medication type. Correction of hypothyroidism is also effective and specific to reduce PRL levels. If prolactin levels are persistently high, they can be effectively treated with a group of medications known as dopamine agonists.

According to our clinical practice patients with macroadenoma suggested to undergo transsphenoidal pituitary surgery. Medical treatment is given to the subjects with microadenoma, persistent postoperative hyperprolactinemia, and to those cases of hyperprolactinemia when it is caused by other medications.

From the available mediactions Bromocriptine 2.5 mg (Parlodel®, Novartis) once or twice a day or cabergoline 0.5 mg (Dostinex®, Pharmacia) once or twice a week is given as prolactin-lowering drug.

9.1. Bromocriptine (Parlodel)

Parlodel is an effective and inexpensive medication for high prolactin levels. Parlodel is usually taken at bedtime with a snack. This is because Parlodel will occasionally cause dizziness or stomach upset, so taking it before sleep and with food will reduce those side effects. Generally with time, the side effects stop anyway.

The prolactin levels can be rechecked in about three weeks. If the levels are still elevated the dose can be increased or a different medication can be tried. The administration of Parlodel can be stopped upon diagnosis of pregnancy. However, if a woman has a macroadenoma, Parlodel should be continued through pregnancy and delivery.

Due to the side effects, some women can not tolerate Parlodel. For these women, they may try alternatives, e.g. vaginal bioadhesive suppositories or inserted the pills vaginally instead of taking them orally.

9.2. Cabergoline (Dostinex)

Because it is more expensive, cabergoline is not usually the first choice for treatment of high prolactin levels. It is usually used when Parlodel is ineffective or a woman cannot tolerate the side effects. Cabergoline is a longer acting medication. It is usually given twice a week instead of every day.

The Endocrine Society has released a new clinical practice guideline for the diagnosis and treatment of patients with hyperprolactinemia (Melmed, 2011). The new recommendations for management of elevated levels of the PRL, which is associated with infertility, low sex drive, and bone loss, are listed.

10. Recommendations for the treatment of prolactinoma

Specific recommendations for management of prolactinoma are as follows (Melmed 2011)::

- Dopamine agonist therapy is recommended to reduce prolactin levels and tumor size and to restore gonadal function in patients with symptomatic prolactin-secreting microadenomas or macroadenomas. Compared with other dopamine agonists, cabergoline is more effective in normalizing prolactin levels and in shrinking pituitary tumours.
- Dopamine agonists are not recommended for asymptomatic patients with microprolactinomas. However, patients with microadenomas who have amenorrhea can be treated with a dopamine agonist or oral contraceptives.
- In patients treated with dopamine agonists for at least 2 years who no longer have elevated serum prolactin levels or visible tumour on MRI, careful clinical and biochemical follow-up therapy may be tapered and perhaps discontinued.

11. Recommendations for resistant, malignant prolactinoma

Specific recommendations for management of resistant and malignant prolactinoma are as follows (Melmed 2011):

- For symptomatic patients in whom normal prolactin levels are not achieved or who have significant shrinking of the tumour size while receiving standard doses of a dopamine agonist, the dose should be increased rather than referring the patient for surgery.
- Patients resistant to bromocriptine should be switched to cabergoline.

- Symptomatic patients with prolactinomas who cannot tolerate high doses of cabergoline or who are unresponsive to dopamine agonist therapy should be offered trans-sphenoidal surgery. Patients intolerant of oral bromocriptine may respond to intravaginal administration. Radiation therapy is recommended for patients in whom surgical treatment fails or for those with aggressive or malignant prolactinomas.
- Temozolomide therapy is recommended for patients with malignant prolactinomas.

12. Recommendations for pregnant women with prolactinoma

Specific recommendations for management of prolactinoma during pregnancy are as follows (Melmed 2011):

- Women with prolactinomas should discontinue dopamine agonist therapy as soon as pregnancy is recognized, except for selected patients with invasive macroadenomas or adenomas abutting the optic chiasm.
- Serum prolactin measurements should not be performed during pregnancy.
- Unless there is clinical evidence for tumour growth, such as visual field impairment, routine use of pituitary MRI during pregnancy is not recommended in patients with microadenomas or intrasellar macroadenomas.
- Women with macroprolactinomas that do not shrink during dopamine agonist therapy or women who cannot tolerate bromocriptine or cabergoline should be counselled regarding the potential benefits of surgical resection before attempting pregnancy.
- Pregnant women with prolactinomas who experience severe headaches and/or visual field changes should have formal visual field assessment followed by MRI without gadolinium.
- Bromocriptine therapy is recommended in patients who experience symptomatic growth of a prolactinoma during pregnancy.

Hyperprolactinemia has been proposed to block ovulation through inhibition of GnRH release. Kisspeptin neurons, which express prolactin receptors, were recently identified as major regulators of GnRH neurons. A recently published study demonstrated that hyperprolactinemia in mice induced anovulation, reduced GnRH and gonadotropin secretion, and diminished kisspeptin expression. Kisspeptin administration restored gonadotropin secretion and ovarian cyclicity, suggesting that kisspeptin neurons play a major role in hyperprolactinemic anovulation. This study indicate that administration of kisspeptin may serve as an alternative therapeutic approach to restore the fertility of hyperprolactinemic women who are resistant or intolerant to dopamine agonists (Sonigo, 2012).

To sum up, the systematic reviews and meta-analyses affirm the use of dopamine agonists in treating hyperprolactinemia and reducing associated morbidity. Cabergoline was found to be more effective than bromocriptine in achieving normoprolactinemia and resolving amenorrhea/oligomenorrhea and galactorrhea. Radiotherapy and surgery are efficacious in patients with resistance or intolerance to dopamine agonists (Wang, 2012).

13. Summary

Hyperprolactinemia is defined as higher-than-normal blood levels of the hormone prolactin. This hormone is made by the pituitary gland, which is located at the base of the brain. The main function of prolactin is to stimulate breast milk production after childbirth. High prolactin levels are normal during pregnancy and breastfeeding. In other cases, prolactin can become too high because of a disease or the use of certain medications. Often, the cause is a prolactin-producing tumour in the pituitary gland, called a *prolactinoma*. This tumour is mostly benign (adenomas), meaning **not** invasive (invasive tumours with multiple recurrences are "atypical adenomas"), and not metastatic (malignant tumours, carcinomas). It is more common in women than men. Rarely, children and adolescents develop prolactinomas. Other brain tumours may also cause the pituitary gland to make too much prolactin.

Prolactin-secreting pituitary tumours are a common cause of amenorrhea and infertility in premenopausal women. The goals of therapy are to normalize prolactin, restore gonadal function and fertility, and reduce tumour size, and dopamine agonists are the preferred therapy. Clinically significant tumour enlargement during pregnancy is uncommon and dependent on tumour size and pre-pregnancy treatment.

Accroding to over 180 clinical study reports (across 3000 patients) treatment with bromocriptine or with cabergoline are both effective in normalization of prolactin levels and also successful in restoration of fertility over 53% of patients. Cabergoline was shown more effective than bromocriptine in persistent hyperprolactinemia, and reducing the symptoms of amenorrhea/oligomenorrhea. At our institution patients with symptomatic prolactinomas, both micro- and macroadenomas, are treated with cabergoline as the first-line approach. In the small group of patients who do not respond to this treatment, or who refuse long-term therapy, surgery is offered. Radiotherapy is given if both pharmacologic therapy and surgery fail.

Author details

Gokalp Oner
Yozgat Bogazlıyan State Hospital, Turkey

14. References

Andersen JR.(1990).Studies of decidual and amniotic prolactin in normal and pathological pregnancy Dan Med Bull 37: 154-165,1990.

Asa SL, Ezzat S. The pathogenesis of pituitary tumours. Nat Rev Cancer 2002; 2:836-49.

Bachelot A, Binart N. Reproductive role of prolactin. Reproduction. 2007 Feb;133(2):361-9. Review.

Baird DT, McNeilly AS, Sawers RS, Sharpe RM. Failure of estrogen-induced discharge of luteinizing hormone in lactating women. J Clin Endocrinol Metab. 1979 Oct;49(4):500-6. PubMed PMID: 479342.

Ben-Jonathan N, Mershon JL, Allen DL & Steinmetz RW 1996 Extrapituitary prolactin: distribution, regulation, functions, and clinical aspects. Endocrine Review 17 639–669.

Binart N, Helloco C, Ormandy CJ, Barra J, Clement-Lacroix P, Baran N & Kelly PA 2000 Rescue of preimplantatory egg development and embryo implantation in prolactin receptor-deficient mice after progesterone administration. Endocrinology 141 2691–2697.

Bracero N, Zacur HA. Polycystic ovary syndrome and hyperprolactinemia. Obstet Gynecol Clin North Am. 2001 Mar;28(1):77-84. Review

Buurman H, Saeger W 2006 Subclinical adenomas in postmortem pituitaries: classification and correlations to clinical data. Eur J Endocrinol 154:753–758

Cepický P, Sulková S, Stroufová A, Roth Z, Burdová I. The correlation of serum prolactin level and psychic stress in women undergoing a chronic hemodialysis programme. Exp Clin Endocrinol. 1992;99(2):71-2. PubMed PMID: 1639120.

Colao A, Loche S, Cappa M, Di Sarno A, Landi ML, Sarnacchiaro F, Facciolli G, Lombardi G. Prolactinomas in children and adolescents. Clinical presentation and long-term follow-up. J Clin Endocrinol Metab 1998; 83: 2777-2780.

Colao A, Vitale G, Di Sarno A, Spiezia S, Guerra E, Ciccarelli A & Lombardi G 2004 Prolactin and prostate hypertrophy: a pilot observational, prospective, case-control study in men with prolactinoma. Journal of Clinical Endocrinology and Metabolism 89 2770–2775.

Crosignani PG. Management of hyperprolactinemia in infertility. J Reprod Med. 1999 Dec;44(12 Suppl):1116-20. PubMed PMID: 10649821.

Daly AF, Rixhon M, Adam C, Dempegioti A, Tichomirowa MA, Beckers A 2006 High prevalence of pituitary adenomas: a cross-sectional study in the province of Liege, Belgium. J Clin Endocrinol Metab 91:4769–4775

Díaz S, Cárdenas H, Brandeis A, Miranda P, Schiappacasse V, Salvatierra AM, Herreros C, Serón-Ferré M, Croxatto HB. Early difference in the endocrine profile of long and short lactational amenorrhea. J Clin Endocrinol Metab. 1991 Jan;72(1):196-201. PubMed PMID: 1824708.

Díaz S, Seron-Ferre M, Croxatto HB, Veldhuis J. Neuroendocrine mechanisms of lactational infertility in women. Biol Res. 1995;28(2):155-63. Review. PubMed PMID: 9251745.

Dworakowska D, Grossman AB. The molecular pathogenesis of pituitary tumors: implications for clinical management. Minerva Endocrinol. 2012 Jun;37(2):157-72. Review. PubMed PMID: 22691889.

Escobar-Morreale HF. Macroprolactinemia in women presenting with hyperandrogenic symptoms: Implications for the management of polycystic ovary syndrome. Fertil Steril. 2004 Dec;82(6):1697-9. PubMed PMID: 15589886

Fahie-Wilson MN, John R, Ellis AR. Macroprolactin; high molecular mass forms of circulating prolactin. Ann Clin Biochem. 2005 May;42(Pt 3):175-92. Review.

Fava GA, Fava M, Kellner R, Serafini E & Mastrogiacomo I. Depression, hostility and anxiety in hyperprolactinemic amenorrhea. Psychotherapy and Psychosomatics 1981 36 122–128.)

Fernandez A, Karavitaki N, Wass JA. Prevalence of pituitary adenomas: a community-based, cross-sectional study in Banbury (Oxfordshire, UK). Clin Endocrinol (Oxf). 2010 Mar;72(3):377-82.

Fideleff HL, Boquete HR, Sequera A, Suárez M, Sobrado P, Giaccio A. Peripubertal prolactinomas: clinical presentation and longterm outcome with different therapeutic approaches. J Pediatr Endocrinol Metab 2000; 13: 261-267.

Filho RB, Domingues L, Naves L, Ferraz E, Alves A, Casulari LA. Polycystic ovary syndrome and hyperprolactinemia are distinct entities. Gynecol Endocrinol. 2007 May;23(5):267-72.

Freeman ME, Kanyicska B, Lerant A & Nagy G. Prolactin: structure, function, and regulation of secretion. Physiological Reviews 2000 80 1523–1631.

Gala RR, and E.M Shevach (1994).Evidence for the release of prolactin like substance by mouse lymphocytes and macrophages. Proc. Soc.Exp. Biol. Med, 205: 12-19.

Garcia MM, Kapcala LP. Growth of a microprolactinoma to a macroprolactinoma during estrogen therapy. J Endocrinol Invest. 1995 Jun;18(6):450-5.

Gellersen B., DiMattia G.E., Friesen H.G. and Bohnet H.G. (1989) Prolactin (PRL) mRNA from human deciduas differs from pituitary PRL mRNA but resembles the IM-9-P3 lymphoblast PRL transcript. Mol. Cell. Endocrinol. 64: 127-130.

Guastamacchia E, Triggiani V, Tafaro E, De Tommasi A, De Tommasi C, Luzzi S, Sabbà C, Resta F, Terreni MR, Losa M. Evolution of a prolactin-secreting pituitary microadenoma into a fatal carcinoma: a case report. Minerva Endocrinol. 2007 Sep;32(3):231-6. PubMed PMID: 17912159.

Harrison RF. Stress spikes of hyperprolactinaemia and infertility. Hum Reprod. 1988 Feb;3(2):173-5. PubMed PMID: 3356771.

Horseman ND, Zhao W, Montecino-Rodriguez E, Tanaka M, Nakashima K, Engle SJ, Smith F, Markoff E & Dorshkind K 1997 Defective mammopoiesis, but normal hematopoiesis, in mice with a targeted disruption of the prolactin gene. EMBO Journal 16 6926–6935.

Isik S, Berker D, Tutuncu YA, Ozuguz U, Gokay F, Erden G, Ozcan HN, Kucukler FK, Aydin Y, Guler S. Clinical and radiological findings in macroprolactinemia. Endocrine. 2012 Apr;41(2):327-33.

Kars M, Souverein PC, Herings RM, Romijn JA, Vandenbroucke JP, de Boer A, Dekkers OM 2009 Estimated age- and sex-specific incidence and prevalence of dopamine agonist-treated hyperprolactinemia. J Clin Endocrinol Metab 94:2729–2734

Klibanski A 2010 Clinical practice. Prolactinomas. N Engl J Med 362:1219–1226

Kruger TH, Leeners B, Naegeli E, Schmidlin S, Schedlowski M, Hartmann U, Egli M. Prolactin secretory rhythm in women: immediate and long-term alterations after sexual contact. Hum Reprod. 2012 Apr;27(4):1139-43.

Kurtz A, Bristol LA, Toth BE, Lazar-Wesley E, Takacs L and Kacsoh B.(1993). Mammary epithelial cells of Lactating rat express prolactin messenger ribonucleic acid. Biol Reprod. 48: 1095-1103.

Lkhider, M., Delpal, S. and Ollivier-Bousquet, M. (1996). Rat prolactin inserum, milk and mammary tissue: characterisation and intracellularlocalisation. Endocrinology 137: 4969-4979.

Marrs RP, Kletzky OA, Mishell DR Jr. A separate mechanism of gonadotropin recovery after pregnancy termination. J Clin Endocrinol Metab. 1981 Mar;52(3):545-8.

Melmed S, Casanueva FF, Hoffman AR, Kleinberg DL, Montori VM, Schlechte JA, Wass JA; Endocrine Society. Diagnosis and treatment of hyperprolactinemia: an Endocrine

Society clinical practice guideline. J Clin Endocrinol Metab. 2011 Feb;96(2):273-88. Review.

Molitch ME 2003 Pituitary tumors and pregnancy. Growth Hormone and IGF Research 13 S38–S44. Suppl A.

Montgomery, D.W. LeFevre, J.A.. Ulrich, E.D., Adamson, C'.R. and Zukoski. CF. (1990) Identification of prolactin like proteins synthesized by normal murine lymphocytes. Endocrinology 127: 2601- 2603.

Muneyyirci-Delale O, Goldstein D, Reyes FI. Diagnosis of stress-related hyperprolactinemia. Evaluation of the hyperprolactinemia rest test. N Y State J Med. 1989 Apr;89(4):205-8.

Oh MC, Tihan T, Kunwar S, Blevins L, Aghi MK. Clinical management of pituitarycarcinomas. Neurosurg Clin N Am. 2012 Oct;23(4):595-606. doi: 10.1016/j.nec.2012.06.009. Epub 2012 Aug 17.

Ono M, Miki N, Amano K, Kawamata T, Seki T, Makino R, Takano K, Izumi S, Okada Y, Hori T. Individualized high-dose cabergoline therapy for hyperprolactinemic infertility in women with micro- and macroprolactinomas. J Clin Endocrinol Metab. 2010 Jun;95(6):2672-9. Epub 2010 Mar 31.

Reis FM, Ribeiro-de-Oliveira A Jr, Guerra RM, Reis AM, Coimbra CC. Blood glucose and prolactin in hyperprolactinemic rats exposed to restraint and surgical stress. Life Sci. 1996;58(2):155-61.

Ružić K, Grahovac T, Graovac M, Dadić-Hero E, Sepić-Grahovac D, Sabljić V. Hyperprolactinaemia with amisulpride. Psychiatr Danub. 2011

Shibli-Rahhal A, Schlechte J. Hyperprolactinemia and infertility. Endocrinol Metab Clin North Am. 2011; 40(4):837-46.

Sobrinho LG, Nunes MCP, Calhaz-Jorge C, Afonso AM, Pereira MC & Santos MA. Hyperprolactinemia in women with paternal deprivation during childhood. Obstetrics and Gynecology 1984 64 465–468.)

Sonigo C, Bouilly J, Carré N, Tolle V, Caraty A, Tello J, Simony-Conesa FJ, Millar R, Young J, Binart N. Hyperprolactinemia-induced ovarian acyclicity is reversed by kisspeptin administration. J Clin Invest. 2012 Oct 1;122(10):3791-5. Epub 2012 Sep 24. PubMed PMID: 23006326.

Sonino N, Navarrini C, Ruini C, Fallo F, Boscaro M, Fava GA. Life events in the pathogenesis of hyperprolactinemia. Eur J Endocrinol. 2004 Jul;151(1):61-5. PubMed PMID: 15248823.

Sonino N, Navarrini C, Ruini C, Fallo F, Boscaro M, Fava GA. Life events in the pathogenesis of hyperprolactinemia. Eur J Endocrinol. 2004 Jul;151(1):61-5. PubMed PMID: 15248823.

Sonino N, Tomba E, Fava GA. Psychosocial approach to endocrine disease. Adv Psychosom Med. 2007;28:21-33. Review. PubMed PMID: 17684318.

Tamer G, Telci A, Mert M, Uzum AK, Aral F, Tanakol R, Yarman S, Boztepe H,Colak N, Alagöl F. Prevalence of pituitary adenomas in macroprolactinemic patients may be higher than it is presumed. Endocrine. 2012 Feb;41(1):138-43.

Taya K, Greenwald GS. Mechanisms of suppression of ovarian follicular development during lactation in the rat. Biol Reprod. 1982 Dec;27(5):1090-101. PubMed PMID: 7159657.

Tetlow LJ, Clayton PE. Tests and normal values in pediatric. In: Brook C, Clayton P, Brown R, editors. Brook's Clinical Pediatric Endocrinology. 5th ed. Blackwell Publishing. 2005; 531-532.

Urman B, Yakin K. Ovulatory disorders and infertility. J Reprod Med. 2006 Apr;51(4):267-82. Review. PubMed PMID: 16737024.

Uzun S, Kozumplik O, Mimica N & Folnegović-Šmalc V. Opis nuspojava psihofarmaka prema pojedinim skupinama lijekova. In: Uzun S, Kozumplik O, Mimica N & Folnegović-Šmalc V, editors. Nuspojave psihofarmaka. 1st ed. Zagreb: Medicinska naklada, Psihijatrijska bolnica Vrapče; 2005; p. 19-28.

Vallette-Kasic S, Morange-Ramos I, Selim A, Gunz G, Morange S, Enjalbert A, et al. Macroprolactinemia revisited: a study on 106 patients. J Clin Endocrinol Metab 2002; 87: 581-8.

Verhelst J & Abs R. Hyperprolactinemia. Pathophysiology and management. Treatments in Endocrinology 2003 2 23–32.

Verhelst J, Abs R. Hyperprolactinemia: pathophysiology and management. Treat Endocrinol. 2003; 2: 23-32.

Wang AT, Mullan RJ, Lane MA, Hazem A, Prasad C, Gathaiya NW, Fernández-Balsells MM, Bagatto A, Coto-Yglesias F, Carey J, Elraiyah TA, Erwin PJ, Gandhi GY, Montori VM, Murad MH. Treatment of hyperprolactinemia: a systematic review and meta-analysis. Syst Rev. 2012; 24: 33.

Wierinckx A, Roche M, Raverot G, Legras-Lachuer C, Croze S, Nazaret N, Rey C, Auger C, Jouanneau E, Chanson P, Trouillas J, Lachuer J. Integrated genomic profiling identifies loss of chromosome 11p impacting transcriptomic activity in aggressive pituitary PRL tumors. Brain Pathol. 2011 Sep;21(5):533-43. doi: 10.1111/j.1750-3639.2011.00476.x. Epub 2011 Feb 23. PubMed PMID: 21251114.

Yoshimura Y, Tada S, Oda T, Nakamura Y, Maruyama K, Ichikawa F, Ebihara T, Hirota Y, Sawada T, Kawakami S, et al. Direct inhibitory ovarian effects of prolactin in the process of ovulation. Nihon Sanka Fujinka Gakkai Zasshi. 1989 Jan;41(1):83-9. PubMed PMID: 2926197.

Yu R, Melmed S. Pathogenesis of pituitary tumors. Prog Brain Res. 2010;182:207-27. PubMed PMID: 20541667.

Yu-Lee LY 1997 Molecular actions of actions of prolactin in the immune system. Proceedings of the society for Experimental Biology Medicine 215 35–51.

Zemmoura I, Wierinckx A, Vasiljevic A, Jan M, Trouillas J, François P. Aggressive and malignant prolactin pituitary tumors: pathological diagnosis and patient management. Pituitary. 2012 Nov 27. [Epub ahead of print] PubMed PMID: 23184261.

Chapter 10

The Regulation of Pituitary Prolactin Secretion: Hypothalamic, Intrapituitary and Intracellular Factors and Signaling Mechanisms

Viktória Reinhoffer, Márk Oláh, Miklós Vecsernyés,
Béla E. Tóth and György M. Nagy

Additional information is available at the end of the chapter

http://dx.doi.org/10.5772/55571

1. Introduction

A consensus view developed over the last decades holds that the basal secretion of PRL from the anterior lobe (AL) is spontaneous (i.e., occurs without stimulation by the hypothalamus) (Neill 1994; Freeman 2000) since PRL is secreted from lactotropes with a high secretory rate for prolonged periods after disconnecting the hypothalamic influence (when it transplanted to a site distant from the hypothalamus under the kidney capsule or when cultured in vitro). Consequently, PRL secretion appears to be severely restrained by the hypothalamus in vivo as the main source prolactin inhibiting factor (PIF). Results of the extensive research of the last decades have clearly demonstrated that the withdrawal of DA tone is not sufficient to account for the surge of PRL secretion observed in response to the suckling (physiological) stimulus during lactation. Similarly, DAerg tone would not completely recover the chronic elevation of PRL during pregnancy, lactation or in other pathophysiological stages. The research has subsequently included the search for putative prolactin-releasing factors (PRF) controlling PRL peaks occurring after mating or triggered by ovarian steroids. These can be termed by central (i.e hypothalamic) or peripheral (within the pituitary gland) sites of actions. However, it may be better to classify them by the levels of control mechanisms to regulate PRL secretion: *(i)* action on hypothalamic DAerg neurons; *(ii)* binding to specific receptors on lactotrophs in the pituitary gland; *(iii)* paracrine/autocrine compounds.

i. The hypothalamic regulating factors acting on *hypothalamic DAergic neurons* may have direct activation or inhibition of their activity, or alter DA, resulting in a consequent changes in PRL secretion (Freeman, 2000; Ben-Jonathan, 2008). The final common pathways of the central stimulatory and inhibitory control are the neuroendocrine neurons producing DA available to be delivered into the hypophyseal portal vessels or to be released to pituitary neurointermediate (NIL) lobe in order to reach ultimately the anterior lobe (AL).

- Prolactin itself, bombesin, gastrin-releasing peptide (GRP), neuromedins B and C, neurotensin, neuropeptide Y, acetylcholine (Ach), PACAP, angiotensin II, calcitonin, atrial natriuretic peptide (ANP) family members demonstrated to stimulate tyrosine-hydroxilase (TH) activity, increase DA release and a consequent depression in PRL secretion.
- Others induce opposite effect, such as opioids, norepinephrine, somatostatin, CCK, serotonin, and GABA act as inhibitors on TH activity of TIDA cells and associated with PRL release.
- Several compounds (e.g. TRH, oxytocin, VIP, neurotensin, neuropeptide Y, histamine, acetylcholine, somatostatin, CCK) may have different central or peripheral effect or exert dual phase actions on PRL release.

ii. The other group of regulators of PRL secretion act *directly on lactotrophs*. These hypothalamic releasing/inhibiting factors bind to specific receptors on pituitary lactotrophs, cause alterations in expression or release of PRL resulting in changes of secretion pattern. PIF and PRF from the neuroendocrine neurons can be released either at the level of median eminence (ME) into the long portal veins or at the level of NIL, which is indirectly connected to the anterior lobe of the pituitary gland by the short portal vessels.

iii. Additional to the hypothalamic PRF and PIF factors, lactotrophs are also influenced by compounds that released from the surrounding cells and act as *a paracrine regulation* or potentially from the *lactotrophs themselves via autocrine regulation*. These putative paracrine or autocrine factors or combined interactions are potentially also responsible for regulation of PRL release, but the robust and dynamic regulation of PRL secretion more likely controlled and strongly relies on hypothalamic factors (*vide supra*).

On the other hand, there is an ever-growing list of peptides with the potential to act as intrapituitary agent to control PRL secretion, and even more of those which may have dual features: enhance or suppress PRL release in the presence/ absence of other factors. That is a challenge for researchers to demonstrate the presence and to prove the precise mode of actions, since data obtained from *in vitro, in vivo* or *ex vivo* experiments may have discrepancies in results. The effect of a putative autocrine-paracrine control is also hard to demonstrate, since the active substance may have an extremely low local level. Detection however, on a single cell level of PRL release; or by presence of those factors using immunocytochemistry and in situ hybridization, or a combination of these techniques has been found successful. The list of proved factors that act as a local regulator on pituitary lactotroph cells considered as a cumulative contributions of "*Pros and Cons*" over the last two-three decades (Freeman 2000; Wenger 1999; Takaya 2000; Brogilo, 2008; Ondo, 1989; Schettini, 1990; Ben-Jonathan, 2008; Toth 2001; Rettori, 2011):

Suppress/ inhibit PRL secretion:

- dopamine (DA),
- somatostatin (SST), cortistatin (CST),
- gamma-aminobutyric acid (GABA),

- calcitonin (in vitro)
- prolactin (PRL),
- TGF-β isoforms,
- endothelin-like peptides, ET1,
- acetylcholine (ACh),
- glucocorticoids,
- cannabinoids,
- adenosine or analogues (in vitro).

Stimulate/enhance PRL secretion:

- VIP,
- TRH (locally in anterior pituitary),
- oxytocin (OT),
- dopamine (DA, in certain low concentrations only)
- cytokines/ IL6, IL1,
- EGF,
- vasopressin (VP),
- angiotensin (ANG) II,
- galanin (GAL),
- Substance P,
- bombesin/ gastrin-releasing peptide (GRP),
- neurotensin (NT),
- serotonin (5-HT),
- GnRH,
- α-MSH,
- estradiol (E2),
- ghrelin and growth hormone secretagogue (GHS),
- adenosine (icv),
- salsolinol,
- ethanol (alcohol).

1.1. Anatomy of hypothalamic structures in control of PRL secretion

The established hypothalamic hypophysiotropic inhibitor of PRL secretion is DA produced by the arcuate-periventricular nucleus and travels from the median eminence (ME) to the anterior lobe (AL) via the long portal vessels. The well known hypophysiotrophic DAergic neurons in the hypothalamus consist of at least two different areas (named as 'A12' and 'A14') by anatomical location. Despite the extensive supportive evidences for this simplistic view, it has recently proven to be incomplete. It has been demonstrated, that the early studies failed to account for an important source of DA reaching the AL through the short portal vessels from the neurointermediate lobe (NIL). It was clarified that these DAergic neurons can be divided into three distinct systems based on functionality due to the anatomical distribution of neurons and the terminals within the pituitary and sensitivity of internal control mechanisms (summarized in Table 1.).

a. Tuberoinfundibular DAergic (TIDA) neurons located mainly in the middle and posterior portion of the arcuate nucleus ('A12'), project to the ME, and the functions are well accepted as a physiological regulator of hypophysial PRL secretion.
b. The periventricular-hypophysial dopaminergic (PHDA, 'A14') neurons' branched axons terminate in the intermediate lobe (IL), (but not in the neural lobe) (Ben-Jonathan 1980; Peters 1981; Ben-Jonathan, 1982; Goudreau, 1995). Taken together that hypothalamic neurons release DA into portal blood flow (rather than into synaptic clefts) and also the fact that no DA autoreceptors found in TIDA neurons, both assist to abolish the effect of the negative feedback by secreted DA on tyrosine-hydroxilase (TH) activity in DA neurons themselves and consequently maintain the high DA output. These cells are not affected by stimuli of nonselective DA agonists, which cells otherwise increase or decrease the DA output and provide consequent change in PRL secretion as a response by selective D1 or D2 agonist's actions, respectively (Ben-Jonathan, 2001).
c. Experimental evidences have been presented to prove that DA derived from the tuberohypophysial DAergic (THDA, 'A12') system also may serve as an important regulator of PRL secretion. Neurons of this THDA system are located in the most rostral part of the arcuate and periventricular nucleus and axons terminate in the NIL of the pituitary gland rather than in the ME of the hypothalamus (Holzbauer, 1978; Holzbauer, 1985; Ben-Jonathan, 1982, Ben-Jonathan, 1985; Neill 1994; Freeman 2000). Due to the anatomical situation that axon terminals branch in NIL, the amount of DA released by THDA neurons would not be present in pituitary stalk blood. These cells carry different functionality and interestingly no differences in activities between males and females were recognized compared these characteristics to neurons of the TIDA system (Higuchi 1992; Freeman 2000).

From the regulatory aspects, DA concentrations reaching the AL, measured in portal blood only may have been underestimated. Indeed, removal (Ben-Jonathan, 1982; Peters, 1981; Ben-Jonathan, 1985) or denervation (Vecsernyes, 1997) of the NIL elevates basal PRL secretion in cycling or lactating females, but also in males. Hypothalamic regions of the main DAergic control (i.e. TIDA neurons) in arcuate nucleus, keep the balance of stimulation and inhibition and maintain the regularly low basal PRL secretion, due to combined action of putative control mechanisms (*vide infra*). On the other hand, elevated PRL levels during pregnancy and lactation mediate actions also in other hypothalamic regions such as the paraventricular nucleus (PVN), rostral preoptic area (rPOA) as demonstrated by Sapsford et al. (2012). The observation that electrochemically detectable DA in the AL is reduced after surgical removal of the NIL was found to be consistent with this finding (Mulchahey, 1985). Thus, DA of hypothalamic origin which is delivered to the AL by way of the long and the short portal vessels (from TIDA or THDA, respectively) together, seems quantitatively sufficient to account for inhibition of PRL release (Nagy, 1992; Freeman, 1993; Nagy, 1990).

The aim of this summary is to review the evidences accumulated to date and outline several new aspects of the regulation and the tonic inhibitory role of DA on PRL secretion in various physiological stages.

1.2. Physiology of responsiveness: The balance

The feedback interaction in which the released PRL controls its own secretion called "short loop feedback", only partially has been characterized. Due to the primary influence as inhibition on PRL release by hypothalamic structures, the mechanism of this feedback is considered fairly complex in process to change the activity of TIDA or PHDA/THDA neurons and trigger effect of immediate reactions, or in course of the physiological regulation, such as estrus cycle or by chronic increase of PRL levels, such as pregnancy or lactation. Elevation of serum PRL levels consequently increases hypothalamic DA synthesis and DA release into hypophysial-portal blood to complete the negative feed-back loop (Gudelsky, 1980). Since hypothalamus is within the brain, PRL that released to circulation should be transferred through the blood-brain barrier (BBB) in order to reach and manifest a feedback to TIDA cells, potentially by an uptake of the choroid plexus (Mangurian, 1992).

For the action of PRL on TIDA neurons several potential mechanisms have been proposed: such as control of TH expression by activation of PRL-receptor in DA neurons (Gonzalez, 1988) or activation of early genes, nerve growth factors (NGF-1), etc (Sagrillo, 1998). Since PRL receptors are found in all the three described subpopulations i.e. TIDA, THDA and PHDA neurons in hypothalamus, the short PRL feedback supported by the relevance of potential activation in all three systems (DeMaria, 1999). Alternatively, PRL can be synthesized *de novo* locally within the hypothalamus, by the stimuli of estrogens may have other functions and questionable the direct action controlling of TIDA neurons (DeVito, 1992; DeVito, 1993; Freeman 2000; Ben-Jonathan 2001). Interestingly, subpopulations of oxytocin neurons in the hypothalamus were also found to be differentially sensitive to PRL, and may have effect controlling PRL secretion, as PRF (Kennett, 2012).

According to the most recent report of Lyons et al. (2012) in which they focused on rapid electrophysiological changes induced by PRL within the hypothalamic TIDA neurons utilizing a whole-cell current- and voltage-clamp recordings. The presence of relatively high doses of PRL in arcuate nucleus resulted in a change to tonic inhibition, manipulating mainly those rapid mechanisms of depolarization on the spontaneously oscillating DA secreting cells. Experiments on slices of hypothalamus, tested to ion substitution and pharmacological manipulations proved that the transparent switch to tonic discharge and consequent APs are composed of low- and high-voltage components: activation of a transient receptor potential-like current and the change of a calcium ion-dependent BK-type K^+-current as a slow component, then broadened APs increase terminal Ca^{2+} influx, and change the vesicular DA release at the terminals in the median eminence. The PRL-induced depolarization is reversible and dose dependent; it involves direct, postsynaptic actions because it persists when AP discharge is blocked by TTX. PRL levels (higher than the physiological range of circadian rhythm) that required for normal reproduction (may be out of the normal range) have been effective in these electrophysiological actions. Accordingly this feedback „option" may primarily play a role during pathophysiological elevations of PRL. (Lyons, 2012)

Perhaps the most intriguing aspect of this neuroendocrine reflex mechanism is the dramatic change in responsiveness of lactotrophs due to a brief application of the suckling stimulus

(Nagy, 1990; Hill, 1991; Nagy, 1991). Previously we have provided experimental evidences that these responsiveness changes (induced by 10 minutes suckling in vivo) can be detected in primary cultures prepared from dissected ALs (Nagy, 1990; Hill, 1991; Nagy, 1991; Murányi, 1997; Murányi, 1998; Horváth, 1999). Pituitary cells from non-suckled rats (separated for 4 hours) exposed to various concentrations of DA exhibit only a dose-dependent inhibitory effect and TRH or Angiotensin II (AII) cannot release PRL. In striking contrast, lactotrophs derived from suckled rats are less responsive to the inhibitory actions of DA as well as more responsive to the stimulatory effects of TRH and AII. The suckling-induced changes in responsiveness related to decrease in protein phosphatase-2A (PP2A) activity which possibly plays a role in the uncoupling of D2 receptors on lactotrophs from the tonic inhibitory influence of DA (Murányi, 1998). Parallel with these, 10 minutes suckling stimulus applied immediately before sacrifice rendered PRL cells to respond with an increase of PRL release to picomolar concentrations (10^{-10} M-10^{-12} M) of DA. Thus, a brief suckling stimulus primes pituitary lactotrophs to respond with an increase of PRL secretion to low dose of DA (Nagy, 1990).

Another distinct advantage of this experimental model (non-suckled and suckled rats) is that it also shows a striking difference in the effectiveness of DA removal-induced increase of PRL release. It is well known, that dissociation of DA from its receptor induces PRL release. AL cells have been dispersed from non-suckled and suckled mothers then subjected to treatment of the inhibitory dose of DA for 2 hours. In the next step DA has been washed out before initiating the plaque assay by infusing the PRL antibody. Withdrawal of DA has clearly induced release of PRL compared to the medium pretreated cells obtained from non-suckled mothers. In contrast, the DA removal signal has been completely missing on cells from suckled animals (Nagy, 1991; Horváth, 1999; Murányi, 1998). Being able to distinguish between dissociation- and stimulation-induced elevation of PRL release is a critical part of the interpretation of these mechanisms.

Salsolinol (SAL), isolated from the NIL is present in the hypothalamic neuroendocrine dopaminergic system, appears to be a selective and potent stimulator of PRL secretion rat *in vivo* and with a moderate effect *in vitro* (Toth, 2001). It seems that SAL does not act through the dopamine D2 receptors, but utilize receptor independent mechanisms to stimulate PRL High affinity binding sites for this putative PRF have been detected in median eminence where TIDA projects and the NIL that are known terminal fields of THDA/PHDA DAergic systems (Toth; 2002; Homicsko, 2003). Reserpine pretreatment (blocking VMAT) prevented the effect of SAL on PRL release. Within the similar experimental model, suckling stimulus increased SAL content of NIL, but there was no change in SAL binding in the anterior lobe. Moreover, structural analogue of SAL (1-methyl-3,4-dihydroisoquinoline) can block salsolinol-induced release of PRL, but does not affect PRL release in response to TRH, TH inhibitors or D2 receptor antagonist domperidone (Homicsko, 2003). Taken together these results suggested that D2 receptor independent mechanisms can play a pivotal role in regulation of PRL secretion in reflection to suckling induced physiological stimuli (Toth, 2002; Bodnar, 2003).

1.3. Tonic inhibition of prolactin secretion

The PRL production and release to circulation is under a predominant inhibitory control of DA. Without the sustained regulation by hypothalamic DA dispersed pituitary cells increase the basal secretion and similarly, disconnected pituitary gland increase the released PRL (Neill, 1982; Leong, 1983; Vecsernyes, 1997; Murányi, 1998). Since most of experimental reports discuss the role of DA in females, it should be noted here that there are marked sexual differences in activity of TIDA (not relevant with PHDA and THDA) neurons and responsiveness to physiological and pharmacological stimuli, even though similar density nerve terminals found in both sexes (See also Table 1.). Higher basal activity of these neurons is seen in females that suppressed by removal of ovaries (OVX) and restored by treatment with E_2. The opposite, i.e. control of lower basal activity of TIDA neurons in males effected by presence of testosterone and may be due also to tonic inhibition by endogenous opioids (Ben-Jonathan 2001, Pan 1996; Freeman 2000).

Name Location	**Termination**	**Function**	**Characteristics / Differences**
TIDA dorsomedial part of the arcuate nucleus (A12)	External zone of the median eminence (EM) around long portal vessels	- Main physiological regulator of PRL secretion. - Daily rhythm by SCN . PRL surges in estrus cycle - Response to suckling stimulus. - Sensitive to feedback to PRL levels.	- Discharge in a highly robust and synchronized oscillations. - Significant difference in activity b/w male and females. - Activity increased by OVX, decreases by orchidectomy.
THDA rostral arcuate nucleus (A12)	Intermediate and the neural lobe (NIL)	- Response to suckling stimulus. - Activated by dehydration. - Release of DA to AL through the short portal vessels.	-No sex differences in activities, - function is independent of gonadal steroids
PHDA periventricular nucleus (A14)	Intermediate lobe (IL)	- tonic inhibition α-MSH and on basal PRL - Release of DA to AL through the short portal vessels.	-No sex differences in activities, - function is independent from gonadal steroids

Table 1. Dopaminergic neurons in control of PRL secretion

All of our recent data clearly indicate that wherever this signal originates and whatever is its nature, suckling-induced desensitization/sensitization of pituitary tissue to PRL-release inhibiting stimuli is manifested at the cellular level of lactotrophs as a proportional increase of subpopulation of those cells less sensitive to inhibition by high doses and more sensitive to stimulatory effect by low doses of DA. The mechanism(s) leading to these suckling-induced changes in DA responsiveness of lactotroph cells is (are) currently only in parts clarified. Efforts have been made to determine the mechanism(s) of this change in responsiveness have indicated that it is mediated through the D2 dopamine receptors (Horváth, 1999; Murányi, 1997). There are certain theories in hormonal- and receptor-level or intracellular signaling cascades-related, which may serve as potential explanation for the complexity of responsiveness to external stimuli and internal controls of pituitary cells during physiological and stress reactions.

TIDA cells form a network that discharges rhythmically in a robust 0.05 Hz synchronized oscillations. Thyrotropin-releasing hormone (TRH), which stimulates PRL release at the level of pituitary, cause transition from phasic pattern to tonic firing at the level of TIDA-cell. The results of these electrophysiology experiments are in concert with earlier findings on dispersed pituitary cell, suggesting a useful model for PRL regulation. TIDA network switches from oscillations to sustained discharge converting DA at high concentrations to a functional agonist as the net DA output decreases. (Lyons, 2010; Nagy, 1991)

Utilizing the analogy that has been reported by Conductier (2011) on hypothalamic neuronal populations, may serve as another potential explanation of this dose-dependent biphasic regulatory process of DA. The theory is based on the observation that certain biological actions believed to be associated with DA are not due to activation of DA receptors, but likely mediated via other receptors (such as α2-noradrenergic) and a subsequent action to open G-protein activated inward rectifier K^+ (GIRK) channels, which leads to hyperpolarization of cells (*vide infra*). It is also possible that DA modulates other hypothalamic inputs in a complex and biphasic manner: at low concentrations DA activates D2-like receptors, promoting presynaptic activity and upregulation, but high concentration of DA activates the D2-like receptors resulting in inhibition, which consequently blocks the presynaptic activity. (Conductier, 2011)

It has been recently discovered that sustained presence of the ligands of G-protein-coupled receptors (GPCRs) can promote specific intracellular signaling adaptation mechanisms parallel with the internalization process of the receptors. The receptor desensitization or "tolerance" is based on these mechanisms. Desensitization has been described in the AL of pituitary gland as well, where dopamine D2 receptors are permanently activated on lactotrophs. Ceasing of the dopaminerg inhibition is essential for the maintenance of the high secretory rate of PRL in lactotrophs during lactation.

2. Receptor mechanisms regulating lactotroph cells

Among those cellular and variety of receptor mediated mechanisms that regulating the pituitary hormone secreting cells only the key elements in this chapter that may have direct impact on PRL release, will be highlighted. DA released from the specific DAerg nerve terminals and bind to its appropriate receptors located at the post-synaptic membrane is the main down-stream process. However, the potential effects of presynaptic receptor mechanisms in regulation can not be completely ruled out. To achieve biological response in cellular level, it is necessary to activate the G-protein-coupled receptors (GPCRs), which described with five distinct but closely related subunits that carry different and versatile subcellular messenger functions. A new concept of GPCR receptor theory describes the options of modified ligand selectivity and alternative intracellular responses on the same receptor type, increasing the down-stream effector mechanisms.

2.1. Dopamine receptors in mammotrop cells

The two major groups of receptors are the D1 and D2 classes: D1 class (D1 and D5 subtypes) has a stimulatory effect on intracellular signaling pathways, while D2 class (D2, D3 and D4 subtypes) has mainly inhibitory influence on cAMP. The predominant D2 type receptor in pituitary lactotroph cells exists in two alternatively spliced isoforms, termed D2-short (D2S) and D2-long (D2L) receptors, which differ from each other in the insertion of 29 amino acids of the third cytoplasmic loop. To date, there are no specific ligands to discriminate the D2S from D2L actions, only KO animal models in use to identify isoform specific effects. (Beaulieu, 2011; Vallone, 2000; Ben-Jonathan, 2001; Radl, 2011). The receptor isoforms exhibit fairly similar pharmacological properties, activation in rat lactotrophs mediates DA suppression of the PRL gene (McChesney, 1991). These two isoforms of D2 dopamine receptor are both present on lactotroph cells. Because each form is selectively coupled to different G proteins, they serve different functions: (i) inhibition of adenylyl cyclase, (ii) activation of voltage-gated calcium channels, and (iii) inhibition of potassium channels in a similar manner but only the D_2S coupled to the phospholipase signaling pathway. (The G_i/G_o family of proteins is not involved in this pathway, since insensitive to PTX) (Senogles, 2000).

D2L is the main isoform present in the anterior pituitary both in rat and in human (Guivarc'h, 1995) and instead of D2S, the D2L isoform is expressed in an elevated manner level during estradiol-induced PRL secretion and cell proliferation in mammotrop cell. However, in cells contained only D2L form, (lactotroph-derived PR1 cells, with no D2S) there was only diminished response to the same stimuli demonstrated. It was concluded that D2S-receptor regulates the Gi3 inhibitory action on Gs; also D2S is more efficient for inhibiting adenylyl cyclase than D2L, thus could serve as mechanism controlling the PRL release and proliferation of mammotrop cells (Sengupta, 2012). The role of D2 receptor is essential to maintain the physiological PRL levels. In receptor knock-out (KO) mice pituitary hyperplasia and persistent hyperprolactinemia is seen. Other data suggest some additional function associated with DA, describing it not just a major inhibitor of PRL secretion and cell proliferation, but also induces apoptosis of mammary cells (Kelly 1997).

Experimental data support the hypothesis that D2S and D2L receptors are functionally distinct in terms of coupling to MAPK pathways, since DA-induced apoptosis in neurons in lactotrophs, via p38 MAPK. Similarly, cabergolin-induces apoptosis of lactotrophs in the presence of E_2. The effect of DA on apoptosis is reverted by a p38 MAPK inhibitor in primary cultures and in PR1-D2S (D2S predominant, transfected pituitary tumor) cells, indicating that p38 MAPK is involved in the apoptosis of lactotrophs induced by D2 receptor activation. Alterations in the proportion of D2L and D2S isoform expression could be involved in the clinical resistance of D2R agonist therapies (i.e. cabergoline). In addition, estrogens sensitize anterior pituitary cells to different proapoptotic behavior. The phosphorylation of p38 MAPK induced by DA seems to be a necessary but not a sufficient event to induce apoptosis of lactotrophs, and moreover the hormonal milieu could affect the action of D2R agonists in patients with prolactinomas (Radl, 2011).

2.2. GIRK channel in lactotroph cells

The theory that a G-protein activated inward rectifier K^+ (GIRK) channel can be considered as a physiological cellular level effector of DA action in pituitary lactotroph cell has been proposed by Gregerson et al (2001). The experiments focused on specific hormonal changes on days of estrus cycle in rat, associated with DA sensitivity and effects of dispersed cell in vitro. In proestrus and not on other days of the reproductive cycle in rats, the functional expression of this DA-activated channel could be observed in lactotrophs isolated from female rats. (Gregerson, 1989, Gregerson, 2001)

This experimental design demonstrated that estradiol (E_2) up-regulates the GIRK channel subunits and controls the functional activation of the D_2R-GIRK pathway on mammotrop cells. The functional D_2R-GIRK pathway is the pertussis toxin (PTX)-sensitive heterotrimeric G-protein complex. The ability of DA to activate the GIRK channel of lactotroph demonstrated on isolated cells prepared from animals on different days of estrus cycle seems to be regulated by the hormonal status and property of the cells obtained only of the day of proestrus. Rising levels of circulating E_2 during the transition from diestrus result in a functional switch in DA signaling to include GIRK channel activation. On the morning of proestrus DA activates membrane hyperpolarization. This negative membrane potential "primes" the lactotroph population by removing inactivation of voltage-gated Ca^{2+} channels (VGCC). The drop of hypothalamic DA levels in portal vessels, i.e. on the afternoon of proestrus, the primed lactotrophs depolarize, initiating increased Ca^{2+} influx through VGCC and a consequent PRL release. (Gregerson, 1989; Gregerson, 2001)

E_2 does not have a direct effect on D2 receptor, but may influence the expression of G protein $\beta\gamma$ subunit isoforms, which are known to bind and potentially activate the GIRK channel. A receptor antagonist that competes with E_2 for binding at both ERα and Erβ blocks the induction of GTPγS-activated GIRK current. It was concluded, that there are 3 „essential components" work in synergy regulating the mammotrop cells during the hormonal changes of estrus cycle:

- D2 receptor, which couples to $G\alpha_i$ and thereby inhibits adenylate cyclase (AC), decrease in density on the afternoon of proestrus or with exposure to high concentrations of E_2. (Enjalbert 1983; Pasqualini 1984)

- D_2R-GIRK pathway: a pertussis toxin-sensitive heterotrimeric G protein complex, where the dissociated $\beta\gamma$ complex directly binds to GIRK proteins to open the K^+ channel. (Krapivinsky 1996; Yamada 1998)
- GIRK channel itself: E_2 significantly increase the percentage of lactotrophs with detectable levels of GIRK transcripts in the rat AP gland, measured by single-cell RT-PCR. (Christensen 2011

2.3. DA transporter (DAT)

This member of the Na+/Cl−-dependent transporter superfamily displays the characteristic twelve transmembrane domains and actively transports DA. It there is a bi-directional mechanism behind, since DAT can not only remove DA from the synaptic cleft but under certain conditions can also pump DAT out of cells which is generally referred to as the "reverse transport" (Barnes 2008). The functionality of dopamine transporter of TIDA neurons that is effective in regulating PRL secretion, but the transporter effective in THDA and PHDA neurons as well. Within the dynamics of DA secretion, the termination of DA action is primarily achieved by its reuptake utilized a dopamine transporter (to inwards) located on the terminals of dopaminergic neurons. Dopamine is translocated from the cytoplasm into the vesicles by the vesicular monoamine transporter (VMAT). DA is stored in synaptic vesicles at extremely high at a 100- to 1000-fold higher concentration than neuropeptides, which is near its limit of solubility. These vesicles intend to store and protect DA from degradation but also prevent leakage and control precise release from the synaptic vesicles (Ben-Jonathan, 2001).

DAT-knock-out mice have increased dopaminergic tone and anterior pituitary hypoplasia, and decreased number of lactotroph cells with down-regulation of the PRL gene (Bosse, 1997). „Clinically" the signs summarized as increased DA, consequent reduction (70-80%) in pituitary PRL content, the lack of milk production (since no PRL) and the inability to lactate (since no suckling-induced PRL release). Interestingly, the DAT-KO mice has the basal PRL level unchanged, which is probably due to activated compensatory mechanisms either in DA terminals, or at the lactotroph level. (Ben-Jonathan, 2001; Ben-Jonathan, 2008)

DAT is a common target of several drugs used in both the therapeutic field of psychiatry (psychostimulants, antidepressants), and subjects of drug abuse (like cocaine or amphetamine). Manipulations with the function of DAT and its potential influence on DA levels might have regulatory potential, but more likely causing side-effect of drugs or in certain cases the drug abuse.

2.4. Non DA related receptor mechanisms

2.4.1. Endothelin receptors

The alternative path in regulation of PRL secretion is the actions of endothelins (ETs) in pituitary cells: all members of the mammalian endothelin family of peptides exert significant effects on PRL release *in vitro* that mediated by ET_A receptors (ET-AR). ET-AR is encoded by an intron-containing gene. Selective ET_A receptor antagonist can block the effects of the ETs in a competitive manner (Samson, 1992). Functional ET_A receptors are expressed in all five secretory pituitary cell types included lactotrophs. The ET receptors are connected to both stimulatory and inhibitory (Gs, Gi/o, Gz) G-protein pathways (Tomic, 2002; Andric, 2005).

Generally in lactotrophs and also in somatotrophs, ETs activate the Ca^{2+} -mobilization pathway and transiently can stimulate hormone release. There is a post transient inhibitory effect of PRL release observed for several hours, underlining the importance of desensitization period. Endothelin, similar to D2 receptors coupled to Gi/o, in a picomolar concentration range inhibits adenylyl cyclase (AC) activity in a dose-dependent manner and consequently the PRL release from cultured anterior pituitary cells (Kanyicska, 1992; Samson, 1990). However, this inhibition of basal cAMP production does not abolish spontaneous firing of PRL cells, and only partially inhibits basal PRL release (Stojilkovic 2009).

2.4.2. *Adenosine receptors*

The presence of adenosine has been identified in the anterior pituitary gland. The experimental results and the direct effect of adenosine are controversial and depend on site of administration or the experimental conditions (Ondo, 1980; Schettini, 1990; We, 1998).

As it was revealed earlier, adenosine inhibits the basal adenylate cyclase activity in a dose-dependent manner and decreased PRL secretion. Adenosine and analogues affects the basal as well as stimulated secretion of PRL in pituitary cells, *in vitro* cell culture. It has a biphasic pattern of effect: low concentrations inhibit both AC activity and that affect the PRL release from primary pituitary cells; high concentrations may restore the action. The mechanisms involve the action on the cAMP coupled adenosine receptors at the level of pituitary gland (Schettini, 1990) or the short-loop negative feedback of released PRL.

The adenosine receptor subtypes (A_1, A_{2a}, A_{2b}, and A_2) are involved in mechanisms of action and in regulation of cell proliferation: A_1 receptors have been shown to activate G_i inhibitory G-proteins that decrease intracellular calcium concentrations which decrease the activity of NOS and lower the NO. NO activatins guanylate cyclase that synthesizes cGMP from GTP, and increase the level, which leads to inhibition of PRL release. Since the A_1 and A_2 receptor blockers did not alter PRL release adenosine plays no role in basal PRL release *in vitro* (We, 1998). There subtypes of purinergic G protein-coupled adenosine receptors (AR), the adenosine nucleotide-controlled receptors (P2YR) and ion-conducting receptor-channels (P2XR) have been characterized in the pituitary by Koshimizu et al. (2000). Lactotrophs cells express three subtypes of P2XR channels, and homomeric and/or heteromeric receptors may utilize also the extremely complex but effective mechanisms to activate the cell- and receptor-specific Ca^{2+} signaling patterns (Koshimizu, 2000; Zemkova 2010).

2.4.3. *Cannabinoid receptors*

Preclinical studies suggest a predominantly inhibitory effect of cannabinoids on PRL secretion and some other pituitary hormones like GH, THS. The cannabinoid receptors (CB-

1R) are found in hypothalamic regions (Murphey, 1998; Wenger 1999) and in pituitary (Yasuo, 2010), co-localized with DA receptors in hypothalamic DA projections and modulate the DA transmission that regulates the PRL secretion (Rodríguez De Fonseca, 2001). Treatment with specific endogenous ligand of cannabinoid receptor anandamide inhibited the postnatal development of hypothalamo-pituitary axis in offspring (Wenger, 1999). Anandamide blocks human breast cancer cell proliferation through CB1-like receptor-mediated inhibition of endogenous PRL action by suppressing the levels of the long form of the PRL receptor (Petrocellis, 1998). In human, however, Δ-9-THC did not change plasma PRL levels across a wide range of relevant doses presented in a study by Ranganathan (2009), however frequent users may have lower baseline plasma PRL levels relative to healthy controls. Accordingly, clinical evidence suggesting effects by dose dependent and the development of tolerance and a long-term adaptation to several cannabinoid effects in association with chronic exposure (Block, 1991).

2.4.4. Ghrelin and GHS receptors

Expression of functional growth hormone secretagogue receptors (GHS-R) and the co-expression of the two GHS-R isoforms (Ia and Ib) was found in GH-, GH-PRL- and PRL-secreting adenomas and in pituitary cells. (Lanfranco, 2010). The PRL mRNA is co-localised with GHS-R mRNA. Triple in-situ hybridization showed co-localization of GHS-R mRNA with messengers of GH and PRL, conjointly or separately, in individual cells of somatotroph, somatomammotroph, and lactotroph adenomas (Barlier, 1999).

The administration ghrelin, serves as an endogenous ligand for the GHS-receptor (and primarily expressed in stomach and hypothalamus), as a direct action on somatomammotroph cells significantly stimulates PRL secretion in in human (Takaya, 2000; Lanfranco, 2010), but may exert inhibitory effects in prepubertal rats (Tena-Sempere, 2004). On the other hand, synthetic cortistatin-derived ghrelin receptor ligand (CST-8) does not modify the stimulatory endocrine responses to acylated ghrelin or hexarelin in humans and seems devoid of any modulatory action on either spontaneous or ghrelin-stimulated lactotrophs (Prodam, 2008).

3. Intracellular regulation of PRL secretion

Over the last two-three decades number papers discussing the signal transduction mechanisms have been presented describing the direct or the indirect regulatory effects of dopaminergic inhibition (or stimulation in certain circumstances) of PRL secretion. DA connected through its D2 receptors to G proteins and subunits to control the cAMP levels, but also activates various ion channels, triggering potassium current; influences voltage-activated calcium and potassium currents that induce changes in membrane depolarization, or cause hyperpolarization (Enjalbert, 1983; Freeman 2000). Most of these plasma membrane channels have been characterized in PRL secreting cells, but the mechanism underlying their extracellular Ca^{2+}-dependent action potentials and pacemaking activity is still not fully understood. The cAMP signaling pathway is probably in control of pacemaking, voltage-gated Ca^{2+} influx and also the PRL release are PKA-independent mechanisms (Gonzalez-Iglesias, 2006). The highlights of key intracellular mechanisms regulating PRL secretion in lactotroph cells discussed below.

3.1. G-protein signaling pathways

The classical dopaminergic inhibition of PRL release from the anterior pituitary mediated through both the adenylate cyclase (AC) and Ca^{2+} mobilization/phosphoinositide pathways. D2 receptors are functionally associated with pertussis toxin (PTX)-sensitive G proteins (i.e. affected by activation of PTX-sensitive blockade). Activation of these receptors via $G_{i\text{-}3}\alpha$ causes inhibition of basal AC activity and consequent inhibition of cAMP production. Concomitantly D2 receptors trigger the voltage-sensitive potassium channels (via $G_o\alpha$) and inhibit the voltage-sensitive calcium channels. The $G\beta\gamma$-subunits can enhance the activity of type II AC, influencing the several other intracellular pathways. These complex intracellular messenger mechanisms alter the cAMP levels and a consequent PKA activity. PKA then in the cascade phosphorylates cytoplasmic and nuclear proteins and this also regulates ion channel function and may cause a desensitization of G protein coupled receptors. Accordingly, both Ca^{2+} and cAMP play important roles also in controlling the fusion of secretory vesicles with the plasma membrane to trigger the release hormones in these endocrine cells. (Lledo 1992; Freeman 2000)

That is in concert with the earlier observations, demonstrated the signaling through G protein-dependent pathways resulting in decreased cAMP levels. The $G_{i/o}$ signaling pathway is involved in DA-related inhibition, since resulted in depressed cAMP production. On the other hand, inhibition of basal cAMP production in pituitary lactotrophs does not completely abolish the spontaneous firing of APs and only partially inhibits basal PRL release (Gonzalez-Iglesias 2006). Similar to D2 DA receptor coupled subunits, the endothelin (ET_A) receptors are also connected to both stimulatory and inhibitory (Gs, Gi/o, Gz) G-protein pathways. (Tomic, 2002; Andric 2005).

The original theory discussed the activated heterotrimeric guanine nucleotide-binding (G) proteins dissociated $G\alpha$ and $G\beta\gamma$ subunits resulting in activate or inhibit various downstream effector molecules, impact the consequence of receptor activation in the same fashion (i.e. G-protein coupling, receptor desensitization, internalization, or trafficking). Utilizing frontiers in scientific approach supported by recent experimental evidences (Nb: not specified all cell types of pituitary gland to date) evolved a new concept for receptor theory of multiple active receptor states. That concept has critical implications since leaves room for alternative mechanisms of signaling; for the optimal receptor conformation of G protein activation that differs between G protein pools and that synthetic ones; or for cases when ligands can selectively promote different coupling conformations of the receptors. It is possible that only subsets of potential G protein partners being activated or induction of G protein coupling happens without triggering desensitization. On the other hand, receptor antagonists can cause receptor desensitization or initiate G protein-*independent* signals without producing detectable activation of heterotrimeric G proteins. As concluded, receptor dimerization and interactions with scaffolding or signaling proteins can specifically modify ligand selectivity and determine the intracellular response from alternatives. Accordingly even within a single cell, multiple copies of the same receptor, may have coupled to different signal transduction cascade (especially if the receptor is susceptible to G protein switching induced by heterologous desensitization or capable of signaling through β-arrestins), so they can activate different down-stream effectors in response to the same ligand. (Maudsley, 2005)

The conclusion of recent reports on activation of G-protein coupled receptors (GPCR) by Stojilkovic et al (2009) outlined the complexity of actions of ET_A and D2 receptors in inhibition of basal PRL release. Pertussis toxin could only partially reverse the action of DA agonist induced inhibition of PRL release indicating the place for the pathway that independent from the $G_{i/o}$ pertussis toxin blocking effect. This PTX insensitive step in agonist-induced inhibition of PRL release is not affected by inhibition of PI3-kinase and GSK-3, but reversed at least partially by down-regulation of the $G_z\alpha$ expression. Moreover, the parallel activation of sensitive and insensitive pathways is affecting the PRL release through actions blocking electrical activity and also by desensitizing calcium-secretion coupling. (Stojilkovic 2009)

3.2. G-protein independent pathways

Update on mechanisms of intracellular events related with D2-dopamine receptor may help to understand several conflicting results that exist in the regulation of pituitary PRL secretion. In 2004, a new, D2-receptor coupled signaling was described in the mouse striatum that involves the ser/thr protein kinase Akt (protein kinase B) and was used to study efficiency of psychotropic drugs and lithium. This alternative vs. "canonical" (Gi-cAMP-PKA) signaling pathway is regulated mainly by β-arrestin2, a ubiquitous molecule of receptorial desensitization. The arrestin type 1 has been associated with the dark-adaptation of the retinal cones. The GPCR-β-arrestin2-Akt-PP2 complex plays a dual role: It can terminate the G-protein-mediated signaling of the receptor and initiates a G-protein independent signaling through different downstream phosphorilation cascades (e.g. Glycogene Synthase Kinase-3, GSK-3) (Beaulieu, 2005; Beaulieu, 2008; Csercsik 2008).

The expression of D2 receptor was found to be associated with filamin-A (FLNA). Recently Pervelli et al (2012) demonstrated reduced FLNA and D2R expression in DA-resistant tumors in human samples in vitro experimental conditions. According to clinical results, a subset of patients is resistant to DA probably D2 receptor alterations. The results indicate that (Peverelli, 2012): *(i)* FNLA is crucial for D2 receptor expression, *(ii)* depression of FNLA expression resulted in loss of inhibitory effect of DA due to decreased D2 receptor expression in 60%, in those prolactinomas that characterized as originally DA-sensitive; *(iii)* in DA-resistant prolactinomas forced FLNA expression restored D2 receptor expression and consequently the responsiveness to DA

3.3. Voltage-gated calcium channels

Dopamine exerts diverse effects on lactotroph, however the two most rapid events are: *(i)* the membrane hyperpolarization leading to inactivation of voltage-gated calcium channels, and resulting in a reduced intracellular free calcium ($[Ca^{2+}]_i$) and a consequent inhibition of PRL release from secretory granules; and *(ii)* suppression of AC activity and inositol phosphate metabolism resulting in diminished of PRL expression of the cells (Ben-Jonathan 2001). All other events associated to DA actions are more redundant on the time-scale, assuming that controls exerted via calcium channels play a critical role in immediate actions of PRL regulations.

The speed that noticed in electrophysiology experiments in the action of DA inhibiting PRL release also underline the involvement of ion channels and harmony in interplay between sodium current, T- and L-type calcium channels and calcium-dependent potassium channels. All of these membrane and ion-concentration related effects contribute to the generation of spontaneous, voltage dependent action potentials (APs) at frequencies between 0.2 and 0.5 Hz and a resting membrane potential -40 to -60 mV. However it should be noted, that a certain population of cells are considered as „quiescent" cells with a stable membrane potential, characterized with lack of changes in electrical activity, compared to „active" cells with higher basal PRL release. As it was reported earlier calcium is required to release PRL from the secretory granules. Action of DA induces a rapid change in cytosolic $[Ca^{2+}]_i$ concentration, particularly in those spontaneously active lactotrophs, as proposed via D2 receptor coupled with voltage-gated calcium channels and consequent phosphorylation/dephosphorylation or via indirect action on GIRK and resulting in a marked decline in intracellular calcium. (Corrette, 1995; Ho, 1996; Curtis, 1985; Nastainczyk, 1987; Ben-Jonathan, 2001; Gregerson, 2001)

As the membrane potential (Vm) of cultured anterior pituitary cells oscillates from a baseline and when it reaches the threshold level, pituitary cells fire action potentials (APs). The types of "active " secretory pituitary cells differ with respect to the pattern of electrical activity and AP-driven calcium signaling and secretion *in vivo* and *in vitro*. Cultured lactotrophs and somatotrophs frequently exhibit larger V_m oscillations, on top of which the depolarizing plateau and bursts of APs are generated, with spikes that do not usually reach the reverse potential. The differences in the patterns of spontaneous firing of APs among secretory pituitary cells are reflected in their respective pattern of calcium signaling. In elegant experiments of Stojilkovic (2009), measuring simultaneously the V_m and intracellular calcium concentration ($[Ca^{2+}]_i$) the lactotrophs cell have been characterized. Generally in lactotroph-somatotroph cells the slow resting V_m oscillations superimposed with bursts of APs, with an average duration of seconds shown high amplitude calcium transients, which reflects the increases in intracellular calcium concentration ($[Ca^{2+}]_i$ (Stojilkovic 2009).

The *in vitro* basal PRL secretion from lacto-somatotroph pituitary cells is high and is dependent on the extracellular calcium concentration. Basal hormone secretion is dependent also on the duration of the AP wave form, since that is the volume to drive calcium through voltage-gated calcium (Ca_v) channels. These non-stimulated cells secrete in a „constitutive and regulated manner", since handled by Ca^{2+} influx and resulted in Ca^{2+}-dependent exocytosis. The voltage-gated calcium influx however, triggers secretion in lactotrophs, resulting in an organized superimposition of APs, so called „plateau-bursting" action potentials that generate high amplitude calcium signals. Since the firing of spontaneous APs depends on the presence of calcium in extracellular medium the transient removal of calcium leads to cease spiking and accompanied by abolition of basal hormone release. These results indicate that a specialty of these „active" lactotroph cells (i.e. the extended duration of the AP wave due to the high amplitude $[Ca^{2+}]_i$ signals) probably is the main reason for their high level of basal PRL secretion profile. (Van Goor 2001)

That is in accordance of earlier results which has been part of experimental protocols also in our laboratory that animals bearing ectopic pituitary grafts (e.g. under kidney capsules) *in vivo*, release high levels of PRL for a prolonged period. It is also plausible that a well-balanced control mechanism is necessary to regulate the PRL release in a precise manner during the different physiological stages, such as needed during the estrus cycle, peaks of diurnal rhythm during pregnancy, suckling induced PRL release, etc. DA serves as the hypothalamic controlling agent, regulating the spontaneous release by the cascades of $G_{i/o}$-coupled receptors for inhibition, controlling ion-channels for immediate action, but in addition to support need for release stimulation via G_s-coupled receptors mobilizing Ca^{2+} is also utilized.

3.4. Cyclic nucleotides in signaling

As discussed above the hypothalamo-hypophyseal system, or more generally the neuroendocrine and also immune systems are prominently regulated by G-protein coupled receptors that utilize the cAMP signal transduction cascade. Increases in cAMP lead to functional activation of PKA by binding to the regulatory subunits and liberating the catalytic subunits, phosphorylates cytoplasmic and nuclear proteins, and desensitize the G protein coupled receptors. Decrease in cAMP suppresses PKA by maintaining it in an inactive conformation and moreover in the presence of secretagogues, that potentially mediates other cellular responses of lactotrophs in relation to DA activation. Involvement of different membrane enzymes in the context of varied levels of activation of G-proteins as well as Ca^{2+}- and protein kinase C-dependent processes are equally important to generate the characteristic cAMP signal and cut-off at certain level by the cAMP-degrading phosphodiesterases. (Antony, 2000; Diamond 1999; Gonzalez-Iglesias, 2006)

The level of Ca^{2+} concentration in cytosol and the cyclic nucleotide signaling pathways are connected in regulation of physiological processes through messenger generation and also influencing additional other signaling pathways and *vice versa*, there is a distinct molecular machinery responsible to modulate the calcium concentration ($[Ca^{2+}]_i$) (Bruce 2003).

- *From one side*, the intracellular calcium concentration influences cAMP levels and balance, may also activates or inhibits some isoforms of adenylyl cyclase (AC), moreover the calcium concentration ($[Ca^{2+}]_i$), and selectively stimulates some phosphodiesterase (PDE) subtypes. Besides the cAMP, calcium also affects cGMP levels, NO synthase, etc through the activation of Ca^{2+}-sensitive phosphodiesterases.

- *From the other side,* the cyclic nucleotide intracellular levels and activity of their kinases can influence membrane potential (V_m) and Ca^{2+} balance by Ca^{2+} influx via channels, and also the Ca^{2+} clearance. (Gonzalez-Iglesias 2006)

This machinery of the cyclic nucleotides and the kinases may serve as a regulator or a pacemaker for hormone secretion of pituitary cells. It was demonstrated by in vitro models, that:

- plasma membrane channels involved in action potential spiking;
- basal cyclic nucleotides could contribute to the modulation of firing activity in lactotrophs;
- both the cyclic nucleotide-dependent and -independent pathways controlling spontaneous VGCI and the level of exocytosis;
- basal cAMP production controls the VGCI and PRL release by modulating electrical activity of the cell;
- VGCI should be accountable for inhibition of intrinsic AC activity, since VGCI attenuates the intrinsic AC activity in intact cells independently of the status of PDEs.

This regulation in lactotroph pituitary cells contributes only to the control of spontaneous electrical activity and basal PRL release, whereas the AC-independent action potential secretion coupling accounts for the majority of basal PRL release. Partial dependence of basal PRL release on cyclic nucleotides and partial inhibition of AC activity by spontaneous VGCI are the findings that consistent with reciprocal modulation of cyclic nucleotides and VGCI in spontaneously firing pituitary lactotrophs. (Gonzalez-Iglesias 2006).

3.5. Role of protein phosphorylation-dephosphorylation in the extracellular signals mediated secretory function of lactotrophs

Since virtually all types of extracellular signals (either those affecting second messenger-dependent activation or inactivation of protein kinases (PKs) or those that use a direct activation or inactivation of an ion channel) converge to a final common system of fundamental importance in biological regulation, called PROTEIN PHOSPHORYLATION, one of the main objectives of this review is to summarize the role of this final messenger system. In recent years, significant advances have been made in our understanding of the role of protein phosphorylation-dephosphorylation in the extracellular signals mediating secretory function of different cells (Murányi 1997; Muranyi 1998; Lefkowitz, 1993; Shenolikar, 1988).

Given the complexity and diversity of intercellular communication between hypothalamic releasing/inhibiting factors and hormone secreting pituitary cells (neuroendocrine communication) or between different cells of the pituitary gland itself (paracrine/autocrine communication), it would not be surprising that many of these systems use reversible protein phosphorylations. In this "third messenger" system, phosphorylation of the appropriate target or substrate proteins is tightly controlled by the activities of phosphorylating PKs and dephosphorylating protein phosphatases (PPs). While the functions of PKs in the pituitary gland have been widely explored (Beretta, 1989; Leighton, 1993; Chneiweiss, 1992), the role of the PPs has been mostly ignored. Significance of dephosphorylation in such regulatory mechanisms has been already demonstrated in the CNS (Leighton, 1993; Chneiweiss, 1992; Nestler, 1983; Shenolikar, 1994; Nestler, 1994) including control of neurotransmitter synthesis and release (Leighton, 1993), signaling through the neurotransmitter receptors (Nestler, 1983; Shenolikar, 1994) and ion channels (Shenolikar, 1994; Nestler, 1994) or various aspect of gene expression (Nestler, 1994; Mumbby, 1993; Wera 1995).

4. Overview: control mechanisms of PRL secretion

The hypophysiotrophic (inhibitory) DAergic neurons in the hypothalamus consist of three distinct groups of neurons: the tuberoinfundibular (TIDA), tuberohypophysial (THDA) and the periventricular-hypophysial (PHDA) dopaminergic systems. DA reaching the AL via short portal vessels from the neurointermediate lobe (NIL) accounts for an alternative regulatory aspect of basal and tonic PRL release besides the main physiological regulator TIDA neurons. The stimulatory and inhibitory factors influencing PRL secretion have multiple sites of action at least in two levels: *(i)* hypothalamic level as neurotransmitter on DA neurons; *(ii)* at the pituitary as a neurohormone acting on lactotrophs, or other factors may act as an autocrine or paracrine modulator. Well defined external effects (circadian patterns, noise, stress, etc) or neuronal stimuli have been identified to modulate PRL secretion, however the main components are endogenous substances that can affect the activity of neuroendocrine dopaminergic and PRF neurons and/or pre-synaptically regulate neural inputs to these neuroendocrine cells; alternatively act directly on pituitary cells.

The predominant dopamine receptor is the D2 type in pituitary lactotroph cells, which exists in two alternatively spliced D2-short (D2S) and D2-long (D2L) isoforms, co-expressed in the same cells. Due to selective coupling to G-proteins, these receptor isoforms serve different functions: *(i)* inhibition of adenylyl cyclase, *(ii)* activation of voltage-gated calcium channels, and *(iii)* inhibition of potassium channels. D2L is the main isoform present in the anterior pituitary both in rat and in human. Alterations in the proportion of D2L/D2S could be the reason of resistance in D2R agonist therapies treating prolactinomas in clinical practice.

The G-protein-coupled receptors carry the mainstream of biological responses, utilizing subunits that carry different and versatile subcellular messenger functions increasing the flexibility of the down-stream effector mechanisms according to the endocrine milieu. $G_{i/o}$ signaling pathway is involved in DA-related inhibition of PRL secretion and results in depressed cAMP production. D2 receptors trigger the voltage-sensitive potassium channels (via $G_o\alpha$) and inhibit the voltage-sensitive calcium channels. Both Ca^{2+} and cAMP play important role to trigger the hormone release. Inhibition of basal cAMP production lactotrophs does not completely abolish the spontaneous firing of APs and only partially effect the basal PRL secretion. The PTX insensitive step in agonist-induced inhibition of PRL release parallel with an activation of the sensitive pathways are affecting the PRL release through actions blocking electrical activity.

The physiology of pituitary cells reflecting to suckling stimulus or separation from pups, controlled by various concentrations of DA: due to suckling stimulus with low dose of DA to PRL release or exhibit dose-dependent inhibitory effect. This experimental model (non-suckled *versus* suckled) serves to demonstrate manipulations on concentrations of DA or receptors of DA *in vivo* or *in vitro* moreover, able to distinguish between ligand dissociation, and stimulation-induced elevation of PRL release. The suckling-induced desensitization/sensitization of pituitary cells is manifested at the cellular level by an increase of subpopulation of those cells less/ more sensitive to high/low dose ranges of DA. The receptor mediated intracellular mechanisms leading to these suckling-induced changes in DA responsiveness of lactotrophs is still not fully understood. It is possible that DA modulates the inputs in a biphasic manner: at low concentrations DA activates D1-like receptors, but higher concentrations activate the D2-like receptors resulting in inhibition. The receptorial desensitization or "tolerance" is based on the mechanisms, in which ligands of G-protein-coupled receptors (GPCRs) can promote specific intracellular signaling adaptation mechanisms parallel with the internalization process of the receptors. Estradiol up-regulates the GIRK channel subunits and controls the functional activation of the D_2R-GIRK pathway on mammotrop cells for the DA action. The negative membrane potential "primes" the lactotroph population by removing inactivation of voltage-gated Ca^{2+} channels.

The intracellular mechanisms of DA activation connected to D2 receptors and G-proteins coupled subunits to control the cAMP levels and various ion channels: triggering potassium current influences voltage-activated calcium and potassium currents. Most of these plasma membrane channels have been characterized, but the mechanism connected to Ca^{2+}-dependent action potentials and pacemaking activity is still not fully understood. The cAMP signaling pathway is probably in control of pacemaking, voltage-gated Ca^{2+} influx and PRL release is a PKA-independent mechanism. The parallel activation of PTX-sensitive and insensitive pathways are affecting the PRL release through changes in electrical activity or modulate voltage-gated calcium channels. A specialty of these „active" lactotroph cells that this voltage-gated calcium influx resulting in an organized superimposition of APs, so called „plateau-bursting" action potentials that generate high amplitude calcium signals triggers secretion in lactotropes.

The complexity and diversity of intercellular and paracellular communication suggests a common theory of a "third messenger" system: phosphorylation of the appropriate target or substrate proteins controlled by the activities of phosphorylating PKs and dephosphorylating by protein phosphatases (PPs). Significance of dephosphorylation has been already demonstrated in the CNS, signaling through the neurotransmitter receptors and ion channels, but role of PPs has been still left some uncertainty. In recent years efforts have been made to understand the role of protein phosphorylation-dephosphorylation in processing extracellular signals to mediate secretory functions.

Author details

György M. Nagy
Neuromorphological and Neuroendocrine Research Laboratory
Department of Human Morphology
Hungarian Academy of Sciences and Semmelweis University, Budapest, Hungary

Viktória Reinhoffer
Neuromorphological and Neuroendocrine Research Laboratory
Department of Human Morphology, Semmelweis University, Budapest, Hungary

Márk Oláh
Department of Human Morphology, Semmelweis University, Budapest, Hungary

Miklós Vecsernyés
Faculty of Pharmacy, University of Debrecen, Debrecen, Hungary

Béla E. Tóth
Director at Academic Research Consulting Group

Acknowledgement

Some of the referred experimental work was supported by OTKA-81522 (for GMN) and by the TÁMOP-4.2.2.A-11/1/KONV-2012-0025 project (for MV).

5. References

Andric SA, Zivadinovic D, Gonzalez-Iglesias AE, Lachowicz A, Tomic M, Stojilkovic SS. Endothelin-induced, long lasting, and Ca2+ influx-independent blockade of intrinsic secretion in pituitary cells by Gz subunits. J Biol Chem. 2005 Jul 22;280(29):26896-903.

Antoni FA. Molecular diversity of cyclic AMP signalling. Front Neuroendocrinol. 2000 Apr;21(2):103-32. Review.

Barlier A, Zamora AJ, Grino M, Gunz G, Pellegrini-Bouiller I, Morange-Ramos I, Figarella-Branger D, Dufour H, Jaquet P, Enjalbert A. Expression of functional growth hormone secretagogue receptors in human pituitary adenomas: polymerase chain reaction, triple in-situ hybridization and cell culture studies. J Neuroendocrinol. 1999 Jul;11(7):491-502.

Beaulieu JM, Marion S, Rodriguiz RM, Medvedev IO, Sotnikova TD, Ghisi V, Wetsel WC, Lefkowitz RJ, Gainetdinov RR, Caron MG (2008) A beta-arrestin 2 signaling complex mediates lithium action on behavior. Cell 2008 132:125–136.

Beaulieu JM, Sotnikova TD, Marion S, Lefkowitz RJ, Gainetdinov RR, Caron MG. An Akt/beta-arrestin 2/PP2A signaling complex mediates dopaminergic neurotransmission and behavior. Cell. 2005 Jul 29;122(2):261-73.

Ben-Jonathan N, Hnasko R. Dopamine as a prolactin (PRL) inhibitor. Endocr Rev. 2001 Dec;22(6):724-63. Review.

Ben-Jonathan N, LaPensee CR, LaPensee EW. What can we learn from rodents about prolactin in humans? Endocr Rev. 2008 Feb;29(1):1-41. Epub 2007 Dec 5. Review.

Ben-Jonathan N, Peters LL. Posterior pituitary lobectomy: differential elevation of plasma prolactin and luteinizing hormone in estrous and lactating rats. Endocrinology 1982 Jun; 110(6): 1861-1865.

Ben-Jonathan N. Catecholamines and pituitary prolactin release. J. Reprod. Fertil. 1980 Mar; 58: 501-512.

Ben-Jonathan N. Dopamine: a prolactin-inhibiting hormone. Endocr. Rev. 1985 Fall;6(4):564-89. Review.

Beretta L, Boutterin MC, Drouva SV, Sobel A. Phosphorylation of a group of proteins related to the physiological, multihormonal regulations of the various cell types in the anterior pituitary gland. Endocrinology. 1989 Sep;125(3):1358-64.

Bhansali A, Walia R, Dutta P, Khandelwal N, Sialy R, Bhadada S. Efficacy of cabergoline on rapid escalation of dose in men with macroprolactinomas. Indian J Med Res. 2010 Apr;131:530-5.

Block RI, Farinpour R, Schlechte JA. Effects of chronic marijuana use on testosterone, luteinizing hormone, follicle stimulating hormone, prolactin and cortisol in men and women. Drug Alcohol Depend. 1991 Aug; 28(2):121-8.

Bodnár I, Mravec B, Kubovcakova L, Toth EB, Fülöp F, Fekete MI, Kvetnansky R, Nagy GM. Stress- as well as suckling-induced prolactin release is blocked by a structural analogue of the putative hypophysiotrophic prolactin-releasing factor, salsolinol. J Neuroendocrinol. 2004 Mar;16(3):208-13.

Bosse R, Fumagalli F, Jaber M, Giros B, Gainetdinov RR, Wetsel WC, Missale C, CaronMG Anterior pituitary hypoplasia and dwarfism in mice lacking the dopamine transporter. 1997 Jul;19(1):127-38.

Broglio F, Grottoli S, Arvat E, Ghigo E. Endocrine actions of cortistatin: in vivo studies. Mol Cell Endocrinol. 2008 May 14;286(1-2):123-7.

Bruce JI, Straub SV, Yule DI. Crosstalk between cAMP and Ca2+ signaling in non-excitable cells. Cell Calcium. 2003 Dec;34(6):431-44. Review.

Caron MG, Beaulieu M, Raymond V, Gagne B, Drouin J, Lefkowitz RJ, Labrie F. Dopaminergic receptors in the anterior pituitary gland: correlation of 3H-dihydroergocryptine binding with the dopaminergic control of prolactin release. J Biol Chem 1978 Apr 10;253(7):2244-53.

Chneiweiss H, Cordier J, Sobel A. Stathmin phosphorylation is regulated in striatal neurons by vasoactive intestinal peptide and monoamines via multiple intracellular pathways. J Neurochem. 1992 Jan;58(1):282-9.

Christensen HR, Zeng Q, Murawsky MK, Gregerson KA. Estrogen regulation of the dopamine-activated GIRK channel in pituitary lactotrophs: implications for regulation of prolactin release during the estrous cycle. Am J Physiol Regul Integr Comp Physiol. 2011 Sep;301(3):R746-56.

Conductier G, Nahon JL, Guyon A. Dopamine depresses melanin concentrating hormone neuronal activity through multiple effects on α2-noradrenergic, D1 and D2-like dopaminergic receptors. Neuroscience. 2011 Mar 31;178:89-100.

Corrette BJ, Bauer CK, Schwarz JR Electrophysiology of anterior pituitary cells. In: Scherubl H, Hescheler J, eds. The electrophysiology of neuroendocrine cells. 1995 London: CRC Press; 101–143.

Cronin MJ, Myers GA, MacLeod RM, Hewlett EL. Pertussis toxin uncouples dopamine agonist inhibition of prolactin release. Am J Physiol. 1983 May;244(5):E499-504.

Csercsik D, Hangos MK, Nagy GM. A simple reaction kinetic model of rapid (G-protein dependent) and slow (beta-arrestin dependent) transmission. J Theor Biol. 2008 Nov 7;255(1):119-28.

Curtis BM, Catterall WA. Phosphorylation of the calcium antagonist receptor of the voltage-sensitive calcium channel by cAMP-dependent protein kinase. Proc Natl Acad Sci 1985 Apr;82(8):2528-32.

De Petrocellis L, Melck D, Palmisano A, Bisogno T, Laezza C, Bifulco M, Di Marzo V. The endogenous cannabinoid anandamide inhibits human breast cancer cell proliferation. Proc Natl Acad Sci USA. 1998 Jul 7;95(14):8375-80.

Delahunty TM, Cronin MJ, Linden J. Regulation of GH3-cell function via adenosine A1 receptors. Inhibition of prolactin release, cyclic AMP production and inositol phosphate generation. Biochem J. 1988 Oct 1;255(1):69-77.

DeMaria JE, Lerant AA, Freeman ME. Prolactin activates all three populations of hypothalamic neuroendocrine dopaminergic neurons in ovariectomized rats. BrainRes. 1999 Aug 7;837(1-2):236-41.

DeVito WJ, Avakian C, Stone S, Ace C. Estradiol increases prolactin synthesis and prolactin messenger ribonucleic acid in selected brain regions in the hypophysectomized female rat. Endocrinology 1992 Nov;131(5):2154-60.

DeVito WJ, Avakian C, Stone S, Okulicz WC. Prolactin stimulated mitogenesis of cultured astrocytes is mediated by a protein kinase C-dependent mechanism. J Neurochem 1993 Mar;60(3):832-42.

Diamond SE, Chiono M, Gutierrez-Hartmann A. Reconstitution of the protein kinase A response of the rat prolactin promoter: differential effects of distinct Pit-1 isoforms and functional interaction with Oct-1. Mol Endocrinol 1999 Feb;13(2):228-38.

Enjalbert A, Bockaert J. Pharmacological characterization of the D2 dopamine receptor negatively coupled with adenylate cyclase in the rat anterior pituitary. Mol Pharmacol 1983 May;23(3):576-84.

Freeman ME, Burris TP. Dopamine as a prolactin-releasing hormone. In: Melmed S.(ed) Molecular and Clinical Advances in Pituitary Disorders. Endocrine Research and Education, Inc., Beverly Hills, CA, 1993 pp. 249-253.

Freeman ME, Kanyicska B, Lerant A, Nagy GM. Prolactin: Structure, function and regulation of secretion. Physiol Rev. 2000 Oct;80(4):1523-631. Review.

Gonzalez HA, Porter JC. Mass and in situ activity of tyrosine hydroxylase in the median eminence: effect of hyperprolactinemia. Endocrinology. 1988 May;122(5):2272-7.

Gonzalez-Iglesias AE, Jiang Y, Tomić M, Kretschmannova K, Andric SA, Zemkova H, Stojilkovic SS. Dependence of electrical activity and calcium influx-controlled prolactin release on adenylyl cyclase signaling pathway in pituitary lactotrophs. Mol Endocrinol. 2006 Sep;20(9):2231-46.

Gonzalez-Iglesias AE, Murano T, Li S, Tomic M, Stojilkovic SS. Dopamine inhibits basal prolactin release in pituitary lactotrophs through pertussis toxin-sensitive and -insensitive signaling pathways. Endocrinology 149: 1470–1479, 2008.

Goudreau JL, Falls WM, Lookingland KJ, Moore KE. Periventricular-hypophysial dopaminergic neurons innervate the intermediate but not the neural lobe of the rat pituitary gland. Neuroendocrinology. 1995 Aug;62(2):147-54.

Gregerson KA, Einhorn L, Oxford GS. Modulation of potassium channels by dopamine in rat pituitary lactotrophs: a role in the regulation of prolactin secretion? Soc Gen Physiol Ser. 1989;44:123-41.

Gregerson KA, Flagg TP, O'Neill TJ, Anderson M, Lauring O, Horel JS, Welling PA. Identification of G protein-coupled inward rectifier potassium channel gene products from the rat anterior pituitary gland. Endocrinology 2001 Jul;142(7):2820-32.

Gregerson KA. Functional expression of the dopamine-activated K+ current in lactotrophs during the estrous cycle in female rats: correlation with prolactin secretory responses. Endocrine 2003 Feb-Mar;20(1-2):67-74.

Gudelsky GA, Porter JC. Release of dopamine from tuberoinfundibular neurons into pituitary stalk blood after prolactin or haloperidol administration. Endocrinology. 1980 Feb;106(2):526-9.

Guivarc'h D, Vernier P, Vincent JD. Sex steroid hormones change the differential distribution of the isoforms of the D2 dopamine receptor messenger RNA in the rat brain. Neuroscience 1995 Nov;69(1):159-66.

Higuchi T, Honda K, Takano S, Negoro H. Estrogen fails to reduce tuberoinfundibular dopaminergic neuronal activity and to cause a prolactin surge in lactating, ovariectomized rats. Brain Res. 1992 Mar 27;576(1):143-6.

Hill JB, Nagy GM, Frawley LS. Suckling unmasks the stimulatory effect of dopamine (DA) on PRL release: possible role for α-melanocyte stimulating hormone (α-MSH) as a mammotrope responsiveness factor. Endocrinology Aug;129(2):843-7.

Ho M-Y, Kao JPY, Gregerson KA. Dopamine withdrawal elicits prolonged calcium rise to support prolactin rebound release. Endocrinology 1996 Aug;137(8):3513-21.

Holzbauer M, Racke K. The dopaminergic innervation of the intermediate lobe and the neural lobe of the pituitary gland. Med. Biol. 1985;63(3):97-116. Review.

Holzbauer M, Sharman DF, Godden U. Observations on the function of the dopaminergic nerves innervating the pituitary gland. Neuroscience 1978;3(12):1251-62.

Homicskó KG, Kertész I, Radnai B, Tóth BE, Tóth G, Fülöp F, Fekete MI, Nagy GM. Binding site of salsolinol: its properties in different regions of the brain and the pituitary gland of the rat. Neurochem Int. 2003 Jan;42(1):19-26.

Horváth KM, Radnai B, Tóth BE, Fekete MIK, and Nagy GM. Inhibition of protein phosphatase 2A (PP2A) mimics suckling-induced sensitization of lactotrophs: Involvement of a pertussis toxin (PTX) sensitive G-protein and the adenylate cyclase (AC). Molecular and Cellular Endocrinology 1999 Mar 25;149(1-2):1-7.

Kanyicska B, Livingstone JD, Freeman ME. Long term exposure to dopamine reverses the inhibitory effect of endothelin-1 on prolactin secretion. Endocrinology. 1995;136:990–4.

Kelly MA, Rubinstein M, Asa SL, Zhang G, Saez C, Bunzow JR, Allen RG, Hnasko R, Ben-Jonathan N, Grandy DK, Low MJ. Pituitary lactotroph hyperplasia and chronic hyperprolactinemia in dopamine D2 receptor-deficient mice. Neuron 1997 Jul;19(1):103-13.

Kennett JE, McKee DT. Oxytocin: an emerging regulator of prolactin secretion in the female rat. J Neuroendocrinol. 2012 Mar;24(3):403-12.

Koshimizu TA, Tomić M, Wong AO, Zivadinovic D, Stojilkovic SS. Characterization of purinergic receptors and receptor-channels expressed in anterior pituitary cells. Endocrinology. 2000 Nov;141(11):4091-9.

Krapivinsky G, Kennedy ME, Nemec J, Medina I, Krapivinsky L, Clapham DE. Gβ binding to GIRK4 subunit is critical for G protein-gated K+ channel activation. J Biol Chem 1998 Jul 3;273(27):16946-52.

Lanfranco F, Motta G, Baldi M, Gasco V, Grottoli S, Benso A, Broglio F, Ghigo E. Ghrelin and anterior pituitary function. Front Horm Res. 2010;38:206-11.

LaPensee EW, Ben-Jonathan N. Novel roles of prolactin and estrogens in breast cancer: resistance to chemotherapy. Endocr Relat Cancer. 2010 Feb 25;17(2):R91-107. Review.

Lefkowitz RJ. G-protein-coupled receptor kinases. Cell 1993 Aug 13;74(3):409-12. Review.

Leighton IA, Curmi P, Campbell DG, Cohen P, Sobel A. The phosphorylation of stathmin by MAP kinase. Mol. Cell. Biochem. 1993 Nov;127-128:151-6.

Leong DA, Frawley LS, Neill JD. Neuroendocrine control of prolactin secretion. Annu Rev Physiol. 1983;45:109-27.

Lledo PM, Homburger V, Bockaert J, Vincent JD. Differential G protein-mediated coupling of D2 dopamine receptors to K+ and Ca2+ currents in rat anterior pituitary cells. Neuron 1992 Mar;8(3):455-63.

Lyons DJ, Hellysaz A, Broberger C. Prolactin regulates tuberoinfundibular dopamine neuron discharge pattern: novel feedback control mechanisms in the lactotrophic axis. J Neurosci. 2012 Jun 6;32(23):8074-83.

Lyons DJ, Horjales-Araujo E, Broberger C. Synchronized network oscillations in rat tuberoinfundibular dopamine neurons: switch to tonic discharge by thyrotropin-releasing hormone. Neuron. 2010 Jan 28;65(2):217-29.

Mangurian LP, Walsh RJ, Posner BI .Prolactin enhancement of its own uptake at the choroid plexus. Endocrinology 1992 Aug;131(2):698-702.

Maudsley S, Martin B, Luttrell LM. The origins of diversity and specificity in G protein-coupled receptor signaling. J Pharmacol Exp Ther. 2005 Aug;314(2):485-94.

McChesney R, Sealfon SC, Tsutsumi M, Dong KW, Roberts JL, Bancroft C. Either isoform of the dopamine D2 receptor can mediate dopaminergic repression of the rat prolactin promoter. Mol Cell Endocrinol 1991 Aug;79(1-3):R1-7.

Missale C, Nash SR, Robinson SW, Jaber M, Caron MG. Dopamine receptors: from structure to function. Physiol Rev 1998 78: 189–225,

Mulchahey JJ, Neill JD. Dopamine levels in the anterior pituitary gland monitored by in vivo electrochemistry. Brain Research 1986 Oct 29;386(1-2):332-40.

Mumbby MC, Walter G. Protein serine/threonine phosphatase: structure, regulation, and functions in cell growth. Physiol. Rev. 1993 Oct;73(4):673-99. Review.

Murányi A, Gergely P, Fekete MI, Nagy GM. Protein phosphatase 2A plays a role in the suckling-induced changes in the responsiveness of pituitary lactotrophs .Endocrinology. 1998 Nov;139(11):4590-7.

Murányi A, Gergely P, Nagy GM, and Fekete MIK. The possible role of protein phosphatase 2A in the sodium sensitivity of the receptor binding of opiate antagonists Naloxone and Naltrindole. Brain Research Bulletin 1997;44(3):273-9.

Murphy LL, Muñoz RM, Adrian BA, Villanúa MA. Function of cannabinoid receptors in the neuroendocrine regulation of hormone secretion. Neurobiol Dis. 1998 Dec;5(6 Pt B):432-46.

Nagy GM, Arendt A, Banky Zs, Halasz B. Dehydration attenuates plasma prolactin response to suckling through a dopaminergic mechanisms. Endocrinology 1992 Feb;130(2):819-24.

Nagy GM, Boockfor FR, Frawley LS. The suckling stimulus increases the responsiveness of lactotrophs located exclusively within the central region of the adenohypophysis. Endocrinology 1991 Feb;128(2):761-4.

Nagy GM, Frawley LS. Suckling increases the proportions of lactotrophs responsive to various prolactin-releasing stimuli. Endocrinology 1990 Nov;127(5):2079-84.

Nastainczyk W, Rohrkasten A, Sieber M, Rudolph C, Schachtele C, Marme D, Hofmann F Phosphorylation of the purified receptor for calcium channel blockers by cAMP kinase and protein kinase C. Eur J Biochem 1987 Nov 16;169(1):137-42.

Neill JD, Frawley LS, Plotsky PM, Peck JD, Leong D. Hypothalamic regulation of prolactin secretion. In: Pituitary Hormones and Releated Peptides, edited by Motta M, Zanisi M, and Piva F. New York: Academic, 1982 pp. 223–241.

Neill JD, Nagy GM. Prolactin secretion and its control. In: E Knobil and JD Neill (eds) The Physiology of Reproduction. Second Edition, Raven Press, New York, 1994 pp. 1833-1860.

Nestler EJ, Greengard P. Protein phosphorylation in the brain. Nature 1983 Oct 13-19;305(5935):583-8. Review.

Nestler EJ, Greengard P. Protein phosphorylation and the regulation of neural function. In: Siegel GJ, Agranoff BW, Albers RW, Molinoff PB (eds), Basic Neurochemistry 5th Edition, Raven Press, Ltd., New York. 1994 Chapter 22. pp. 449-474.

Ondo JG, Walker MW, Wheeler DD. Central actions of adenosine on pituitary secretion of prolactin, luteinizing hormone and thyrotropin. Neuroendocrinology. 1989 Jun;49(6):654-8.

Pan J-T Neuroendocrine functions of dopamine. In: Stone TW, (ed). CNS neurotransmitters and neuromodulators: dopamine. Boca Raton, FL: CRC Press; 1996 pp. 213–231.

Pasqualini C, Lenoir V, el Abed A, Kerdolhue B. Anterior pituitary dopamine receptors during the rat estrous cycle. A detailed analysis of proestrus changes. Neuroendocrinology 38: 39–44, 1984.

Peters LA, Hoefer MT, Ben-Jonathan N. The posterior pituitary: regulation of anterior pituitary prolactin secretion. Science 1981 213: 659-661.

Peverelli E, Mantovani G, Vitali E, Elli FM, Olgiati L, Ferrero S, Laws ER, Della Mina P, Villa A, Beck-Peccoz P, Spada A, Lania AG. Filamin-A is essential for dopamine d2 receptor expression and signaling in tumorous lactotrophs. J Clin Endocrinol Metab. 2012 Mar;97(3):967-77.

Prodam F, Benso A, Gramaglia E, Lucatello B, Riganti F, van der Lely AJ, Deghenghi R, Muccioli G, Ghigo E, Broglio F. Cortistatin-8, a synthetic cortistatin-derived ghrelin receptor ligand, does not modify the endocrine responses to acylated ghrelin or hexarelin in humans. Neuropeptides. 2008 Feb;42(1):89-93.

Radl DB, Ferraris J, Boti V, Seilicovich A, Sarkar DK, Pisera D. Dopamine-induced apoptosis of lactotropes is mediated by the short isoform of D2 receptor. PLoS One. 2011 Mar 25;6(3):e18097.

Ranganathan M, Braley G, Pittman B, Cooper T, Perry E, Krystal J, D'Souza DC. The effects of cannabinoids on serum cortisol and prolactin in humans. Psychopharmacology (Berl). 2009 May;203(4):737-44.

Rettori V, De Laurentiis A, Fernandez-Solari J. Alcohol and endocannabinoids: neuroendocrine interactions in the reproductive axis. Exp Neurol. 2010 Jul;224(1):15-22.

Rodríguez De Fonseca F, Gorriti MA, Bilbao A, Escuredo L, García-Segura LM, Piomelli D, Navarro M. Role of the endogenous cannabinoid system as a modulator of dopamine transmission: implications for Parkinson's disease and schizophrenia. Neurotox Res. 2001 Jan;3(1):23-35.

Sagrillo CA, Selmanoff M. Effects of prolactin on expression of the mRNAs encoding the immediate early genes zif/268 (NGF1-A), nur/77 (NGF1-B), c-fos and c-jun in the hypothalamus. Brain Res Mol Brain Res 1998 Oct 30;61(1-2):62-8.

Samson WK, et al. Pituitary site of action of endothelin: selective inhibition of prolactin release in vitro. Biochem Biophys Res Commun. 1990;169:737–43.

Sapsford TJ, Kokay IC, Ostberg L, Bridges RS, Grattan DR. Differential sensitivity of specific neuronal populations of the rat hypothalamus to prolactin action. J Comp Neurol. 2012 Apr 1;520(5):1062-77.

Schettini G, Landolfi E, Meucci O, Florio T, Grimaldi M, Ventra C, Marino A. Adenosine and its analogue (-)-N6-R-phenyl-isopropyladenosine modulate anterior pituitary adenylate cyclase activity and prolactin secretion in the rat. J Mol Endocrinol. 1990 Aug;5(1):69-76.

Sengupta A, Sarkar DK. Estrogen inhibits D2S receptor-regulated Gi3 and Gsprotein interactions to stimulate prolactin production and cell proliferation in lactotropic cells. J Endocrinol. 2012 Jul;214(1):67-78. doi: 10.1530/JOE-12-0125.

Shenolikar S. Protein phosphorylation: hormones, drugs, and bioregulation. FASEB Journ. 1988 Sep;2(12):2753-64. Review.

Shenolikar S. Protein serine/threonine phosphatase - new avenues for cell regulation. Annu. Rev. Cell Biol. 1994;10:55-86. Review.

Stojilkovic SS, Iida T, Merelli F, Catt KJ. Calcium signaling and secretory responses in endothelin-stimulated anterior pituitary cells. Mol Pharmacol. 1991 Jun;39(6):762-70.

Stojilkovic SS, Murano T, Gonzalez-Iglesias AE, Andric SA, Popovic MA, Van Goor F, Tomić M. Multiple roles of Gi/o protein-coupled receptors in control of action potential secretion coupling in pituitary lactotrophs. Ann N Y Acad Sci. 2009 Jan;1152:174-86. Review.

Takaya K, Ariyasu H, Kanamoto N, Iwakura H, Yoshimoto A, Harada M, Mori K, Komatsu Y, Usui T, Shimatsu A, Ogawa Y, Hosoda K, Akamizu T, Kojima M, Kangawa K, Nakao K. Ghrelin strongly stimulates growth hormone release in humans. J Clin Endocrinol Metab. 2000 Dec;85(12):4908-11.

Tena-Sempere M, Aguilar E, Fernandez-Fernandez R, Pinilla L. Ghrelin inhibits prolactin secretion in prepubertal rats. Neuroendocrinology. 2004 Mar;79(3):133-41.

Tomic M, et al. Ca(2+)-mobilizing endothelin-A receptors inhibit voltage-gated Ca(2+) influx through G(i/o) signaling pathway in pituitary lactotrophs. Mol Pharmacol. 2002;61:1329–39.

Toth BE, Bodnar I, Homicsko KG, Fülöp F, Fekete MI, Nagy GM. Physiological role of salsolinol: its hypophysiotrophic function in the regulation of pituitary prolactin secretion. Neurotoxicol Teratol. 2002 Sep-Oct;24(5):655-66. Review.

Toth BE, Homicsko K, Radnai B, Maruyama W, DeMaria JE, Vecsernyes M, Fekete MI, Fülöp F, Naoi M, Freeman ME, Nagy GM. Salsolinol is a putative endogenous neuro-intermediate lobe prolactin-releasing factor. J Neuroendocrinol. 2001 Dec;13(12):1042-50.

Van Goor F, Zivadinovic D, Martinez-Fuentes AJ, Stojilkovic SS. Dependence of pituitary hormone secretion on the pattern of spontaneous voltage-gated calcium influx. Cell type-specific action potential secretion coupling. J Biol Chem. 2001 Sep 7;276(36):33840-6.

Vecsernyes M, Krempels K, Toth EB, Julesz J, Makara GB, Nagy GM. Effect of posterior pituitary denervation (PPD) on prolactin (PRL) and α-melanocyte-stimulating hormone (αMSH) secretion of lactating rats. Brain Research Bulletin 1997;43(3):313-9.

Wenger T, Toth BE, Juanéda C, Leonardelli J, Tramu G. The effects of cannabinoids on the regulation of reproduction. Life Sci. 1999;65(6-7):695-701. Review.

Wera S, Hemmings BA. Serine/threonine phosphatases. Biochem. Journal 1995 Oct 1;311 (Pt 1):17-29. Review.

Yamada M, Inanobe A, Kurachi Y. G protein regulation of potassium ion channels. Pharmacol Rev 1998 Dec;50(4):723-60. Review.

Yasuo S, Unfried C, Kettner M, Geisslinger G, Korf HW. Localization of an endocannabinoid system in the hypophysial pars tuberalis and pars distalis of man. Cell Tissue Res. 2010 Nov;342(2):273-81.

Yu WH, Kimura M, Walczewska A, Porter JC, McCann SM. Adenosine acts by A1 receptors to stimulate release of prolactin from anterior-pituitaries in vitro. Proc Natl Acad Sci U S A. 1998 Jun 23;95(13):7795-8.

Zemkova H, Kucka M, Li S, Gonzalez-Iglesias AE, Tomic M, Stojilkovic SS. Characterization of purinergic P2X4 receptor channels expressed in anterior pituitary cells. Am J Physiol Endocrinol Metab. 2010 Mar;298(3):E644-51.

Chapter 11

Prolactin Receptor Isoforms in Human Breast Cancer

Erika Ginsburg, Christopher D. Heger,
Paul Goldsmith and Barbara K. Vonderhaar

Additional information is available at the end of the chapter

http://dx.doi.org/10.5772/54217

1. Introduction

Prolactin (PRL) is a polypeptide hormone secreted by the anterior pituitary responsible for the growth and differentiation of the normal mammary gland and plays a role in breast cancer. It functions systemically as an endocrine factor, but PRL may also act in an autocrine/paracrine fashion in a number of other tissues. Studies in both pre- and post-menopausal women have determined a significant increased risk for breast cancer for those with serum PRL in the highest quartile [6, 7]. PRL, acting through its receptors, has been shown to increase cell proliferation and decrease apoptosis in breast cancer cells *in vitro* [3, 8]. PRL also acts as a pro-angiogenic factor in mammary tissues [9]. PRL exerts its effects by binding to its receptors on the surface of normal human breast epithelial and cancer cells, initiating the Jak2/Stat5, PI3K, and mitogen-activated protein kinase (MAPK) signaling pathways [3].

The PRL receptor (PRLR) is a member of the class I cytokine/hematopoietic receptor superfamily. A single hydrophobic transmembrane region separates the extracellular ligand-binding domain from the intracellular signaling domain. Five cell-associated PRLR isoforms differ only in their C-terminal cytoplasmic domains [1, 3]. The three major isoforms (long, LF; short 1a and 1b, SF1a and SF1b, respectively) are regulated by PRL itself. LF signals for many functions including growth and differentiation, whereas SF1a and SF1b act as dominant-negatives for differentiation [1, 2]. The role of the short forms in breast cell growth remains to be determined.

2. Problem statement

Studies from our laboratory [1] and from others [2] have demonstrated that three specific isoforms of the PRLR are expressed in both normal and cancerous breast cells and tissues. We recently developed and characterized PRLR isoform specific polyclonal antibodies that revealed that the three isoforms, LF, SF1a, and SF1b, are differentially expressed in ductal and lobular carcinomas [5]. These two most common histological types of breast cancer originate from the terminal ductal lobular unit and may be difficult to classify. However, distinct differences were observed in PRLR expression in normal, benign, and malignant breast tissue which may have prognostic significance [10, 11]. The development and characterization of PRLR isoform specific monoclonal antibodies will provide a near limitless supply of reagent to continue to examine how and where these isoforms interact both in normal breast development and in breast cancer.

3. Application area

The identification of estrogen receptor (ER) and progesterone receptor (PR) in the current testing of breast cancer has advanced the field. Other hormones/growth factors are also involved; for example, PRL and its receptor isoforms. If their roles are more clearly identified with the use of specific antibodies then there may be a practical need for them in the diagnosis of this disease. Examining normal breast development could give clues to the relevance of PRLR isoforms in cancer. Not only do these apply to the breast, but may also be of value to studying ovarian and prostate cancers where PRL may play a role/function. PRLR isoform specific antibodies could be powerful tools in this quest.

4. Methods

4.1. Preparation of the PRLR isoform specific monoclonal antibodies

Synthetic peptides were designed based on the regions of unique intracellular sequences of the PRLR splice variants and synthesized (AnaSpec, Inc., San Jose, CA) by the solid-phase method. Peptides (4 mg) were conjugated to bovine serum albumin (10 mg) with 1mM DSS overnight at room temperature and sent to Epitomics (Burlingame, CA) for immunization of rabbits. Initially, a total of 76 clones were received (54 clones for SF1a, 22 clones for SF1b) and screened for reactivity to their respective antigens by Western blot analysis. Briefly, lysates of CHO-K1 cells expressing either SF1a or SF1b were separated by SDS-PAGE, and transferred to PVDF. Membranes were blocked for 1 hr at room temperature in 5% non-fat dairy milk diluted in TBST+0.1% sodium azide. Subsequently, the clonal supernatants were diluted 1:1 in 10% non-fat dairy milk (diluted in TBST+0.1% sodium azide) and incubated for 3 hr at room temperature. Membranes were washed and probed with goat anti-rabbit Alexa680 (1:4000) prior to visualization using a LiCOR Odyssey reader. Supernatants from positively reacting clones were re-screened prior to selection for subcloning. In total, four SF1a and six SF1b rabbit monoclonal antibodies were put into production. The rabbit sera were initially purified by MEP Hypercel (PAL) chromatography, followed by size-exclusion chromatography to further purify the antibodies. Final pools of antibody were produced and protein concentration determined by the Pierce 660nm assay.

For LF, 6 mg peptide was conjugated to 3 mg keyhole limpet hemocyanin overnight at room temperature using glutaraldehyde. Peptide conjugates were sent to Green Mountain

Antibodies (Burlington, VT) for generation of mouse monoclonal antibodies. Initially, 120 clones were screened by Western blot as described above using CHO-K1 cells expressing LF with the exception that the antibodies were diluted 1:100 in 5% non-fat dairy milk (diluted in TBST+0.1% sodium azide) and incubated overnight at 4° C. Secondary antibody and imaging were essentially as described above. Supernatants of positively reacting clones were re-screened by Western blot and examined by fluorescence microscopy (to confirm appropriate localization) prior to selection for production. In total, 10 positive clones were selected for this process, 8 of which produced IgG. Antisera was purified as described for SF1a and SF1b antibodies. Final pools of antibody were produced and protein concentration determined by the Pierce 660nm assay.

4.2. Cell culture and transfection

Chinese hamster ovary cells (CHO-K1, ATCC, Manassas, VA) were maintained in α-MEM (Invitrogen, Gaithersburg, MD) supplemented with 5% fetal bovine serum (FBS, Invitrogen) and penicillin/streptomycin (100 U/ml and 100 μg/ml respectively, Invitrogen). Transfections were performed using FuGENE 6 (Roche Applied Science, Indianapolis, IN) at a ratio of 1 μg DNA to 3 μl FuGENE. The PRLR isoform specific cDNA constructs were previously described [1]. Cells were transfected for 48 hr, then allowed to grow for an additional 48 hr.

T47D, ZR75-1, MDA-MB-231, MDA-MB-468, MCF7, and SK-BR-3 breast cancer cell lines were obtained from ATCC. T47D, ZR75-1, MDA-MB231, and MDA-MB468 cells were maintained in RPMI1640 (Invitrogen). MCF7 cells were grown in DMEM and SK-BR-3 cells were maintained in McCoys 5a media. All media were supplemented with 5% heat inactivated FBS, 10 μg/ml bovine insulin (Sigma, St. Louis, MO), and penicillin-streptomycin (100 U/ml and 100 μg/ml respectively, Invitrogen). Where indicated, breast cancer cell lines were plated on 8-well glass chamber slides (Nunc, Rochester, NY) in normal growth media, and allowed to attach overnight. The media were replaced and the cells were treated for the indicated times with 500 ng/ml recombinant human PRL in media where the FBS was replaced with 1% charcoal stripped serum, then fixed in 10% normal buffered formalin prior to Duolink assay.

All cells were maintained at 37 °C in a humidified atmosphere with 5% CO2. Cells were passaged using trypsinization (0.05% trypsin-EDTA, Invitrogen) and counted on a hemocytometer using trypan blue exclusion

4.3. Western blot analysis

Transfected CHO cells were collected and whole cell lysates were prepared in Complete Buffer (Roche Applied Science) according to the manufacturer's instructions. Total protein was estimated according to Bradford [12]. Protein (100 μg) was subjected to 10-20% SDS-PAGE (Invitrogen). Proteins were transferred to nitrocellulose membrane and probed with PRLR isoform specific antibodies (10 μg/ml for LF, 6 μg/ml for SF1a or SF1b). Reactivity was detected using ECL Plus (GE Healthcare Life Science, Pittsburgh, PA). Molecular size determinations were made using BenchMark Protein Ladder (Invitrogen).

4.4. Fluorescent immunocytochemistry

CHO cells were plated on 8-well glass chamber slides (Nunc) and transfected as above. After blocking with 5% normal goat serum (Jackson Laboratories, Bar Harbor, ME) prepared in PBS-0.1% Triton, slides were incubated with the PRLR isoform specific monoclonal antibodies (10 µg/ml for LF, 6 µg/ml for SF1a or SF1b) overnight at 4° C. In all cases no primary antibody served as the negative control. Slides were washed four times with PBS-0.1% Triton followed by incubation for 1 hr with either red fluorescent tagged goat anti-mouse secondary antibody for the PRLR-LF or red fluorescent tagged goat anti-rabbit secondary antibody for the PRLR-SF (AlexaFluor 594, 1:500, Invitrogen) in the dark. After extensive washing with PBS containing Triton, slides were mounted with Prolong Gold antifade reagent with DAPI (Invitrogen). The fluorescent staining pattern of the receptor isoforms was evaluated using an Olympus BX40 fluorescence microscope (Olympus America, Center Valley, PA).

4.5. Fluorescent immunohistochemistry

Fresh breast samples were supplied by either the Cooperative Human Tissue Network, a NCI supported resource that supplies human biospecimens to IRB approved researchers, or from patient samples collected in accordance with the guidelines of the National Cancer Institute Review Board, protocol 02-C-0144. Breast tissue was obtained from 15 pre-menopausal reduction mammoplasty patients; each sample was determined free from hyperplastic growth by a pathologist. Samples were fixed in 10% normal buffered formalin, embedded, cut into four micron sections, deparaffinized, and stained as above. For dual labeling studies, sections were incubated overnight at 4° C with LF (10 µg/ml) and either SF1a or SF1b (6 µg/ml) monoclonal antibodies. Red fluorescent anti-mouse secondary antibody (AlexaFluor 594, 1:500) was used for LF; green fluorescent anti-rabbit secondary antibody (AlexaFluor 588, 1:500) was used for SF1a and SF1b.

An additional eight samples were also snap-frozen and stored at -80° C for OCT embedding and sectioning. Frozen tissue sections were thawed for 30 to 60 sec and fixed in ice-cold methanol:acetone (1:1) for 10 min. After washing twice with PBS, sections were blocked for 30 min with 10% normal goat serum in IF buffer (PBS containing 0.05 mg/ml sodium azide, 0.1 mg/ml BSA, 0.02% Triton X, and 0.05% Tween 20). Sections were incubated with either LF (10 µg/ml) and SF1a or SF1b (6 µg/ml) PRLR isoform specific monoclonal antibodies overnight at 4° C. Sections were extensively washed with PBS, then incubated with red fluorescent anti-mouse secondary antibody (AlexaFluor 594, 1:500) for LF and green fluorescent anti-rabbit secondary antibody (AlexaFluor 588, 1:500) for SF1a and SF1b. Sections were washed again and mounted with Prolong Gold antifade reagent with DAPI.

The fluorescent staining patterns of the PRLR isoforms were assessed using an Olympus BX40 fluorescent microscope. For both paraffin-embedded and frozen tissue sections, photographs were immediately taken under the violet, green, and blue channels to detect DAPI, red, and green fluorescence, respectively. Images were merged in order to observe PRLR isoform localization patterns.

Nine samples of paraffin-embedded breast tumor tissue were stained and analyzed as above.

4.6. Measurement of fluorescence intensity

Because serial sections for the breast specimens were used, the same region of each tissue could be measured for fluorescence intensity using Adobe Photoshop (Adobe Systems Inc., Beaverton, OR). Nearly every cell in positive samples showed some level of PRLR isoform expression; as a result, red fluorescence intensity was used to compare levels of isoform expression between samples. In order to do this, the same fluorescent areas were selected from each serial section using the lasso and rectangular marquee tools. Selected sections were analyzed using the histogram function through the red channel, which gave the mean red intensity of the selected section. Photoshop assigns intensity values between 0 and 255 to each pixel in the selected area and then averages these intensities. The distribution of these means was analyzed and used to divide samples into four intensity classes: negative (less than 10 intensity), low (between 11 and 30 intensity), medium (between 31 and 50 intensity), and high (greater than 51 intensity).

4.7. Generation of ProbeMaker probes for Duolink

Antibodies against the various PRLR isoforms were directly conjugated using the ProbeMaker protocol as described by the manufacturer (OLINK BioScience, Upsala, Sweden). Briefly, 2 µl ProbeMaker conjugation buffer was added to 20 µg of each antibody (starting antibody concentration, 1 mg/ml) prior to addition of the antibody to the lyophilized oligonucleotides (PLUS and MINUS probes). Incubation with oligonucleotides proceeded overnight at room temperature, followed by addition of 2 µl of ProbeMaker Stop Reagent and incubation for 30 min at room temperature to conclude the labeling reactions. Unreacted oligonucleotides were rendered inactive during this step, preventing spurious signals from being generated. For storage of the antibody-oligonucleotide conjugates, 24 µl ProbeMaker storage buffer was added. The final concentration of the antibody-oligonucleotide conjugates were ~0.4 mg/ml and stored at 4° C until use.

4.8. *In situ* proximity ligation assay

Cultured cells were plated onto 8-well chamber slides (Millipore) in media for one day prior to stimulation as described above. Cells were stimulated for 0, 5, 10, or 60 min with PRL, washed twice in PBS, then fixed in 4% paraformaldehyde for 10 min. Fixed cells were subsequently washed twice with PBS, dried and frozen at -20° C.

On the day of the experiment, slides were thawed at room temperature and rehydrated in PBS for 10 min at room temperature. All steps of the Duolink protocol were performed as open droplet reactions on the chamber slides, using 30 µl volume per chamber to ensure complete coverage of the cells. Cells were then permeabilized in PBS+0.1% Triton X-100 for 10 min at room temperature, washed twice in PBS, and blocked in 1X Duolink Blocking solution for 30 min at 37° C in a humidity chamber to prevent evaporation. PRLR primary antibody-oligonucleotide conjugates were diluted in PLA Probe Diluent to 5 μg/ml, and applied to slides overnight at 4° C in a cooled humidity chamber. On the second day, slides were washed 3 times in 1X Duolink Wash Buffer A to remove excess antibody-oligonucleotide conjugates. Bound antibody-oligonucleotide conjugates were ligated together for 30 min at 37° C according to the manufacturer's instructions. Subsequently, ligated templates were amplified for 2 hr at 37° C according to the manufacturer's protocol, washed twice for 10 min in Duolink 1X Wash Buffer B, and once for 1 min in 0.1X Wash Buffer B prior to mounting with Duolink Fluorescence mounting media (which also contains DAPI for nuclear counterstaining) and observation under a fluorescent microscope.

Image acquisition was performed using a Zeiss Axioscope M1 under 40X magnification and an AxioCam HR. Image analysis was performed using the Duolink ImageTool software according to the instructions provided by OLINK®.

5. Results

5.1. Characterization of PRLR isoform specific monoclonal antibodies

We have recently prepared and characterized PRLR isoform specific polyclonal antibodies [5]. However, a limitless source of polyclonal antibody is restricted because it is generated by repeated immunization of a rabbit. Each antibody preparation has the potential to vary in its specificity as well. Monoclonal antibodies are more homogeneous and can produce a near inexhaustible supply of reagent. We used the same peptide sequence as for the preparation of isoform specific polyclonal antibodies and, again, demonstrate specificity for the individual isoforms. CHO cells were transiently transfected with cDNA containing the individual PRLR isoforms; western blot analysis from cell lysates indicate that the antibodies detect the corresponding protein without cross-reactivity (Figure 1A).

By immunocytochemical analysis using transiently transfected CHO cells, we were able to positively stain for isoform specific PRLR. As shown in Figure 1B, no cross-reactivity was identified using the antibodies on cells transfected with non-corresponding PRLR cDNA. By both western and immunochemical analysis we were able to demonstrate the specificity of the PRLR isoform specific monoclonal antibodies.

5.2. Immunofluorescent staining of human breast tissue

Once we determined the specificity of the isoform specific monoclonal antibodies on transfected cells, we tested them on histosections obtained from reduction mammoplasty specimens. In order to examine the localization patterns of the PRLR, we stained the tissues simultaneously with LF and either SF1a or SF1b antibodies. Similar, striking, distribution of isoform expression was observed, regardless of whether paraffin-embedded or frozen sections were used. As seen in Figure 2, LF expression appeared primarily basal, whereas SF localized more luminally.

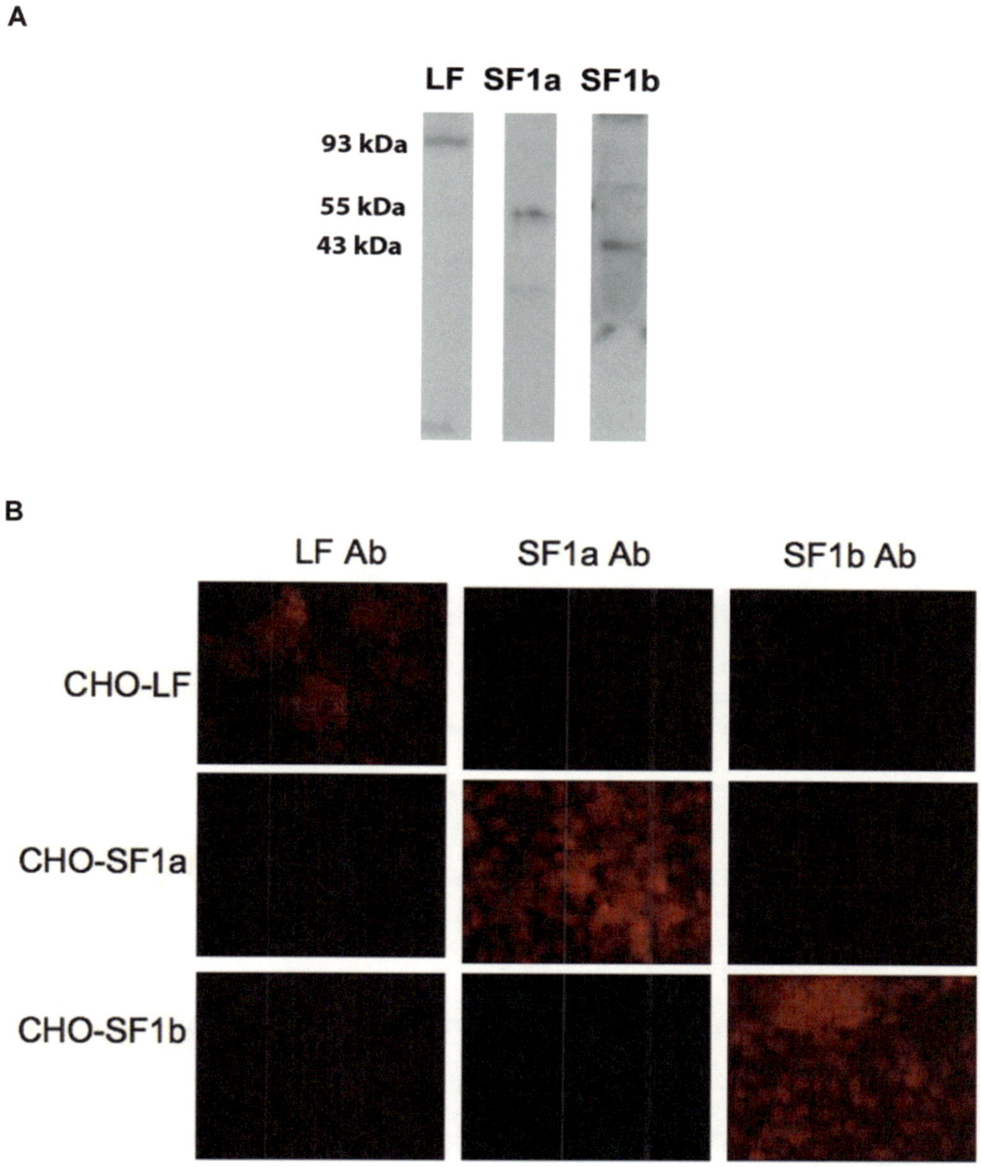

Figure 1. Characterization of PRLR isoform antibodies. **A**. Western blot analysis indicating specificity of monoclonal antibodies. CHO cells were transiently transfected with isoform specific PRLR cDNA as described. Cell lysates were prepared and proteins separated by PAGE. Each isoform specific lysate was probed with each isoform specific antibody. Western blot analysis was performed twice with separate lysates. Data shown are a representative autoradiogram. Molecular weights are marked as indicated: LF = 93kDa, SF1a = 55kDa, SF1b = 43kDa. **B**. Fluorescent immunocytochemical analysis. CHO cells were transiently transfected with isoform specific PRLR cDNA as described. Specific staining was observed. The negative control lacks primary antibody. Data shown are representative of triplicate experiments. Magnification 20X.

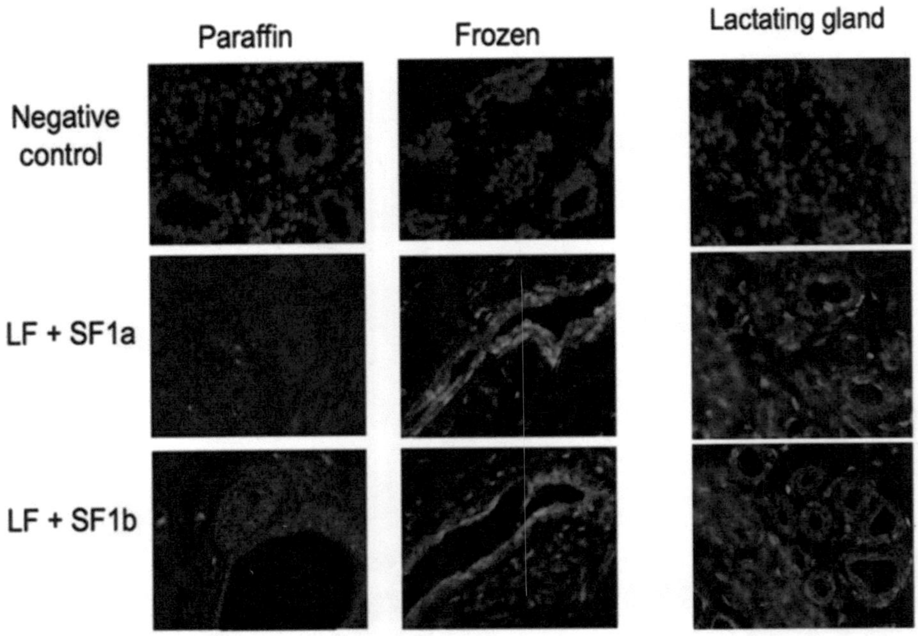

Figure 2. Fluorescent immunohistochemical analysis from normal breast tissues. Representative photos taken from breast reduction mammoplasty specimens. Images in left panels are taken from paraffin embedded tissues; middle panels are imaged from frozen sections; right panels are taken from paraffin embedded normal lactating mammary tissues. Negative control indicates no primary antibody used. LF is indicated by green fluorescence; SF is indicated by red fluorescence. LF = long form; SF = short form. Magnification 40X.

However, the expression patterns localized quite differently in cancer tissue. The PRLR isoforms appeared to colocalize, but were only present in specific areas (Figure 3). The pattern seemed more random, concentrated in "hot spots," particularly for SF1a.

5.3. *In situ* proximity ligation assay monitors PRLR dimerization

The Duolink reagents allow for specific protein-protein interactions to be examined *in situ*. Using antibodies to PRLR-LF, SF1a and SF1b we generated PRLR isoform-specific PLA probes in order to monitor every possible dimer combination using the OLINK ProbeMaker kit. This kit allows for the direct conjugation of the oligonucleotide (PLUS or MINUS end) to the primary antibody, which is essential for examining homodimers. Using these probes, we examined the six possible dimer pairings (LF/LF, SF1a/SF1a, SF1b/SF1b, LF/SF1a, LF/SF1b, SF1a/SF1b) in six established breast cancer cell lines: T47D, ZR75-1, MDA-MB-231, MDA-MB-468, MCF7, and SK-BR-3 in the absence and presence of PRL stimulation. In addition to the specific antibodies, we included non-specific isotyped control antibodies as negative controls (i.e. LF/NSR, where NSR is a non-specific rabbit IgG in place of a specific rabbit antibody against PRLR). After the proximity ligation reaction has taken place, a single fluorescent red dot is observed. This dot represents a single molecular interaction between the two proteins being interrogated.

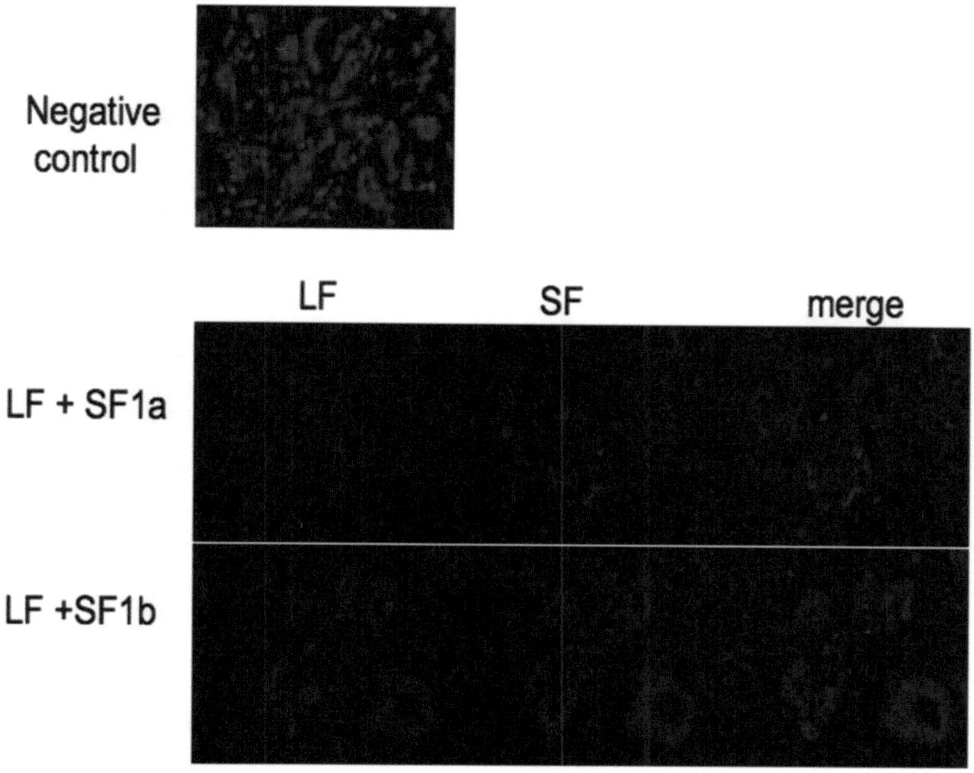

Figure 3. Fluorescent immunohistochemical analysis from breast cancer tissues. Representative photos taken from breast tumor specimens. LF is indicated by green fluorescence; SF is indicated by red fluorescence. LF = long form; SF = short form. Magnification 40X.

With the exception of the MDA-MB-231 cells, similar patterns of expression were observed in all breast cell lines tested. In the ER positive MCF7 cells, dimers of all six potential combinations were observed in the absence of stimulation, and were maintained throughout the stimulation with PRL (Figure 4A). However, in the ER negative MDA-MB-231 cells, a much more complex pattern appeared (Figure 4B). We observed changes in the levels of several dimers over the course of PRL stimulation, suggesting that the different dimer pairings may be utilized by the cell to mitigate responses to prolonged PRL stimulation.

While performing these experiments, we noticed a significant amount of PRLR dimers at either the perinuclear or nuclear region of the cell. Several receptors in the mammary gland have been shown to undergo nuclear translocation including EGFR, FGFR, and GHR [13]. However, there is little information known about the nuclear localization of PRLR. Several reports in the literature have offered contradicting evidence for PRLR nuclear translocation [19-21].

In a preliminary study of PRLR isoform nuclear translocation, MDA-MB-231 cells were stimulated with PRL

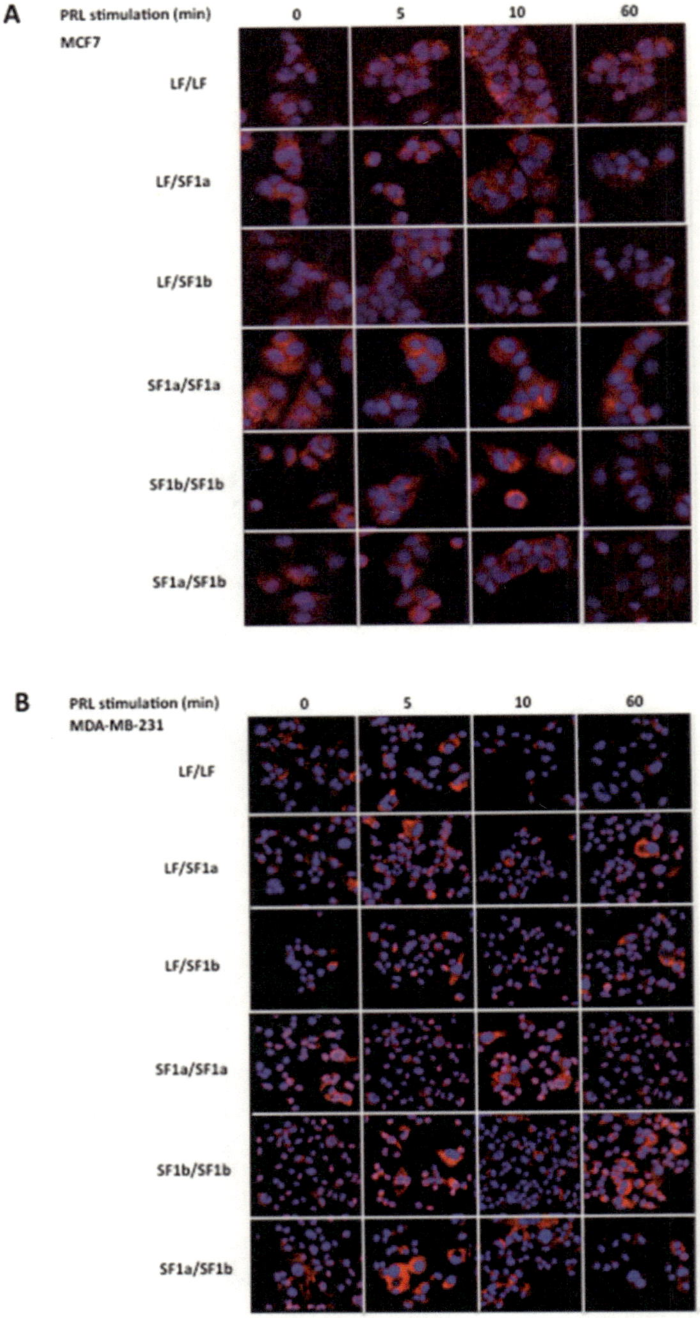

Figure 4. Duolink analysis of breast cancer cell lines for PRL-dependent PRLR dimerization. Representative images are shown for each dimer pairing in both MCF7 (panel A) and MDA-MB-231 (panel B) cells at 0, 5, 10 and 60 min post-stimulation with PRL. Magnification 40X. Nuclei stained (shown in blue) with DAPI, Duolink signal shown in red. Each red dot represents a single dimerization event.

6 hr prior to Duolink analysis to examine steady-state nuclear localization of PRLR dimer formation using confocal microscopy (Figure 5). Of the various combinations of PRLR isoform dimers that were examined, nearly all exhibited some nuclear localization. The exception was for SF1a/SF1a homodimers, which formed perinuclear rings but showed little to no nuclear localization (Figure 5B). Homodimers of the two short forms or a heterodimer of the two short forms (Figure 5B, SF1a/SF1a; Figure 5C SF1b/SF1b; Figure 5D, SF1a/SF1b) exhibited significantly higher levels of nuclear localization while LF homodimers (Figure 5A) and the two LF-short form heterodimers (Figure 5E, LF/SF1a; Figure 5F, LF/SF1b) showed modest levels of nuclear localization. These results confirm that nuclear localization exists for the human prolactin receptor isoforms and may suggest a new role for them as potential transcriptional regulators. Pathways indicating the intranuclear transport and function of PRL and its receptor targeting intracellular actions, such as transcription, have been demonstrated [13]. Increases in transcription may effect cell proliferation and/or differentiation. However, the function of perinuclear localization has yet to be explored.

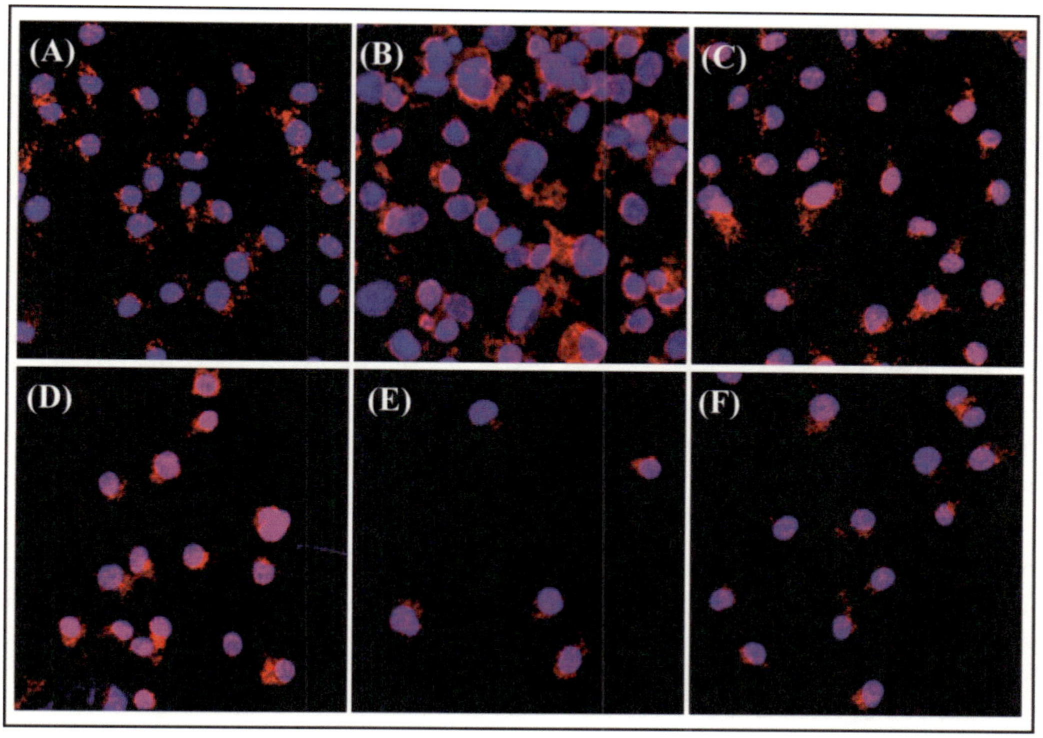

Figure 5. PRLR isoform dimers exhibit different localization patterns. MDA-MB-231 cells were stimulated for 6 hr with 500 ng/ml recombinant human PRL, fixed and examined by confocal microscopy for PRLR dimer localization using Duolink. Dimer combinations: A. LF/LF; B. SF1a/SF1a; C. SF1b/SF1b; D. SF1a/SF1b; E. LF/SF1a; F. LF/SF1b. Images were acquired using a 20X objective with a 2X zoom.

6. Discussion and further research

Prolactin signaling through the LF of the PRLR has been well studied [13]. Two short forms of the PRLR (SF1a and SF1b) share common extracellular and transmembrane domains with the LF, yet contain different cytoplasmic sequences due to alternative splicing of exon 11 [1,2]. The role of these short forms in PRLR function remains elusive, in part due to a lack of specific reagents. Both SF1a and SF1b contain the Box1 binding site for Jak2 and MAPK proteins, yet lack the Box 2 site (and downstream phosphorylation sites) required for STAT binding [2, 14]. By lacking part of intracellular signaling domain, the short forms of the PRLR act as dominant negatives of the LF in transfected cells and its effects most likely occur through heterodimerization with LF [5]. While both short forms can function as a dominant negative, SF1b is the more potent negative regulator of LF function.

To facilitate the study of the PRLR short forms, we generated isoform-specific polyclonal antibodies and demonstrated a breast cancer specific pattern of expression. While all tumor biopsies expressed both LF and SF1b equally, the presence of SF1a was detected mainly in ductal breast carcinoma biopsies and not in those derived from lobular carcinomas [5]. These data suggest diagnostic potential for the PRLR short forms.

The mere expression profiles of these proteins may not serve as sufficient biomarkers, as PRLR dimers are the functional unit for PRL-mediated events. Therefore, an analysis of the ratios of the various potential dimers may be needed to generate a more complete understanding of PRLR signaling. Techniques such as BRET and FRET have been used to examine PRLR dimer formation [14-17]. However, these techniques collectively constrain the user to cells that express tagged constructs and prevent analysis of tissue samples. Co-immunoprecipitation has been used with moderate success for PRLR dimer analysis and avoids the need for tagged constructs, but lacks quantitation, requires specific antibodies, and is devoid of any cellular localization information. To overcome these technical challenges, we employed an *in situ* proximity ligation assay developed by OLINK®. This technique allows for the sensitive detection of protein-protein interactions in unmodified cells and tissue. Using the newly generated rabbit and mouse monoclonal PRLR isoform-specific antibodies, we examined PRLR dimer formation in breast cancer cell lines in the absence and presence of PRL stimulation. Due to the flexibility of the method, we were able to monitor all possible homo- and hetero-dimers concurrently.

We were able to confirm that PRLR homo- and hetero-dimers form in the absence of PRL, similar to reports by others [14, 17]. Similar reports have shown that members of the EGFR family can form dimers in the absence of ligand [18]. In total, we observed homodimers of LF/LF, SF1a/SF1a, and SF1b/SF1b and heterodimers of LF/SF1a, LF/SF1b, and SF1a/SF1b in two different, but well-established breast cancer cell lines, MCF7 and MDA-MB-231. While SF homodimerization has been shown, heterodimerization of the short forms has been examined but not proven [16]. However, these assays utilized PRLR receptors C-terminally tagged with GFP or Rluc to perform BRET analysis, which may somehow block the detection of the SF heterodimer. The functional consequence of the SF1a/SF1b heterodimer is not known. Given that both short forms lack the majority of the intracellular domain, this dimer may be formed to limit the inhibitory activity of each monomer towards the LF by a yet-to-be discovered mechanism.

In addition to confirming the existence of all possible dimer pairings, we were able to show that the different PRLR dimers peaked at different times during the PRL time course. These data suggest that upon stimulation with PRL, regulatory events occur within the cell to favor a particular signaling outcome. For example, an increase in LF/SF1b dimers is predicted to sequester otherwise functional LF monomers into inactive dimers with SF1b. These dimers (and similarly LF/SF1a dimers) would be capable of binding PRL, but would most likely be unable to transmit the signal from ligand binding to the intracellular milieu. Thus, the dominant negative nature of the PRLR short forms could occur by isolating PRLR LF monomers and also result in diminished effects of PRL on cells. Further studies would be required to better understand the dimerization time course for PRLR in these and other breast cancer cell lines.

The confirmation of the nuclear localization of PRLR dimers is an important finding. Conflicting reports were found in the literature [13, 19, 20], however our study confirms that PRLR dimers can be found in the nucleus of cultured breast cancer cells. Interestingly, the amount of nuclear localized PRLR was different for the various dimer pairings tested in MDA-MB-231 cells. In general, the SF dimer combinations (SF1a/SF1a, SF1a/SF1b, and SF1b/SF1b) exhibited higher levels of nuclear localization than dimers containing at least one monomer of LF. In addition, only SF1a homodimers localized to a perinuclear region, and appeared as rings around the nucleus. Together these data suggest a potential transcriptional role for PRLR. Recent work performed in the Walker laboratory [21] demonstrated that, in prostate cancer, the expression of SF1b was upregulated after treatment with the PRL inhibitor S179D. This increase in repression also led to an upregulation of p21 and the vitamin D receptor (VDR), both known to affect differentiation and apoptosis. *In vitro* studies also confirmed that long-term overexpression to SF1b decreased the growth and migration of prostate cancer cells, in addition to enhancing cell-matrix interactions and cell-cell aggregation [22]. Abnormalities in the vitamin D endocrine system have been linked to many disorders, including cancer [23]. Strong epidemiological associations were made between vitamin D deficiency and breast and prostate cancers. The VDR system may arrest the tumor cell cycle at G1/G0 through several mechanisms such as by induction of p21 gene transcription [24] or by inducing the synthesis and/or stabilization of p27 [25]. Recent work in tumor-derived endothelial cells has implicated VDR as an anti-proliferative factor inducing cell cycle arrest in G1/G0 and tumor angiogenesis [26]. Loss of VDR in this system or in mammary epithelial cells may affect differentiation and apoptosis or modulate intracellular signaling routes. These changes in the tumor microenvironment could potentially result in aberrant angiogenic signaling pathways, possibly even enhancing angiogenesis for a more efficient delivery of chemotherapeutic drugs. PRL and its signaling pathways could be exploited to search for more effective therapies in prostate and breast cancer [27]. Potential synergy with various chemotherapeutics may be another aspect of the importance of dimerization and localization of PRL and its receptors in breast cancer.

As discussed herein, our laboratory has recently published the utility of PRLR isoform-specific antibodies in characterizing breast cancer samples as either lobular or ductal in nature [5]. The generation of monoclonal antibodies to the various PRLR isoforms provides a more renewable and reliable supply of these antibodies, and were crucial to the dimerization studies. To our knowledge, this is the first time that the Duolink *in situ* proximity ligation assay enabled detection of all possible PRLR dimer combinations. The technique is robust, quantitative and relatively easy to use.

With the advent of the tissue microarray (TMA) [28, 29], researchers are able to examine large populations of tissues from patients on a single glass slide. There are many commercially available TMAs as well, including arrays for breast cancer patients. These arrays have typically been evaluated for ER/PR/HER2 status and, in many cases, have both normal and diseased tissue for each patient. Given that OLINK® provides a Brightfield Duolink kit, several studies could be envisioned. First, since the Duolink assay can also be used to obtain quantitative total expression of a target, the application of this technique to TMAs would provide a significantly better means of analyzing the expression levels of targets (rather than high, medium, and low expression). These data could also be combined with expression profiles of the PRLR dimer complexes and ultimately compared with other markers to identify more specific breast cancer signatures. Further correlations could be made with the levels of the hormone PRL itself, which could help further diagnose patients.

The "hormonal responsiveness" of breast cancer has been known for a long time. Unfortunately, this phrase has only been used to indicate responsiveness to estrogen (E) and progesterone (P). However, several other hormones including PRL, growth hormone, and thyroid hormone have been shown to play roles in normal breast development and function and their various roles in breast cancer are being investigated. The complex interplay of the three major hormones involved in normal breast development, E, P, and PRL, is well documented. In model systems that include human breast cancer cells in culture as well as rodent models, E, P, and PRL have all been shown to stimulate growth. In fact, when compared directly with E acting on MCF-7 human breast cancer cells, PRL is a more potent mitogen than E [8].

Additionally, these model systems have demonstrated that each of these hormones acts as more than just a mitogen. Complex systems of inter-regulation exist between these steroids, PRL and their receptors. PRL stimulates growth through both an endocrine as well as an autocrine/paracrine mechanism. The expression of autocrine PRL in human breast cancer cells is regulated by E through action on the PRL promoter [30]. Expression of the PRL gene is regulated by two promoters, the proximal promoter utilized primarily in the pituitary and the distal promoter utilized in breast cancer cells. E directly induces hPRL gene expression in T47D human breast cancer cells through the action of a functional non-canonical E response element (ERE) and an AP1 site on the distal promoter. Both the ERE and AP1 sites are required for full induction of promoter activity through the alpha form of the ER.

Similarly, the interplay of P and PRL is well established in various models. PR and PRLR are co-expressed temporally and spatially in the developing mouse mammary gland. In mammary glands from ovariectomized female mice lacking both E and P, neither P nor PRL stimulate DNA synthesis in epithelial or adjacent stromal cells. However, simultaneous injection of P and PRL results in a significant synergistic effect on DNA synthesis in both cell types [31]. Similarly, disruption of expression and distribution of PR in the mammary gland results in a parallel disruption of expression and distribution of the PRLR suggesting inter-regulation of these receptors [32]. Expression of the PRLR in human cells is regulated through a complex system of promoters. The PRLR gene in humans has six exon 1s, the most generic of which (PRLR promoter region III) is functional in human breast cancer cells. T47D human breast cancer cells treated with P overexpress the PRLR and activate PRLR promoter III. This promoter lacks a classical P response element. Thus P acts through the cooperative interaction of the PR with the transcription factors C/EBP and an adjacent Sp1A site to confer P responsiveness leading to increased expression of the PRLR [33].

These examples of the complex interactions of E, P, and PRL underscore the importance of understanding all three hormones' actions and their receptor interactions, distribution, and functions in the normal human breast and in breast cancer. Effective tools for these studies are now available.

7. Conclusion

Just as the identification of the ER and PR are now routinely performed on all clinical breast cancer samples, screening for PRLR status and isoform profile may also one day become a routine procedure in the characterization of breast cancers. Isoform specific antibodies to the PRLR can be powerful tools in detection and characterization of breast and other cancers and provide valuable insights into the important PRLR signaling pathways that could be effective targets for prevention and treatment.

Author details

Erika Ginsburg, Christopher D. Heger, Paul Goldsmith and Barbara K. Vonderhaar
Center for Cancer Research, National Cancer Institute, National Institutes of Health, USA

Acknowledgement

This research was supported by the Intramural Research Program of the NIH, National Cancer Institute. We thank Sarah J. Tarplin for her assistance with the immunostaining and to Dr. Jodie M. Fleming for helpful discussions. The authors have no competing interests.

8. References

[1] Trott JF, Hovey RC, Koduri S, Vonderhaar BK (2003) Alternative splicing to exon 11 of human prolactin receptor gene results in multiple isoforms including a secreted prolactin-binding protein. *J Mol Endocrinol* 30(1):31-47.

[2] Hu ZZ, Meng J, Dufau ML (2001) Isolation and characterization of two novel forms of the human prolactin receptor generated by alternative splicing of a newly identified exon 11. *J Biol Chem* 276(44):41086-41094.

[3] Clevenger CV, Furth PA, Hankinson SE, Schuler, LA (2003) The role of prolactin in mammary carcinoma. *Endocrine Rev* 24(1): 1-24.

[4] Meng J, Tsai-Morris CH, Dufau ML (2004) Human prolactin receptor variants in breast cancer: low ratio of short forms to the long-form human prolactin receptor associated with mammary carcinoma. *Cancer Res* 64(16):5677-5682.

[5] Ginsburg E, Alexander S, Lieber S, Tarplin S, Jenkins L, Pang L, Heger CD, Goldsmith P, Vonderhaar BK (2010) Characterization of ductal and lobular breast carcinomas using novel prolactin receptor isoform specific antibodies. *BMC Cancer* 10:678.

[6] Hankinson SE, Wilett WC, Michaud DS, Manson JE, Colditz GA, Longcope C, Rosner B, Speizer FE (1999) Plasma prolactin levels and subsequent risk of breast cancer in postmenopausal women. *J Natl Cancer Inst* 91:629-634.

[7] Tworoger SS, Eliassen AH, Sluss P, Hankinson SE (2007) A prospective study of plasma prolactin concentration and risk of premenopausal and postmenopausal breast cancer. *J Clin Oncol* 25(12):1482-1488.

[8] Biswas R, Vonderhaar, BK (1987) Role of serum in prolactin responsiveness of MCF-7 human breast cancer cells in long term tissue culture. *Cancer Res* 47:3509-3514.

[9] Faupel-Badger JM, Ginsburg E, Fleming JM, Susser L, Doucet T, Vonderhaar BK (2010) 16-kDa prolactin reduces angiogenesis, but not growth of human breast cancer tumors in vivo. *Horm Canc* 1(2):71-79.

[10] Gill S, Peston D, Vonderhaar BK, Shousha S (2001) Expression of prolactin receptors in normal, benign and malignant breast tissue: an immunohistological study. *J Clin Pathol* 54(12):956-960.

[11] Bonneterre J, Peyrat JP, Vandewalle B, Beuscart R, Vie MC, Cappelaere P (1982) Prolactin receptors in human breast cancer. *Eur J Cancer Clin Oncol* 18:1157-1162.

[12] Bradford MM (1976) A rapid and sensitive method for the quantitation of microgram quantities of protein utilizing the principle of protein-dye binding. *Anal Biochem* 72:248-254.

[13] Clevenger CV (2003) Nuclear localization and function of polypeptide ligands andtheir receptors: a new paradigm for hormone specificity within the mammary gland? *Breast Cancer Res* 5:181-187.

[14] Qazi AM, Tsai-Morris CH, Dufau ML. Ligand-independent homo- and heterodimerization of human prolactin receptor variants: inhibitory action of the short forms by heterodimerization. *Mol Endocrinol* 2006;20(8):1912–1923.

[15] Biener E, Martin C, Daniel N, Frank SJ, Centonze VE, Herman B, Djiane J, Gertler A (2003) Ovine placental lactogen-induced heterodimerization of ovine growth hormone and prolactin receptors in living cells is demonstrated by fluorescence resonance energy transfer microscopy and leads to prolonged phosphorylation of signal transducer and activator of transcription (STAT) 1 and STAT3. *Endocrinology* 144(8): 3532-3540.

[16] Tan D, Johnson DA, Wu W, Zeng L, Chen YH, Chen WY, Vonderhaar BK, Walker AM (2005) Unmodified prolactin (PRL) and S179D PRL-initiated bioluminescence resonance

energy transfer between homo- and hetero-pairs of long and short human PRL receptors in living cells. *Mol Endocrinol* 19(5): 1291-1303.

[17] Gadd SL, Clevenger CV (2006) Ligand-independent dimerization of the human prolactin receptor isoforms: functional implications. *Mol Endocrinol* 20(11) 2734-2746.

[18] Yu X, Sharma KD, Takahashi T, Iwamoto R, Mekada E (2002) Ligand-independent dimer formation of epidermal growth factor receptor (EGFR) is a step separable from ligand-induced EGFR signaling. *Mol Biol Cell* 13(7): 2547-2557.

[19] Perrot-Applanat M, Gualillo O, Buteau H, Edery M Kelly, PA (1997) Internalization of prolactin receptor and prolactin in transfected cells does not involve nuclear translocation. *J Cell Sci* 110:1123-1132.

[20] Rao YP, Buckley DJ, Buckley, AR (1995) The nuclear prolactin receptor: a 62- kDa chromatin-associated protein in rat Nb2 lymphoma cells. *Arch Biochem Biophys* 322:506-515.

[21] Wu W, Ginsburg E, Vonderhaar BK, Walker AM (2005) S179D prolactin increases vitamin D receptor and p21 through up-regulation of short 1b prolactin receptor in human prostate cancer cells. *Cancer Res* 65(16):7509-7515.

[22] Huang KT, Walker AM (2010) Long term increased expression of the short form 1b prolactin receptor in PC-3 human prostate cancer cells decreases cell growth and migration, and causes multiple changes in gene expression consistent with reduced invasive capacity. *Prostate* 70(1):37-47.

[23] Dusso AS, Brown AJ, Slatopolsky E (2005) Vitamin D. *Am J Physiol Renal Physiol* 289:F8-F28.

[24] Liu M, Lee M-H, Cohen M, Bommakanti M, Freedman LP (1996) Transcriptional activation of the cdk inhibitor p21 by vitamin D3 leads to the induced differentiation of the myelomonocytic cell line U937. *Genes & Dev* 10:142-153.

[25] Li P, Li, C, Zhao X, Zhang X, Nicosia SV (2004) $p27^{kip1}$ stabilization and G_1 arrest by 1,25-dihydroxyvitamin D_3 in ovarian cancer cells mediated through down-regulation of cyclin E/cyclin-dependent kinase 2 and skp1-cullin-F-box protein/skp2 ubiquitin ligase. *J Biol Chem* 279(24): 25260-25267.

[26] Chung I, Han G, Seshadri M, Gillard BM, Yu W, Foster BA, Trump DL, Johnson CS (2009) Role of vitamin D receptor in the antiproliferative effects of calcitrol in tumor-derived endothelial cells and tumor angiogenesis in vivo. *Cancer Res* 69(3): 967-975.

[27] Jacobson EM, Hugo ER, Borcherding DC, Ben-Jonathan N (2011) Prolactin in breast abd prostate cancer : Molecular and genetic perspectives. *Discov Med* 11(59):315-324.

[28] Battifora H, Mehta P (1990) The checkerboard tissue block. An improved multitissue control block. *Lab Invest* 63:722-724.

[29] Kononen J, Bubendorf L, Kallioniemi A, Barlund M, Schraml P, Leighton S, Torhorst J, Mihatsch MJ, Sauter G, Kallioniemi OP (1998) Tissue microarrays for high-throughput molecular profiling of tumor specimens. *Nat Med* 4:844-847.

[30] Duan R, Ginsburg E, Vonderhaar BK (2008) Estrogen stimulates transcription from the human prolactin distal promoter through AP1 and estrogen responsive elements in T47D human breast cancer cells. *Mol Cell Endocrinol* 281(1-2):9-18.

[31] Hovey RC, Trott JF, Ginsburg E, Sasaki MM, Fountain SJ, Sundararajan K, Vonderhaar BK (2001) Transcriptional and spatiotemporal regulation of prolactin receptor mRNA and cooperativity with progesterone receptor function during ductal branch growth in the mammary gland. *Dev Dyn* 222(2):192-205.

[32] Grimm SL, Seagroves TN, Kabotyanski EB, Hovey RC, Vonderhaar BK, Lydon JP, Miyoshi K, Hennighausen L, Ormandy CJ, Lee AV, Stull MA, Wood TL, Rosen JM (2002) Disruption of steroid and prolactin receptor patterning in the mammary gland correlates with a block in lobuloalveolar development. *Mol Endocrinol* 16(12):2675-2691.

[33] Goldhar AS, Duan R, Ginsburg E, Vonderhaar BK (2011) Progesterone induces expression of the prolactin receptor gene through cooperative action of Sp1 and C/EBP. *Mol Cell Endocrinol* 335(2):148-157.

Chapter 12

Physiological and Pathological Hyperprolactinemia: Can We Minimize Errors in the Clinical Practice?

Miguel Ángel Castaño López, José Luís Robles Rodríguez and Marta Robles García

Additional information is available at the end of the chapter

http://dx.doi.org/10.5772/54758

1. Introduction

Human prolactin is a single-chain polypeptide hormone. It has a molecular weight of approximately 22,500 Da (figure 1). It takes part in lactation through physiological and biochemical events.

Its polypeptide chain consists of 198-200 amino acid remainders which complete sequence is unknown. Over 80% of the first 50 amino acids are identical or equivalent to the bovine prolactin.

The prolactin molecule is arranged in a single chain of amino acids with three intra molecular disulfide bonded between six cysteine residues (Cys4-Cys11, Cys58-Cys174, Cys191-Cys199 in humans). The sequence homology can vary from the striking 97% among primates to as low as 56% in rodents (1)

The sequence of the first 23 amino acid remainders corresponding to the N-terminal extreme

NH2-leu-pro-ile-cys-pro-gly-ala-ala-arg-cys-gln-val-thr-leu-arg-asp-leu-phe-asp-arg-ala-val

It's secreted by the anterior part of the hypophysis, the adenohypophysis (figure 2) that stimulates the milk production in the mammary glands and the progesterone synthesis in the corpus luteum.

Although the major form of prolactin found in the pituitary gland is 23 kDa, variants of prolactin have been characterized in many mammals, including humans. Prolactin variants can be results of alternative splicing of the primary transcript, proteolytic cleavage and other posttranslational modifications of the amino acid chain (1)

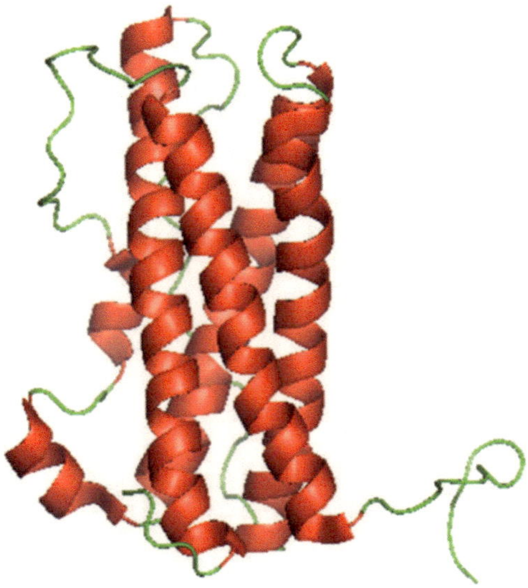

Source: Originally from en.wikipedia; description page is/was here.
Author: Original uploader was BorisTM at en.wikipedia
Permission (Reusing this file): Released into the public domain (by the author); PDB

Figure 1. Prolactin´s structure

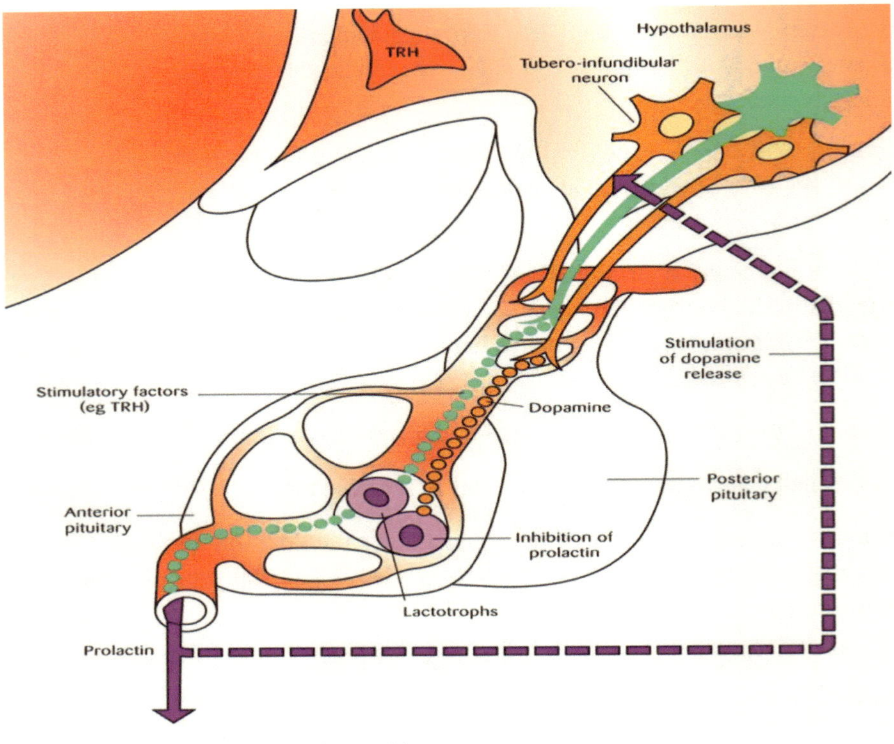

This image is propriety of our laboratory and created by us.

Figure 2. Prolactin's secretion.

It was discovered in 1928 in a cow's hypophysis and it is phylogenetically considerated as the oldest known hormone in the animal kingdom. It has been detected in insects, amphibian, fish and mammals. Its luteotrophic activity was not discovered until 1945 (2-4).

Its isolation was difficult due to its structure, which is similar (in a 16%) to the growth hormone (GH) structure. Both are located in the hypophysis, but the GH is present in higher concentration. Its existence was demonstrated through a trial series performed between 1965 and 1971, it was discovered, as well, the way its secretion is performed, where some physiological factors are positive and negative hypothalamic neurohormonal compounds (5-6).

Studies on the secondary structure of prolactin have shown that 50% of the amino acid chain is arranged in α-helices, while the rest of it forms loops. Although it was predicted earlier, there are still no direct data about the three-dimensional structure of prolactin. The tertiary structure of prolactin was predicted by homology modeling approach, based on the structural similarities between prolactin and other helix bundle proteins, especially growth hormone.

According to the current three-dimensional model, prolactin contains four long α-helices arranged in antiparallel fashion (1).

It shows a synergic effect with the following hormones: estrogens, progesterone and GH.

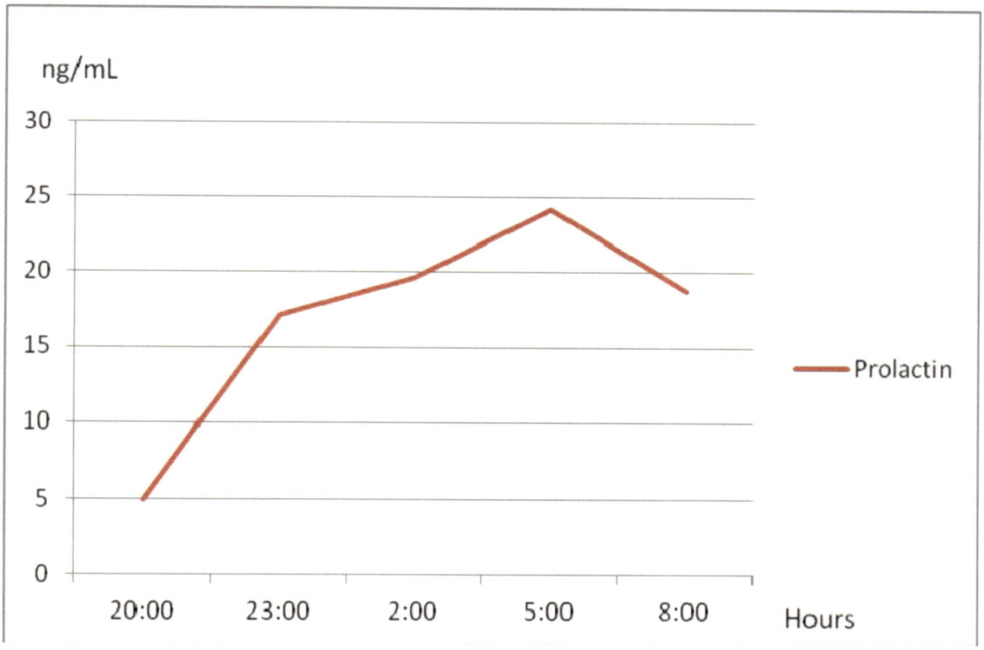

This image is propriety of our laboratory and created by us. The data was taken from Benavides IZ, Castillo AP, Montemayor I, DeEstrada R,Onatra W, Posso H. Biorritmo de prolactina en mujeres de edad reproductiva vs.Perimenopáusicas.Rev Coloma Menop.2003;9:153–8.[16 Sep 2009].

Figure 3. Prolactin's circadian rhythm

The nipple suction during breastfeeding favors a bigger amount of hormone synthesis. Besides, it's one of the few physiological systems that have positive feedback, so the presence of prolactin in the organism favors this peptide production.

Nipple and areola´s terminal nerves are stimulated when suction occurs. This stimulus travels via afferent nerve pathways to the hypothalamus, proving the prolactin release, by inhibition of the release of dopamine. (5-9)

Prolactin levels during pregnancy rise from its normal value up to 200 or 400 ng/ml. This increase starts around the 8th week in a simultaneous way with the estrogen increasing. The rising in prolactin secretion is due to the suppression that estrogens provoke over dopamine and the direct stimulation of the transcription of the prolactin gene in the hypophysis. (8)

Prolactin shows a circadian and pulsatile rhythm (figure 3) that starts raising 90 minutes after sleep beginning, with maximum peaks at 4-5 hours and it can stay high two hours after waking up (7-9).

It is known that its discharges are 20-30 minutes intervals and the mean life is 20-30 minutes (7-11).

The main circulating form is the monomeric prolactin (little prolactin) or native prolactin which is a non-glycosylated monomer that makes up the 80-90% of the total amount of prolactin in a normal individual.

Another circulating form in the big prolactin (big PRL) which consist in glycosylated dimers or trimers of 40.000-50000 daltons molecular weight, which is supposed to be a deposit form which is rarely detected in serum and which biological activity is nearly non-existent. However, it is detected in hyperprolactinemia without any pathological clinical signs.

Finally, big-big prolactin or macroprolactin wich is a dimer form of the big-PRL joined to IgG immunoglobulin with a molecular weight over 100000 daltons and without any biological activity (10-12).

2. Effects

The prolactin´s main function in women is to stimulate and maintain the puerperal breastfeeding, direct action over acidophilic cells known as lactotrophs cells of the mammary glands (6, 13). Estrogens, GH, corticoids, placental lactogenic hormones and prolactin are needed to increase the ductal system. Estrogens, progesterone and prolactin are needed to develop the lobuloalveolar system, so levels of these hormones should be considered in pathological states as fibrocystic mastopathy, mastodynia (breast pain), mammary carcinoma, etc.

Among its effects over the mammary alveolar cells there is an increase of the lactose synthesis and a higher production of lactose proteins as casein and lactalbumin.

It is related with the reproductive cycle, the pregnancy maintenance and the fetal growth, through an effect over the mother metabolism acting over different effector organs to facilitate its functions through synergy or inhibition of other hormones.

It shows a synergism with the gonadal steroid hormones in the continuance of the corpus luteum and progesterone production, with action in the reproductive processes, according to some researches that revealed the presence of specific prolactin receptors in the mammal's ovaries, transferring part of the progesterone function which, among other functions, stimulates the formation of membrane receptors for the follicle stimulating hormone (FSH) and the luteinizing hormone (LH) for the follicle growth and the estradiol synthesis. It was found, in the little antral follicles, a prolactin concentration 6 times higher than in circulation, when the follicle is 6-8 mm of diameter the levels drop, getting close to the basal blood levels near the ovulation (3, 4, 12, 14).

Some secondary functions or less powerful have been reported, being related to androgenesis that takes part in the suprarenal cortex reticular area, where some specific receptors for prolactin have been found, the joint with those receptors stimulates the secretion of **dehydroepiandrosterone** and its sulfate.

Prolactin has also an inhibitory effect over the gonadotropin secretion, so its hypersecretion can cause oligomenorrhea or amenorrhea in women (3,4, 14).

In men, the prolactin behavior can affect the adrenal function, the electrolytic balance, gynecomastia, galactorrhea sometimes, libido decreasing and sexual impotence and some other actions in prostate, seminal vesicles and testicles (15-17).

Prolactin serum levels have daily and circadian variations, its secretion is pulsatile, as described by Sassin et al, measuring blood levels every 20 minutes with raises up to 50% (13).

It shows a circadian rhythm with increases or secretory peaks during the sleep, started between 10 minutes and one hour after sleep beginning and reaching the highest values mainly in the deepest stages. These values do not go down in the next two hours after waking up and decrease slowly by the end of the afternoon, without any tendency to be repeated in the same individual in the days after, once in circulation prolactin mean life is estimated around 14 minutes.

It seems that variation during time and sleep are due to the hypothalamus dopaminergic stimulus modifications, the circadian fluctuation is not affected by the use of oral contraceptives (10-15).

3. Limits of reference

In blood, prolactin can be found from the 16th week of fetal life, increasing its levels due to active secretion, as in birth it shows higher amounts to the ones recorded in the mother.

The normal described limits (figure 4 y 5) for healthy population are the following:

- Men: 2 - 18 ng/mL
- Non-pregnant women: 1 - 46 ng/mL
- Pregnant women: 35 - 600 ng/mL

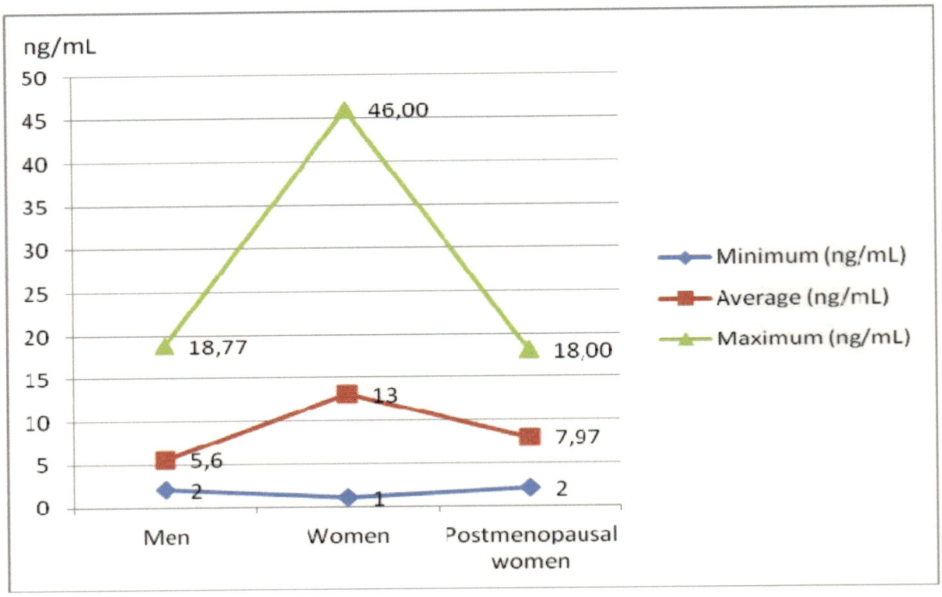

This image is propriety of our laboratory and created by us.The data was taken from Fuchs, F. y Koppler A. Endocrinología de la Gestación. 1982. Segunda edición. Salvat Editores,S.A. Capítulo 12. Pag. 249-72

Figure 4. Prolactin's limits of reference (I)

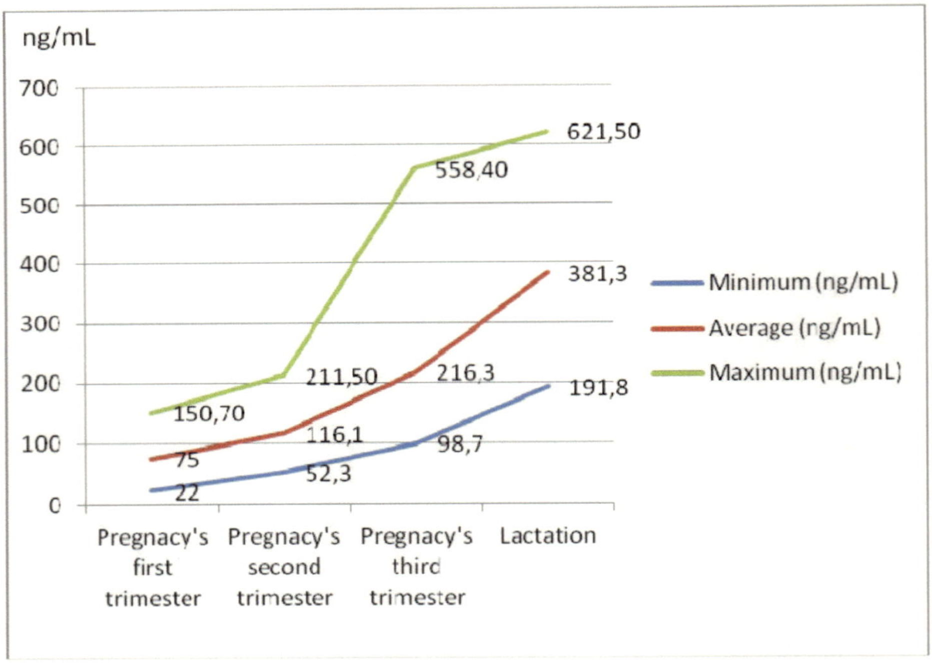

This image is propriety of our laboratory and created by us. The data was taken from Tyson JE, Hwang P, Guyda H, Friesen Hg. Studies of prolactin secretion in human pregnancy. Am J Obstet Gynecol 1972;113:14-20.

Figure 5. Prolactin's limits of reference (II)

The limits of reference change according to the studied population showing very pronounced individual variations, even in age and sex groups.

In fertile women the levels show a light elevation during ovulation and the luteinic phase, concerning to the follicular phase, corresponding to the endogenous estrogens liberated by the ovaries, which reduce the prolactin inhibitory factor in the hypothalamus increasing the amount of lactotroph cells as demonstrated in rats by stimulation although that effect depends on the dose and duration of the application, but it used to be shown by 24 hours (3, 12-15).

In postmenopausal woman and elderly men, levels go down, it is not clear if it is due pituitary deficiency or gonadal insufficiency, showing some role in gonadal function and aging.

The presence of different nonspecific stimulus, as the coitus, exercises, stress situations as surgery, insulin hypoglycemia course….can cause variations in prolactin secretion, some of the can have an adaptive nature, as them one occurred in hypoglycemia (12).

Because of what we mentioned previously, it is recommended to take from 2 to 3 samples to determine the prolactin level after 9 am to avoid late effects at night and hypoglycemia.

4. Hyperprolactinemia

As it has been described before, prolactin is secreted by lactotroph cells from the anterior hypophysis and it is subjected to the dopamine inhibitory effect in the hypothalamus. Any cause which interferes in its synthesis, the transport to the pituitary gland or the action over the dopamine receptors can produce hyperprolactinemia (Table 1).

Physiological Pregnancy and lactation Breast stimulation Stress
Hypothalamic diseases Craniopharyngioma Meningioma Dysgerminoma Sarcoidosis Eosinophilic granuloma Irradiation Vascular causes Pituitary stalk section
Pituitary pathology Prolactinoma Acromegaly Nonsecretory pituitary adenoma

Empty-sella syndrome Cushing disease Lymphocytic hypophysitis
Drugs Estrogens Antipsychotics: phenothiazine (chlorpromazine, perphenazine, fluphenazine, thorazine, promazine, fluoperazine, trifluoperazine, etc.), haloperidol, butyrophenone. Other dopaminergic blockers: metoclopramide, sulpiride, domperidone, cisperidone, cisapride. Antidepressant: monoamine oxidase inhibitors (imipramine), amoxapine, Tryciclic antidepressants. Antihypertensives: reserpine, methyldopa. Verapamil Fluoxetine Protease inhibitors Opiates: cocaine, morphine, heroine. Benzodiazepine Cimetidine (iv) Beta endorphins GABA Serotonin Noradrenaline HRT Adrenergic receptor antagonists (medroxalol)
Neurogenic causes Thoracic wall lesions Spinal cord lesions Breast stimulation
Other Primary hypothyroidism Chronic renal insufficiency Liver cirrhosis Suprarenal insufficiency Polycystic ovary syndrome Convulsions Idiopathic macroprolactinemia

GABA: Gamma-aminobutyric acid
HRT: Homone replacement therapy
Iv: intra-venous

Table 1. Hyperprolactinemia causes

The most important cause of hyperprolactinemia is the secretory pituitary adenoma. Nevertheless, the most common cause are drugs and, when it is possible, the serum prolactin determination should be done once those are suspended.

5. Physiological causes

1. Pregnancy

Serum prolactin rises in a progressive way during gestation, but in a variable manner (18-19). At the end, the mean value is around 200 ng/ml but the range is 35-600.

Around the 6th week from the labor the normoprolactinemia is restored. Although the prolactin concentration is high before the labor, the milk secretion only takes place after it, because the high presence of estrogens and progesterone in pregnant women has an inhibitory effect over the milk secretion. When these hormones levels drop after the labor, lactation is produced.

During gestation the prolactin levels in the amniotic liquid can reach the 1000 ng/ml, higher concentration that any other organic fluid, this happens around the 15th and the 20th week of gestation and it drops slowly until the end of the pregnancy to 450 ng/ml. It is supposed to be produced by the fetal and the mother´s hypophysis, with a possible function of fetal osmoregulation to survive in the intrauterine liquid environment, helping and contributing to the pulmonary maturing raising the content of phospholipids and changes in the lecithin-sphingomyelin ratio (20).

2. Breast stimulation

Nipple suction, probably by neural via, during breastfeeding, rises the serum values of prolactin, especially in the first weeks after giving birth in direct relation to the lactotroph hypertrophy by the estrogenic stimulus of the pregnancy (18-20)

3. Stress

Any kind of stress, physical or psychical, can cause hyperprolactinemia, which is normally slight, and rarely over 40 ng/ml.

4. Sexual contact

There is a dopamine decreasing after orgasm, immediately, the prolactin rises, in men and women, acting as a sexual satiation mechanism (21). In men, without any doubt contributes to the "turn around and snore" phenomenon. In women, its effects can be delayed.

Kruger TH et al have demonstrated that sexual intercourse with orgasm induced not only the well-established immediate prolactin increasing of 300% but also an additional prolactin elevation around noon of the next day. These fluctuations were measured on top of regular circadian rhythm (22).

6. Pathological causes

Pathological hyperprolactinemia can be caused by: lactotroph hyperplasia, lactotroph cells adenoma (prolactinoma) and miscellaneous.

1. Lactotroph hyperplasia

   Lactotroph hyperplasia derives, in most cases, from the decrease of the dopamine inhibitory tone over the lactotroph cells. Hypothalamic and pituitary stalk lesions can cause light or moderated hyperprolactinemia, normally less than 150 ng/ml (18-19, 23).

   The most common cause of hyperprolactinemia are the drugs. Any substance that acts over the central nervous system can, potentially, change the prolactin serum levels. Generally, the serum prolactin concentration increase a few hours or days after the drug administration and it gets normal from 2 to 4 days after its suspension.

   Drugs can be divided in two big groups: drugs that act over the hypothalamus altering the dopamine metabolism and the drugs that act directly over the hypophysis. These last ones are more powerful and its action mechanism is dopamine antagonist, displacing it from its receptor in the lactotroph cell. Examples of these are the metoclopramide, sulpiride and domperidone. The Antihypertensives as reserpine and methyldopa act in the hypothalamus. Cimetidine and similar substances stimulate the receptor H2 and provoke the hyperprolactinemia.

   The hyperprolactine grade depends on the drug, for example, haloperidol can provoke rises lower than 20 ng/ml, but the risperidone can raise it over 100 ng/ml (19).

   Estrogens rise the prolactin secretion and explain the higher response of prolactin in women in the presence of the different physiological stimulus.

   Besides, up to a 30% of the patients with polycystic ovary syndrome show a light hyperprolactinemia, and the treatment with dopaminergic agonists can, in some cases, normalize the menstrual cycle.

   The primary hypothyroidism is associated with a slight increase of the prolactin serum concentration in a 40% of the patients, but values over 25 ng/ml appear in less of the 10% (19, 23).

2. Lactotroph cells adenoma: prolactinoma

   It is the most frequent secretory pituitary tumor and it represents a 60% of the operating tumors. The 90% of the prolactinomas are intrasellar microadenomas (<10 nm).

   In women, over 90% are microadenomas, especially between 20 and 40 years old (2, 3). In male, the 60% are macroadenomas and it is because the poor symptoms, the delay of the medical visit for erectile dysfunction or a higher growth rate (19).

   Prolactinomas are the most common pituitary tumors and they are, normally, benign. They are more frequent in women, but they can also appear in men. The symptoms that they cause, if the symptoms appear, are related to prolactin excess and so, the milk production in non-pregnant women, which is called galactorrhea.

Prolactinoma, the same as other pituitary neoplasms, comes from a monoclonal expansion of a cell that has mutated (18, 19, 23). It is usually sporadic and benign and it is rarely malign and metastatic.

Sometimes, it takes part of the type one multiple endocrine neoplasms (MEN). It is the only pituitary tumor with an effective medical treatment.

The prolactinoma natural history shows that over 90% of the microadenomas do not grow and they do not progress to macroadenomas, that suggest that these have a different biological behavior to the microadenomas (19, 24-27), Most of the times the lactotroph cells are the only ones affected but up to a 10% can alter, as well, the somatotropes or the mamosomatotropes, and a prolactin and growth hormone (GH) co-secretion is produced.

Prolactinoma can lead to:

- Interruption of the pulsatile secretion of the gonadotropin releasing hormone (GnRH) with inhibition of the gonadal steroids production and can provoke infertility and hypogonadism.
- Compression over adjacent structures.
- Deleterious effects over the organism, specifically the skeleton.

Prolactin secretion by the prolactinoma is characterized by:

1. Its efficiency: even small tumors, smaller than 1 cm, can produce significant hyperprolactinemia.
2. Its proportionality: usually, the prolactin serum concentration rises in direct relation to the adenoma size:
- < 1cm is associated with serum prolactin values under 200 ng/ml.
- Between 1 and 2 cm usually leads to values between 200 and 1000 ng/ml.
- > 2 cm leads to prolactinemia over 1.000 ng/ml.

Discrepancies are frequent:

1. Big tumors with light hyperprolactinemia: they are usually atipic prolactinomas, worse differentiated and, so, less sensitive to therapy with dopaminergic agonists and more susceptible to surgical treatment.
2. Hook effect: very high levels of prolactin secreted by the macroadenoma saturate the assays and lead to an apparently low value (between 20 and 200 ng/ml), which could confuse the macroprolactinoma with a non-secretory macroadenoma. It is produced by interferences in the enzime inmunoassays for prolactin and it can be settled by serum dilution to 1:100, which will show the real prolactin serum values secreted by the tumor (19, 28-29).

7. Miscellaneous

1. Decrease of the prolactin clearing:
   a. Chronic renal insufficiency. (CRI)

   The hyperprolactinemia appears in most of the patients with CRI and dialysated. When these patients take medication that can alter the hypothalamic regulation of the prolactin, this can take to serum values over 2000 ng/ml. It is produced by a decrease of the glomerular filter, although a pituitary primary defect associated to a renal failing cannot be dismissed.

b. Macroprolactinemia.

In some patients with hyperprolactinemia without a perceptible cause or idiopathic, this could be due to an excess of macromolecules of prolactin, known as macroprolactin or big prolactin. The macroprolactin is a complex of prolactin joined to an IgG antibody with a low bioactivity but with a higher mean life than normal prolactin, of 23 kDa, which condition its lower clearing and the consequent accumulation of high serum concentrations.

To distinguish it from other causes, some samples of serum with polyethylene glycol should be precipitated (13, 19-20).

This prolactin variety can be present in over 10% of the patients with hyperprolactinemia, and its presence should be suspected in every hyperprolactinemia without a defined etiology, with poor or nonexistent symptomatology, despite of the high prolactin serum concentrations and with poor or nonexistent response to normal therapy with dopaminergic agonists (13,19-20, 28-30).

This situation can lead to unsuitable diagnosis and treatments in patients with hyperprolactinemia, but usually without clinical significance. Every hyperprolactinemia assay should consider the possible presence of macroprolactinemia (19, 30).

When the cause is not found and the imaging tests are negative, the hyperprolactinemia is defined as idiopathic. In most of the cases they are small microadenomas. A 10% of them will be visible between 2 and 6 years. In other cases it is a transitory and self-limited disorder that can be solved spontaneously (19,31).

2. Hyperprolactinemia related to psychotropic drugs

Prolactin determinations will not be needed in individual under psychotropic treatment, but if there is indicative clinical symptoms of hyperprolactinemia.

However, in a patient with hyperprolactinemia under psychotropic drugs, among others, subsequent studies (hormonal and imaging) will be performed only if:

- There are clinical symptoms derived from hyperprolactinemia.
- There are prolactin serum concentrations over 6 times the normal value.

The assessment of the new patient should be done ideally 3 months after the medication suppression or, if not possible, the possibility of a substitutive medication that does not provoke hyperprolactinemia should be assessed, always under psychiatric control.

It is normally not recommended the dopaminergic agonists use in a combined form to psychotropic or dopaminergic antagonist drugs because of the undesirable effects. (19,20).

8. Assessment and diagnosis of the hyperprolactinemia

Because the secretion of the prolactin is pulsatile, it is advisable to determine the serum prolactin in, at least, 2 times or more.

To the most of the clinical laboratories, the normal serum concentration is less than 25 ng/ml in women and 20 ng/ml in men.

(Note: conversion factor: mU/l × 0,0472 =ng/ml; ng/ml × 21,2 = mU/l.)

The determination should be done, ideally, in a basal situation, under rest conditions and after suppression of any medication that can interfere in its quantification.

The clinical records are determinant to the hyperprolactinemia treatment:

- The data collection, especially about drugs, must be meticulous.
- Other non-pituitary causes should be dismissed: pregnancy, thyroid, renal, hepatic and adrenal dysfunction.
- We should investigate the existence of compressive symptomatology like cephalalgia, chiasmatic syndrome, liquorrhea and pituitary dysfunction data related to the pituitary tumor presence.

Values of serum prolactin can lead to the diagnosis (figure 6):

- Serum concentrations slightly raised (20-40 ng/ml) require confirmation before cataloguing the hyperprolactinemia state.
- Prolactin serum values between 20 and 200 ng/ml can appear in iatrogenic or extrapituitary hyperprolactinemia.
- Serum values between 40 and 100 ng/ml appear in secondary and idiopathic causes and less frequently in some microprolactinomas.
- Serum concentrations between 100 and 200 ng/ml, ruled out the pregnancy, are characteristic of a prolactinoma.
- Values over 200 ng/ml appear in macroprolactinomas.

It is convenient to insist in the importance of differentiate between the big pituitary non-secretory macroadenomas, that apply compression to the pituitary stalk and can curse with prolactin serum values that are not too high, generally lower than 200 ng/ml (pseudo-prolactinoma) from the real macroprolactinomas, which usually show prolactin serum concentrations over 200 ng/ml.

The first ones are susceptible of surgical treatment, while the prolactinomas are treated, most of them, with medical treatment. In a same way, low prolactin serum concentrations can coexist with uncovered small tumors in an incidental way, and they can lead to false diagnosis of microprolactinoma (19, 33).

Nevertheless, values between 20 and 200 ng/ml, in presence of a macro-lesion, obliged to reassess the samples using a dilution of 1:100 to dismiss the hook effect described previously and according to it very high values of serum prolactin saturate the assays and lead to an apparently low value, that could confuse the macroprolatinoma with a non-secretory macroadenoma (31).

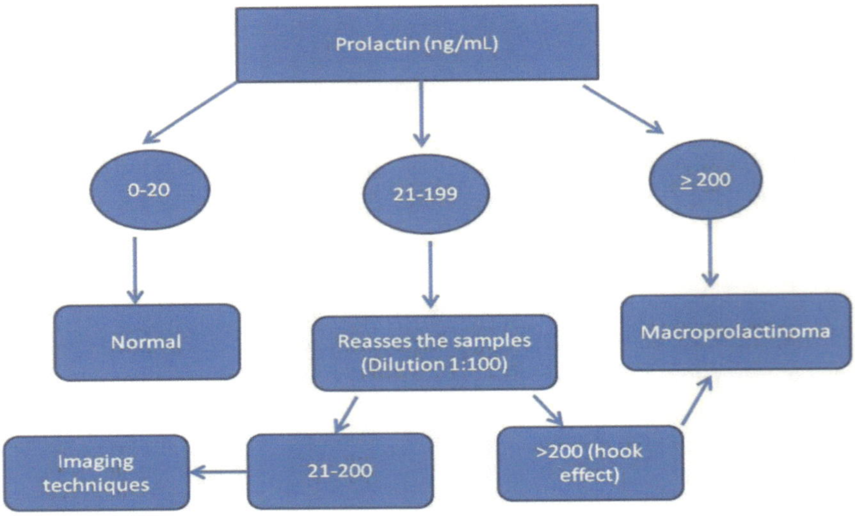

This image is propriety of our laboratory and created by us.

Figure 6. Diagnosis of the hyperprolactinemia

The dynamic tools of suppression or stimulation of prolactin (TRH, L-dopa, etc.) offer inconsistent results and should be rejected (19). In the study of the pituitary gland functionalism, in the case os a microadenoma, the determination of the basal pituitary hormones would be normally enough.

On the other hand, the presence of a macroadenoma would make advisable a deepest anterior hypophysis study.

9. Protocol of samples extraction to determine the serum prolactin

Prolactin measurement is subjected to a very careful extraction protocol, because most of the errors happen in the pre-analytic stage (between 53-75%) (20, 32).

Due to some physiological stimulus that rise prolactin levels, it is recommended to use 2-3 samples obtained at different times to assure that a patient suffers hyperprolactinemia (19-20).

Some clinical guides as the "Pituitary Society Guidelines" (35) recommend the macroprolactin screening under certain conditions (moderate increase of prolactin levels and the patient should not show typical symptoms associated to hyperprolactinemia). Other authors recommend the macroprolactin screening performing to all those samples that show high prolactin concentrations (19, 20, 36).

Our work team has developed a protocol to optimize the samples extraction and the monomeric prolactin measurement, when values are above the reference limits (19). This procedure has shown to reduce the amount of false hyperprolactinemias if compared to the direct puncture technique, because this eliminates the possible increase of prolactin due to stress puncture.

In our protocol (figure 7), patient visit us at 8.00 a.m., following the pre-analitic requirements for prolactin measurement (table 2). Then we place a micro-diffusor (canalizing the vein, which stays permeable, salinizing the blood vessel puncture). Once it has been 60 minutes since the micro-diffuser placement, we will extract the blood sample.

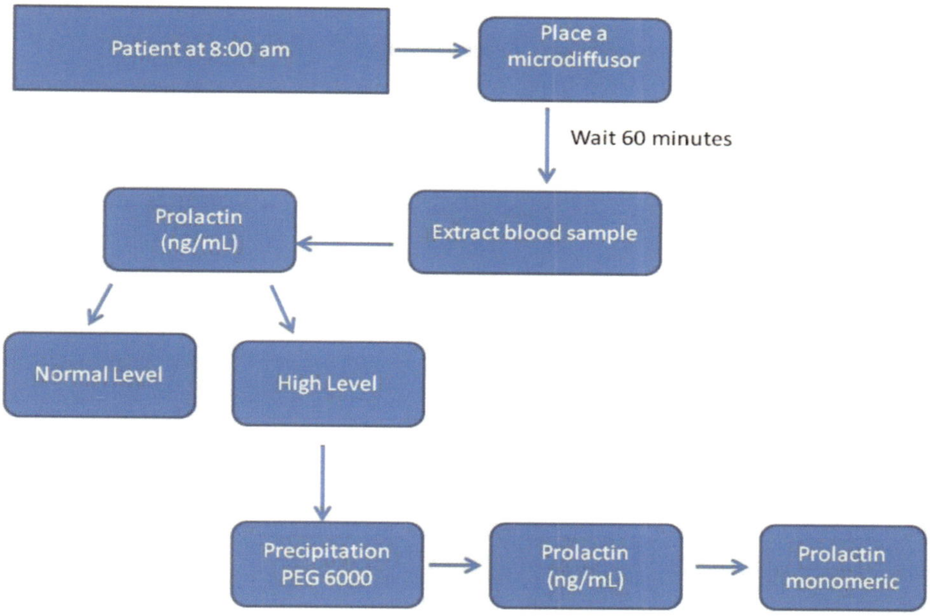

This image is propriety of our laboratory and created by us.

Figure 7. Protocol of extraction samples to determine the serum prolactin

- Being awake 2 hours before extraction and without making any physical effort.
- Avoid high-protein diet from the day before the extraction
- Avoid high-fat diet from the day before the extraction.
- Avoid breast stimulation from the day before the extraction.
- Be 8-10 hours of fasting prior to extraction.
- Do not take medications that may increase or decrease prolactin.
- Be relaxed and rested for at least 30 min before extraction.
- Do not be under stress.

Table 2. Conditions for the extraction of prolactin

The monomeric fraction determination was performed when we found high prolactin levels after 60 minutes, then we perform the macroprolactin precipitation through PEG 6000 (20, 36)

Polyethylene glycol was mixed in equal parts with the patient serum, then it was stirred and centrifuged. Prolactin was measured in the supernatant (monomeric prolactin).

We show in our report the prolactin measure at 60 minutes, the percentage of recuperation after precipitation with PEG 6000 and the monomeric prolactin (we add in a note this is the fraction that has biological activity).

10. Imaging techniques

Neuro-imaging studies must be performed with any hyperprolactinemia degree that cannot be explained with the purpose of dismiss the hypothalamic-pituitary diseade.

The Magnetic resonance imaging (MRI) with gadolinium gives the most precise anatomical details, and let us measure the tumor size and its relation to the optical chiasma and the cavernosus sinus, that is why this is, nowadays, the best imaging technique (19, 32). If MRI is normal, after excluding other hyperprolactinemia causes, we should talk about idiopathic hyperprolactinemia.

Computed tomography with intravenous contrast is less efficient than MRI in small adenomas diagnosis and the definition of big tumors, but it can be used if MRI cannot be used or if it is contraindicated. The rest of the image techniques that are more usual like X-Rays and isotope techniques are not recommended. (37).

Author details

Miguel Ángel Castaño López, José Luís Robles Rodríguez and Marta Robles García
Hospital "Juan Ramón Jiménez", Spain

11. References

[1] Freeman ME, Kanyicska B, Lerant A, Nagy G. Prolactin:structure, function and regulation of secretion. Physiol Rev 2000; 80: 1523-631.

[2] Azíz D.C. Use and Interpretation of Tests in Endocrinology. 1997. Specialty Laboratories. Capítulo 10 Desordenes pituitarios Páginas 129-130

[3] Benson R.C. Diagnóstico y Tratamiento Ginecoobstétricos. 1990. Editorial el Manual Moderno,S.A. Capítulo 3 Fisiología del sistema reproductor de la mujer. Pagina 64 y Capítulo 37 El puerperio Paginas 818-820.

[4] Comparato M.R. Terapéutica Hormonal en Ginecología. 1988. Editorial "El Ateneo". Capítulo 2 Hormonas sexuales. Páginas 36-37 Capítulo 13 Terapéutica hormonal en endocrinología ginecológica Páginas 207-216.

[5] Farreras P.Valenti y Rozman C. Medicina Interna.1982. Décima Edición. Ediciones Doyma. Capítulo 15 Endocrinología. Páginas 1805, 1806, 1811, 1812, 1814.

[6] Douze H,Guell R,Ventura S,Chueca MP.Comisión de interferencias y efectos de los fármacos. Sociedad Española de Química Clínica. Recomendaciones sobre las interferencias de prolactina en la medición de prolactina. QuimClin. 2006;25:45–8.

[7] Benavides IZ, Castillo AP, Montemayor I, DeEstrada R,Onatra W, Posso H. Biorritmo de prolactina en mujeres de edad reproductiva vs.Perimenopáusicas.Rev Coloma Menop.2003;9:153–8.[16 Sep 2009]. Disponible en: http://www.encolombia.com/medicina/menopausia/Meno9303-Biorritmo1.htm.

[8] Hazard J, Perlemuter L. Manual de Endocrinología. Barcelona: Ed. Toray-Masson; 1981.p.87–9.

[9] Melmed S, Kleinberg D. Anterior pituitary. In: Kronenberg HM, Melmed S, Polonsky KS, Larsen PR, eds. *Williams Textbook of Endocrinology*. 11th ed. Philadelphia, PA: Saunders Elsevier; 2008:chap 8.

[10] Molitch ME. Anterior pituitary. In: Goldman L, Schafer AI, eds. *Cecil Medicine*. 24th ed. Philadelphia, Pa: Saunders Elsevier; 2011:chap 231.

[11] Robles JL. Optimización de la extracción de PRL.An Clin. 1995;20:71–8.

[12] Sapin R,Gasser F,Fischbach E,Grucker D.Détection de la macro-prolactine:une nouvelle approche. Ann Biol Clin. 2000;58:729–34.

[13] Fuchs, F. y Koppler A. Endocrinología de la Gestación. 1982. Segunda edición. Salvat Editores,S.A. Capítulo 12 Prolactina Humana. Páginas 249-272.

[14] Santana F, Fernández GM, Padrón RS. Hiperprolactinemia en el hombre: Estudio de 9 casos. Rev Cubana Endocrinol 1997; 9 (1): 29-33.

[15] Falaschi P, Frajese G, Sciarra F, et al. Influence of hyperprolactinemia due to metodopamide on gonadal function in men. Clin Endocrinol 1978; 8:427-34.

[16] Costello LC, Franklin RB. Effect of prolactin on prostate. Prostate 1994;24:162-6.

[17] Molitch ME. Disorders of prolactin secretion. Endocrinol Metab Clin North Am 2001: 30:585-610

[18] Moreno B, Obiols G, Páramo C, Zugasti A. Guía clínica del manejo del prolactinoma y otros estados de hiperprolactinemia. Endocrinol Nutr 2005; 52: 9-17

[19] Robles JL, Castaño MA. Empleo de un nuevo protocolo de extracción y disminución de las falsas hiperprolactinemias. Endocrinol Nutr 2010.doi:10.1016/j.endonu.2010.04.004

[20] Kruger TH, Haake P, Chereath D, Knapp W, Janssen OE, Exton MS et al. Specificity of the neuroendocrine response to orgasm during sexual arousal in men. Journal of Endocrinology 2003, 177:57-64.

[21] Kruger TH, Leeners B, Naegeli E, Schmidlin S, Schedlowski M, Hartmann U et al. Prolactin secretory rhythm in women: immediate and long-term alterations after sexual contact. Hum Reprod 2012; 27:1139-43.

[22] Molitch ME. Prolactinomas En: Melmed S, editor. The pituitary, 2nd ed Cambridge: Blackwell; 2002. p. 455-95.

[23] Schlechte Jk Sherman B, Halmi N, Van Gilde J, Chaplor F, Dolan K, et al. Prolactin-secreting pituitary tumor in amenorrheic women: a comprehensive study. Endocr Rev. 1980; 1: 295-308.

[24] Schlechte J, Dolan K, Sherma B, Chapler F, Luciano A. The natural history of untreated hyperprolactinemia: a prospective analysis. J Clin Endocrinol Metab. 1989; 68; 412-8.

[25] Sisam D, Sheehan JP, Sheehan LR. The natural history of untreated microprolactinomas. Fertil Steril 1987; 48:67-71.

[26] March C, Kletzky O, Davajan V, Teal J, Werss M, Apiuzzo MH et al. Longitudinal evaluation of patients with untreated prolactin-secretingpituitary adenomas. Am J Obstet Gynecol. 1981; 139: 835-44

[27] De Shepper J, Schiettecatte J, Velkeniers B, Blumenfeld Z, Shteinberg M, Devroey P, et al. Clinical and biological characterization of macroprolactinemia with and without prolactin-IgG complexes. Eur J Endocrinol 2003;149:201-7.

[28] Casamitjana R. Macroprolactinemia: interpretación diagnostic. Endocrinol Nutr 2003;50: 313-6.

[29] Amadori P, Dilberis C, Marcolla A. All the studies on hyperprolactinemia should not forged the possible presence of macroprolactinemia. Eur J Endocrinol 2004; 150: 93-4.

[30] Lucas T. Problemas en el diagnóstico diferencial de las hiperprolactinemias. Endocrinol Nutr 2004; 51: 241-4.

[31] Naidich MJ, Russell EJ. Current approaches to imaging of the sellar region and pituitary. Endocrinol Metab Clin North Am 1999; 28: 45-79.

[32] Torres Y, Acebes JJ, Soler J. Incidentaloma hipofisario: evaluación y abordaje terapéutico en la actualidad. Endocrinol Nutr 2003; 50: 153-5.

[33] Cattaneo F, Kappeler D, Müller B. Macroprolactinaemia, the major unknown in the differential diagnosis of hyperprolactinaemia. Swis Med Wkly.2001;131:122–6

[34] Casanueva FF, Molitch ME, Schlechte JA, Abs R, Bonert V, Bronstein MD, et al. Guidelines of the pituitary society for the diagnosis and management of prolactinomas. Clin Endocrinol (Oxf). 2006; 65: 265–73.

[35] Goldschmidt HMJ, Lent RW. Gross errors and work flow analysis in the clinical laboratory.Clin Biochem Metab.1995; 3: 131–40.

[36] Fahie-Wilson M, Bieglmayer C, Kratzsch J, Nusbaumer C, Roth HJ, Zaninotto M, et al. Roche Elecsys Prolactin II assay: reactivity with macroprolactin compared with eight commercial assays for prolactin and determination of monomeric prolactin by pre-capitation with polyethyleneglycol. Clin Lab. 2007; 53: 485–92.

[37] Casanueva FF, Molitch ME, Sclechte JA, ABS R, Bonert V,Bronstein MD et al. Guías de la Pituitary Society para el diagnóstico y tratamiento de los prolactinomas. Endocrinol Nutr. 2007; 54:438.e1-e10